AF393585

MEDICAL RADIOLOGY

Diagnostic Imaging and Radiation Oncology

Springer

Berlin
Heidelberg
New York
Barcelona
Budapest
Hong Kong
London
Milan
Paris
Santa Clara
Singapore
Tokyo

C. Masciocchi (Ed.)

Radiological Imaging of Sports Injuries

With Contributions by

A. Barile · K. Bohndorf · M. Breitenseher · N. Chemla · A. Chevrot · A.M. Davies
N. De Stefano · S. Dragoni · J.L. Drape · A.M. Dupont · C. Fabbriciani
C. Faletti · R.C. Fritz · F. Gires · D. Godefroy · A. Greco · J. Haller · H. Imhof
F. Kainberger · L. Lucania · M.V. Maffey · C. Masciocchi · M. Mastantuono
M.T. McNamara · G. Milano · A. Minoui · W.R. Obermann · R. Passariello · E. Pessis
M. Reiser · F. Rossi · L. Sarazin · A. Schiavone Panni · S. Sintzoff · M. Steinborn
E.R. Tijn A Ton · S. Trattnig · P.N.M. Tyrrell

Foreword by

A.L. Baert

Preface by

C. Masciocchi

With 265 Figures in 462 Separate Illustrations

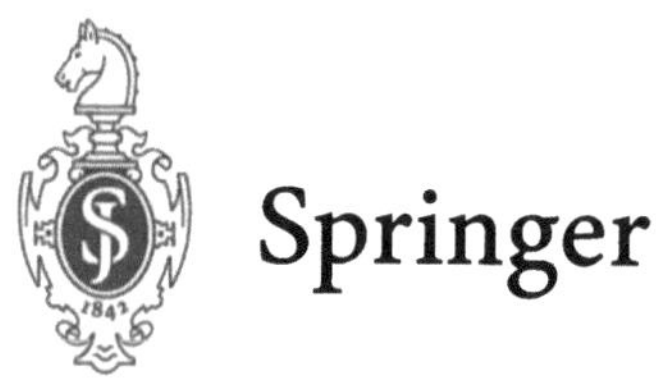

Springer

Professor Dr. Carlo Masciocchi
Department of Radiology
University of L'Aquila
Collemaggio Hospital
67100 L'Aquila
Italy

MEDICAL RADIOLOGY · Diagnostic Imaging and Radiation Oncology

Continuation of
Handbuch der medizinischen Radiologie
Encyclopedia of Medical Radiology

ISBN-13: 978-3-642-64322-4   e-ISBN-13: 978-3-642-60256-6
DOI: 10.1007/978-3-642-60256-6

Library of Congress Cataloging-in-Publication Data. Radiological imaging of sports injuries / C. Masciocchi, ed. ; with contributions by A. Barile ... [et al.] ; foreword by A. L. Baert. p. cm. -- (Medical radiology) Includes bibliographical references and index. ISBN 3-540-60870-2 (alk. paper) 1. Sports injuries--Imaging. 2. Sports injuries--Diagnosis. I. Masciocchi, C. (Carlo), 1956- . II. Barile, A. (Antonio) III. Series. [DNLM: 1. Athletic Injuries--diagnosis. 2. Diagnostic Imaging--methods. 3. Sports Medicine--methods. QT 261 R129 1997] RD97.R33 1997 617.1'0757--dc21 DNLM/DLC for Library of Congress 97-12401 CIP

Cover design: de'blik, Berlin

Typesetting: Best-set Typesetter Ltd., Hong Kong

SPIN: 10526113   21/3155 – 5 4 3 2 1 0 – Printed on acid-free paper

Foreword

Sport has become a more and more pervasive part of modern life. The public media and society in general are paying increasing attention to professional sporting activity. Professional athletes are forced to reach for the limits of physical endurance, thereby putting extreme strain on their muscoloskeletal system. In the ease of lower than expected performance, or when confronted with obvious musculotendinous damage, they quite logically seek medical help, involving, first of all, exact diagnosis of potential lesions.

There is, however, another rapidly growing segment of the population where sport is practised mainly for relaxation as a leisure pastime and as a means to improve health. In our modern society it is increasingly considered one of the basic rights of the citizen, indeed part of our culture, to regularly spend time participating in sporting activities. The practice of sports without appropriate physical training and preparation, frequently the case for non-professionals, has led to an increasing number of complaints related to strain or damage of the locomotor system.

During recent years we have seen tremendous progress in our capacity to diagnose sports lesions. The new cross-sectional modalities such as ultrasonography, computed tomography and magnetic resonance imaging permit much improve visualization of the musculoskeletal anatomy in the living person. Consequently, we are now able to visualize morphological changes in lesions of the soft tissues, notably muscles, ligaments and tendons, that we are unable to see before. Therefore, there is a great demand on the part of radiologists, orthopedic surgeons and sports medicine physicians in general for more information concerning the diagnosis of these types of lesions and injuries.

Professor C. Masciocchi has been very successful in bringing together an outstanding group of specialists in the imaging of sports injuries. As a result this book constitutes a comprehensive and up-to-date volume which I hope will be much appreciated by all those interested in sports medicine.

Leuven

ALBERT L. BAERT

Preface

The number of people participating more or less regularly in sporting activity has grown impressively in recent decades. This phenomenon, more widely diffused in the affluent societies, justifies the growth of medical interest in physical activities in general and competitive sports in particular. The result is a constantly developing awareness of the scientific importance of research in this field and of the social impact of application of the results. The proliferation of scientific volumes that include contributions from the different fields of physiology, biomechanics, orthopaedics and sports traumatology, cardiology and radiology bears witness to the attention now devoted to sports-related injuries in athletes and in the general population.

Of course, the growing interest in sports medicine also originates from the revolutionary technological developments in diagnostic imaging brought about by the diffusion of ultrasonic tomography, computer tomography and magnetic resonance imaging, now clinically employed by radiologists and orthopaedists on a large scale. This volume was conceived with the aim of demonstrating the potential of the diagnostic techniques now available for the study of both rare and commonly observed injuries related to medium- and high-level sporting activity.

L'Aquila

CARLO MASCIOCCHI

Contents

1 Epidemiological Aspects of Sports Injuries

S. Dragoni

CONTENTS

1.1
Introduction

Over recent decades, both interest and levels of participation in both recreational and competitive sports activities have significantly increased. An important factor in this development has been people's need for personally and socially significant experiences.

One of the more noble aspects of sport is the drive to achieve one's maximum potential; this desire, however, often leads athletes to ignore the potential risk factors involved in sporting activities. The increasing numbers of participants at various levels expose a greater number of athletes to potential injury, provoking a concomitant increase in sports-related injuries which often require specific medical consultations and absence from school and/or work, with direct and indirect economic costs (Sorensen and Sonne-Holm 1980; Tolpin et al. 1981; de Loes 1990).

It has become axiomatic that the corollary of "sports for all" is "sports injuries for all" (Sperryn 1983). On the other hand, it is well known that every form of human activity involves some risk of accidental injury and that different games and sports

involve different degrees of risk. In common speech, the terms "tennis elbow" and "jumper's knee" suggest that some injuries are associated with particular sports activities.

In light of the frequency of injuries, it is necessary to classify the potential risk factors involved with each individual sport. The knowledge of these risk factors will aid coaches and physicians in identifying events or activities needing closer supervision, as well as provide a means to improve technique within each individual sport. This will establish models of relationship between risk factors and protective factors suited to addressing injury prevention through well-designed intervention and evolution. The application of this knowledge, directed towards development, implementation and evaluation of preventive measures, will promote awareness of the proper use of equipment and training necessary for each sport (Williams 1976; Grisogono 1986). Moreover, specific steps can be taken to help reduce the number of acute injuries and prevent chronic disability.

Many questions may be resolved by epidemiological studies dealing with occurrence and distribution of injuries that may result from exposure to a specific set of conditions. In fact, epidemiology can be defined as the study of the distribution of injuries and their causative agents (Caine et al. 1989).

This brief overview introduces basic concepts of the relationship between sports activities and injuries.

1.1.1
The Definition of Sports Injury

Standardization in defining sports injury is fundamental to the accomplishment of a uniform global standard of care directed by current research.

Scientific evaluation of the problems related to epidemiologic studies of sports injuries is hampered by considerable variation in study participants, study design (retrospective versus prospective), data collection, injury definition and application of

S. Dragoni, MD, Istituto di Scienza dello Sport del CONI, Dipartimento di Medicina dello Sport Via dei Campi Sportivi 46 00197 Rome, Italy

findings. Several authors have stressed the difficulties of finding common denominators among studies (KRANENBORG 1982; WALTER et al. 1985; VAN MECHELEN et al. 1992; MEEUSEN and BORMS 1992).

However, it is not always easy to distinguish all the elements necessary to construct a single objective definition for sports injury. For example, some studies define an injury as something that alters athletic performance and/or produces a time loss from participation; the problem with this is that an injury may impair or alter performance in one sport while not affecting performance in another. Moreover, time lost due to injury is difficult to define. One player might play when injured, while another with the same injury might not (NOYES et al. 1988). For other authors, the definition of sports injury is reserved for cases which require medical treatment or for which an insurance claim has been submitted (GERBERICH 1985).

EKSTRAND and GILLQUIST (1982, 1983a,b) and NIELSEN and YDE (1989) define an injury as a lesion that prevents the athlete from participating in a game or training session, excluding injuries sustained from nonsporting activities. Another approach is pathoanatomical classification allowing incorporation of objective medical examination findings applicable to every activity; here too, however, problems are evident. Apart from fractures, confirmation by advanced imaging techniques (MRI, CT), and surgical exploration, objective establishment and documentation of injuries is difficult (WALLACE and CLARK 1988).

Moreover, an injury can present different characteristics depending upon the experience and knowledge of the evaluator performing the examination (physician, trainer, physiotherapist). The time elapsing between injury and examination also influences the findings.

In general, sports injuries encompass every type of injury that may occur as a result of sports activity.

Some definitions, however, include specific time criteria; in fact, "the reportable injury is one that limits athletic participation for at least the day after the day of onset" (VINGER 1981) or requires professional attention by a physician or trainer.

1.1.2
Severity of Sports Injuries

The US National Athletic Injury Registration System (NAIRS) subdivides injuries into "minor" (1–7 days), "moderately serious" (8–21 days) and "serious" (over 21 days, including permanent damage). A similar classification has been accepted by the US National Athletic Trainers Association (NATA).

The severity of injuries can also be classified by using the Abbreviated Injury Scale (Committee on Injury Scaling 1985), which grades injuries from 1 to 6, where 6 is maximum injury (virtually unsurvivable). Another measure of severity is related to the absence from sports activity due to injury (EKSTRAND and GILLQUIST 1983b). It has three grades:

– Minor = absence of less than 1 week
– Moderate = absence of more than 1 week but less than 1 month
– Major = absence of more than 1 month

The Council of Europe proposed (VAN VULPEN 1989) a definition of sports injury that takes into account any damage resulting from participation in sports with one or more of the following consequences: (a) a reduction in the amount or level of sports activity; (b) a need for medical advice or treatment; (c) adverse social or economic effects.

An important aspect of data collection for sports injuries is the adoption of a precise medical terminology in which a term holds the same meaning for all involved in the study.

The NAIRS medical terminology notebook (CLARKE 1976) gives the following first-level classification regarding the pathological condition of body parts:

1. Acute injuries
   a) General trauma
   b) Neurotrauma
   c) Burn
   d) Sprain
   e) Strain
   f) Fracture
2. Illnesses/conditions
   a) Miscellaneous musculoskeletal disorders
   b) Drug/chemical illness
   c) Illness, others
3. Catastrophic injuries/illnesses
   a) Severe permanent disability

Each of these primary conditions is followed by second-level listing with diagnosis codes which allow the recording of large amounts of detail as well as the production of summary data and in-depth analysis.

1.1.3
Aetiology of Sports Injuries

It is highly important to examine causes and reasons for sports injuries. We can divide causes into *endogenous* and *exogenous*. Endogenous factors are those that strictly are linked not to the sports discipline practiced, but rather to the psychological and physical condition of the subject, such as:

- Age, sex, and general health, with particular emphasis on those parts of the body more exposed to the risks resulting from motor activity (locomotor apparatus)
- Anthropometric characteristics (height, weight, body fat)
- Physical and psychological approach to the sports discipline practiced; particularly important is the gradual progression of the physical activity
- Level of physical fitness, which should always be correlated to the intensity and amount of effort expended
- Awareness of the risks arising from sporting activity and level of preparation, both physical and psychological.

Exogenous causes include type of activity (individual or team sport), environmental conditions (playing surface, lighting), equipment (clothes and accessories), use of protective devices, and observance of the rules.

It should also be considered that there are a number of general risk factors, such as:

- Malfunctioning of instruments or apparatus (for example, a flat tire in cycling)
- Traffic accidents such as in cycling (especially amateur) or motor racing
- Adverse weather conditions

If we differentiate sports disciplines on the basis of direct causes and effects of injuries as a result of the sport or type of activity involved, we obtain the following three main groups:

1. Sports disciplines not characterized by direct contact with the opponent, in which accidents are more frequently the result of intense and prolonged activity (track and field, swimming, tennis, rowing etc.).
2. Sports involving direct contact with opponents, where to contusions, strains, dislocations and fractures can result (e.g. soccer, rugby, boxing fencing, and, more generally, all team sports).

3. All activities carried out with the help of an animal or mechanical means, such as motorcycling, cycling, and equestrianism; accidents are related to the means used.

1.2
Sports Injuries Incidence

1.2.1
Measurement of Sports Injuries

In epidemiologic studies, one of the most fundamental units of measurement is the quotient, which consists of a numerator and a denominator whose determination may be simple or difficult, depending on the sophistication of the study. A general injury rate can be derived, for example, from the number of injured players and the number of players at risk (LINDENFELD et al. 1988):

$$\text{Injury rate} = \frac{\text{Number injured (numerator)}}{\text{Number exposed (denominator)}}$$

Naturally, the quality of the study depends on the accuracy with which the data are collected and on the amount of data.

In the study of sports injuries, the denominator can be defined as those who are at risk of sustaining an injury during participation in sports while the numerator can be defined as the type of lesions, the total number of reported injuries (case rate) or the total number of athletes injured (injury rate). In general, the injury rate is lower than the case rate because some athletes are injured more than once during the period of time considered (SCHOOTMAN et al. 1994).

Incidence and prevalence can be utilized. Incidence is a dynamic measure than can be defined for our purposes as the number of new sports injuries occurring during a specified period of time in a specified population and that can be calculated by dividing the number of new cases in the population by the total population at risk at the beginning of the period (HUNTER and MARTIN LEVY 1988).

In contrast, prevalence is a static measure indicating the total amount of injured athletes at a particular time. Prevalence (P) depends on the incidence (I) and duration (D) of the pathologic condition (POWELL et al. 1986) according to the following ratio:

$$P = I \times D \text{ (year/part of year)}$$

To correctly interpret and compare data, it is important to consider how the duration of exposure to risk can influence the epidemiologic study. Results precisely describing all the risks linked to the practice of a sports activity are more reliable when the time variable refers not to, say, a sporting season or a year, but to the real time needed to carry out the sporting activity (time of exposure to accident risk); in this case, KELLER's formula (1987) can be adopted in order to obtain the frequency of injuries:

$$\text{lesions players}^{-1} \text{ exposure time}^{-1} (1000\,h)$$

Another possibility of calculating the incidence rate that takes into account exposure time and the length of the season is the equation of CHAMBERS (1979), modified by DE LOES and GOLDIE (1988):

$$\text{injury incidence} = \frac{\text{injuries per year} \times 10^4}{\begin{array}{c}(\text{participants}) \times (\text{average} \\ \text{hours of participation/week}) \\ \times (\text{weeks of season/year})\end{array}}$$

The risk of sports accidents can be evaluated on the basis of two main factors: the average number of accidents and the mean value of the damage produced. The first factor shows the degree of risk involved in the sport, while the second shows the consequences and the intensity of damage.

With regard to the dangerousness of different sports, the frequency of injuries is often expressed as the number of accidents per 100 (or 1000 or 10 000) athletes; in this way, the different exposure of athletes to trauma is shown along an ideal scale, and it is possible to classify sports according to the degree of danger.

Obviously, this "risk index" is not sufficient to establish which sports are more dangerous; other factors also have to be considered, such as the seriousness of the injuries, their cause and their evolution (complete recovery, permanent disability or death).

Risk values for different disciplines can be obtained by relating the absolute frequency of accidents taking place in a specific time interval (generally a year) to the mean population in the interval.

This index can be calculated using the formula

$$F_i = I/P_m$$

where F_i is the frequency of injuries, I represents the number of accidents and P_m indicates the mean population during the period considered.

1.3
Sports Injuries Data

1.3.1
Overall Sports Injuries Incidence Rates

Several studies, especially by Dutch authors, have provided detailed epidemiologic data about overall sports injury incidence rates, although it is difficult to compare data because of the different methods of evaluation used.

BOERSMA-SLUTTER et al. (1979), for example, recorded 560 000 medically treated injuries per year, while KRANENBORG (1980) reported 1 200 000 injuries, both medically treated and otherwise, corresponding respectively to yearly rates of 20% and 46.5%.

A more recent study (VAN GALEN and DIEDERIKS 1990) carried out in The Netherlands on a total population of some 15 million showed an overall sports injuries incidence of 3.3 injuries per 1000 h spent on sports, of which 1.4/1000 h required medical treatment.

In Germany, VON STEINBRUCK and COTTA (1983) found out that sports injuries represented 10%–15% of all accidents medically treated by the Orthopedics Department of Heidelberg University. They also produced a list of the sporting disciplines involving major traumatic risks.

In Sweden, a prospective study revealed that acute sports injuries represented 17% of the total amount of medical examinations of injuries over the course of a year. (DE LOES 1990); a similar study in Finland (SANDELIN et al. 1987), investigating 1.5 million acute medically treated injuries, fixed the frequency of sports injuries at about 14% of the total amount.

Obviously, these studies refer only to highly acute medically treated injuries; the exposure time to sport, which can effect the risk of sustaining an injury, is not considered.

In Great Britain, a study of new patients attending an emergency department of a hospital found that 7.1% had injured themselves playing sport. The majority had played football and sustained soft tissue injuries (JONES and TAGGART 1994). WEIGHTMAN and BROWNE (1974) found that approximately 5% of all patients seen in accident departments of British hospitals attended due to sporting injuries. It has been estimated that the annual injury rate throughout the United Kingdom is 2 000 000 accidents of sufficient severity to preclude the victim from participating in sport for at least 1 week (WILLIAMS 1976).

In 1985, a survey by the Dutch Ministry of Health, Welfare and Cultural Affairs concerning the risk of sports injures (without taking into account the time spent in sporting activities) found an increased risk in soccer (4.2 per 100 participants). In Denmark, a prospective study conducted for 1 year in a well-defined geographical area with 124 321 inhabitants revealed a total of 1839 sports injuries. The incidence was 61 per 100 active sports players per year and 15 per 10 000 inhabitants (LINDBLAD et al. 1991).

In Switzerland, an epidemiological study including all acute injuries that occurred in the "Youth and Sports" organization and taking into account the number of participants and the time of exposure was carried out by the Military Insurance. Per year there were close to 350 000 participants (age 14–20 years), for a total of 13.2 million person hours, suffering more than 5000 injuries. The overall injury rate was significantly higher in males than in females. The highest incidence in males was found in ice hockey, handball and soccer, while in females the ranking order was handball, soccer and basketball (DE LOES 1995).

KANNUS et al. (1987) found that in adults taking part in high school athletics, the incidence of injuries in men was significantly higher than in women, which a ratio of nearly 2:1. MEEUWISSE and FOWLER (1988) demonstrated an injury rate of 38% for men and 32% for women in a group of 712 intercollegiate athletes performing 24 different sports; in this study, the knee was the anatomic region most frequently injured. McLAIN and REYNOLDS (1989) reviewed 1283 student athletes involved in organized high school athletics, finding that sprains and strains accounted for 57% of all injuries.

Many other epidemiological studies have been undertaken during recent years on sports injuries to identify the incidence and consequently the risk of various sports activities.

In Hong Kong, a prospective survey carried out on 2293 patients (nonprofessional and nonelite athletes) attending the Sports Injury Clinic in the Prince of Wales Hospital over a period of 6 years showed that soccer, basketball, volleyball, long-distance running and cycling were, in descending order, the five most common sports to cause injuries. In this study, sprain was the most common injury of all (44.6%; CHAN et al. 1993).

DE LOES and GOLDIE (1988), taking into account the exposure time to risk, carried out a prospective study for 1 year in a total population of 31 620 inhabitants, finding a total of 571 injuries 28 different sports. Soccer had the majority of injuries, but the

ranking order differed when calculating exposure time and so ice hockey and handball were found to have the highest risk, followed by soccer.

Many studies are dedicated to particular sports in a particular geographic zone (for example, Alpine skiing and ice hockey injuries in Northern Europe, Canada and the USA; soccer in Italy; rugby in Great Britain, New Zealand and Australia) while other studies discuss the epidemiology of some sports-related injuries involving a particular body structure.

1.3.2
Sports Injuries Incidence in Italy

Some interesting data for overall epidemiologic evaluation of sports injuries can be found in the statistics gathered by the National Sports Insurance Fund for Athletes (1996), whose activity can be described under the following headings:

- Insurance against personal injuries occurring during the practice of a competitive sport or in training
- Third party insurance for damage caused as a consequence of events during sporting activity for which the insured party can be proven responsible

The data gathered by the National Sports Insurance Fund demonstrate that from 1983 to 1992, the total number of athletes considered has diminished; the number of insured athletes fell from 7 446 729 in 1983 to 7 051 089 in 1992.

Bearing in mind the insurance objectives, the insured population can be divided into three main groups:

- Athletes belonging to National Sports Federations, which constitute the most qualified nucleus of active athletes, since they comprise all the members of the Federations grouped under CONI (Italian National Olympic Committee).
- The second group, consisting of members of "youth activities", has fallen by nearly 30% in the past 10 years, attributed to the fact that selection criteria for the "Youth Games" have become stricter during this period.
- The third group comprises the members of "sports promotion bodies", organizations that carry out intense athletic and publicity activity, uniting enthusiasts of different sports activities in various associations.

Within a population at risk consisting of more than 7 million participants at various levels of sports activities, when taking due account of the limits related to exposure time, there has been systematic and ordered noting of the cases and accidents reported to the Fund by the insured and of the compensation paid out; the cases reported make it possible to note, among other things:

- The distribution of acute injuries for each sporting activity
- The sex and age of the injured athletes
- The time of the accident (competition or training)
- The type and site of the lesion
- The outcome of the lesion and any permanent disability

The evaluation of average annual frequency of accidents per 10 000 insurees in the various sports activities shows a wide range of variability (from 1 to about 945 per 10 000 insurees) and that at the top of the list, following motorcycling events, boxing and cycling, were those that demand violent motor activity, such as rugby and soccer (Fig. 1.1).

An analysis of the frequency of injuries elucidates a number of interesting points. One general conclusion is that there are more dangerous sports activities performed in teams than individually, and that activities with animal or machine participation and those with direct contact with opponents pose an increased risk.

Individual activities are less dangerous in general, although intense and prolonged motor activities (track and field, tennis, swimming) are more so than less strenuous sporting activities (table tennis, bowls, fishing, golf, trapshooting and skeet, archery).

With reference to the entire insured sporting population, the cause of injury was:

- 33% direct contact with an opponent
- 31% falls (bicycles, motorcycles or horses)
- 14% extraneous contact
- 22% other causes

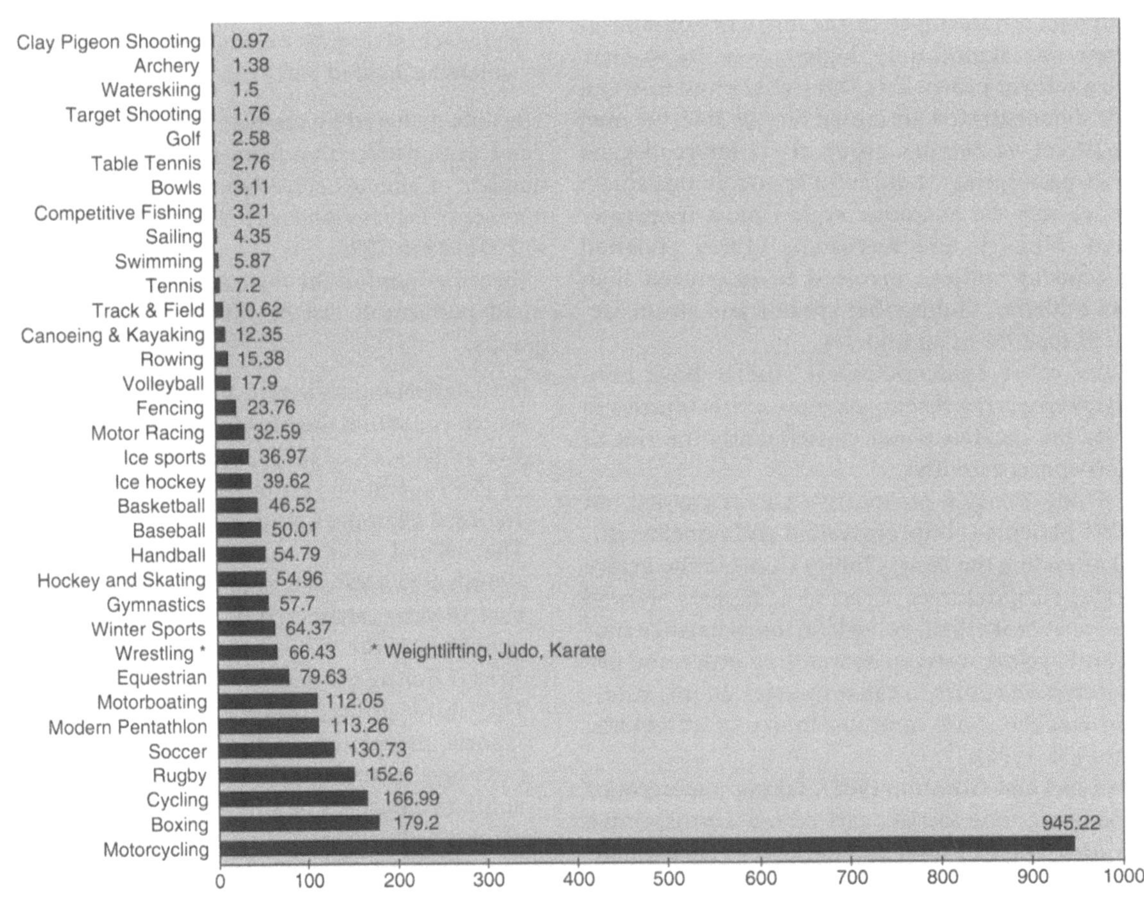

Fig. 1.1.

The percentage distribution of accidents according to sex shows a high prevalence of men (92% overall). These values vary considerably from one sport to another; in fact, there are some sports (soccer, rugby, wrestling) in which men account for all injuries, while in others the percentage of women reaches 80% (gymnastics) or 50% (equestrianism volleyball). With regard to distribution by age, excluding organized youth activities, the greatest incidence of injuries (45%) occurs below the age of 20, while 28% of those injured are between 20 and 24, 15% between 25 and 29, and only 12% beyond 30 years of age.

The highest incidence of injuries is found in winter and spring, in accordance with the seasons of the most widely practiced sports (soccer, rugby, basketball, volleyball). During certain months of the year, such as July, August and September, there is less activity and usually only athletics and swimming take place.

The majority (66%) of injuries take place during competition, 31% during training sessions.

Analysis of the percentage distribution of types of lesions according to discipline, shows that fractures have the highest incidence (48.4% of the total), followed by sprains (22.69%), muscle-tendon injuries (9.16%) and contusions (8.03), while dislocations and wounds are less frequent (Fig. 1.2). With regard to the site of lesions, almost 50% of injuries occur in the lower limbs, especially in the joints (24% knee, 16% ankle). Upper limbs are involved in 30% of accidents, mostly involving the shoulder (10% of these injuries are dislocations). Injuries to the skull, thorax, pelvis and to multiple sites are less frequent.

It is interesting, especially for preventive purposes, to consider some individual sports. For example:

- In motorcycling, 73% of injuries are due to falls, with frequent damage to the shoulders (20%), the knees (11%) and the legs (9%).
- In athletics, about 55% of injuries are to the lower limbs, especially the ankles and knees; injuries to the upper limbs account for about 20% of the total, while 12% concern the head and face. With regard to the types of injuries, fractures and sprains occur more frequently in the lower limbs, while in the upper limbs fractures are followed by dislocations.
- In cycling, the most frequent site of injury is the shoulder (about 25% of accidents), with a high frequency of fractures and dislocations; there is also a high incidence of multiple lesions as a result of falls.
- In winter sports, the most common injuries are sprains and fractures of the lower limbs, representing 26% and 18% of accidents, respectively.
- In boxing, typical injuries are those to the wrist and hand, accounting for 42% of the total reported.

If we analyze the proportion of accidents resulting in permanent disabilities, we see that higher incidences are recorded among disciplines that present the greatest number of accidents, i.e. motorcycling (49.58%), motorboating (30.38%), pentathlon (27.02%), rugby (22.27%), boxing (20.95%), equestrian sports (19.39%), cycling (18.89%) and soccer (11.06%).

1.4
Conclusions

Because of the many variations in the definition of sports injuries, methods of data collection and application of findings, no reliable and comparable conclusions can be drawn about incidence and severity of sports-related injuries. Although there are difficulties in defining the epidemiology of these problems, it is clear that there is some degree of relationship between injury and the provoking activity, allowing us to take, in some cases, the necessary steps to offset the risk. However, even with the adoption of preventive measures to reduced the amount of sports injuries, it should be kept in mind that injuries are a likely consequence of many sporting activities.

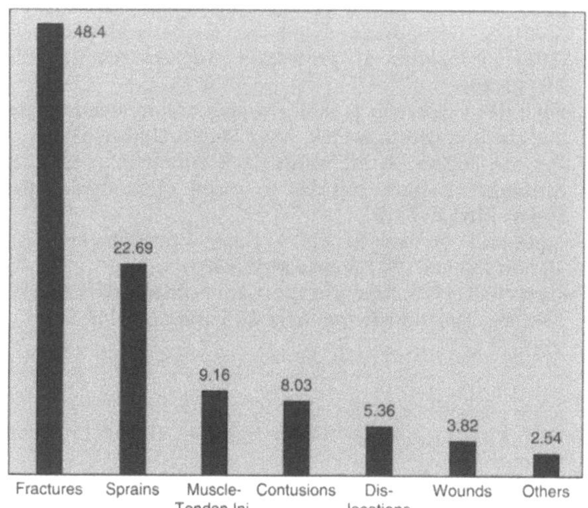

Fig. 1.2.

References

Boersma-Slutter W, Brodkman A, Lagra HA, Minderaa PH (1979) Sport, one risky activity. Gen Sport 12:41–49 (in Dutch)

Caine DJ, Cochrane B, Caine C, Zemper E (1989) An epidemiologic investigation of injuries affecting young competitive female gymnasts. Am J Sports Med 17:811–820

Chambers RB (1979) Orthopedic injuries in athletes (age 6 to 17). Comparison of injuries occurring in six sports. Am J Sports Med 7:195–197

Chan KM, Yuan Y, Li CK, Chien P, Tsang G (1993) Sports causing most injuries in Hong Kong. Br J Sports Med 27:263–267

Clarke KS (1976) The National Athletic/Illness Reporting System, NAIRS recorder handbook. Pennsylvania State University, University Park

Committee on injury scaling (1985) The abbreviated injury scale. Am Assoc Automot Med, Arlington Heights, Ill

de Loes M (1990) Medical treatment and costs of sports-related injuries in a total population. Int J Sports Med 11:66–72

de Loes M (1995) Epidemiology of sports injuries in the Swiss organization "Youth and Sports" 1987–1989. Injuries, exposure and risks of main diagnoses. Int J Sports Med 16:134–138

de Loes M, Goldie I (1988) Incidence rate of injuries during sport activity and physical exercise in a rural Swedish municipality: incidence rates in 17 sports. Int J Sports Med 9:461–467

Ekstrand J, Gillquist J (1982) The frequency of muscle tightness and injuries in soccer players. Am J Sports Med 10:75–78

Ekstrand J, Gillquist J (1983a) The avoidability of soccer injuries. Int J Sports Med 4:124–128

Ekstrand J, Gillquist J (1983b) Soccer injuries and their mechanism: a prospective study. Med Sci Sports Exerc 15:267–270

Gerberich SG (1985) Sports injuries: implications for prevention. Public Health Rep 100:570–571

Grisogono V (1986) Prevention and prophylaxis. In: Helal B, King J, Grange W (eds) Sports injuries and their treatment. Chapman and Hall, London, p 1

Hunter RE, Martin Levy I (1988) Vignettes. Am J Sports Med 16:25–37

Jones RS, Taggart T (1994) Sport related injuries attending the accident and emergency department. Br J Sports Med 28:110–111

Kannus P, Niittymaki S, Jarvinen M (1987) Sports injuries in women: a one-year prospective follow-up study at an outpatient sports clinic. Br J Sports Med 21:37–39

Keller CS, Noyes FR, Buncher CR (1987) The medical aspects of soccer injury epidemiology. Am J Sports Med 15:230–237

Kranenborg N (1980) Sports participation and injuries. Gen Sport 13:89–93 (in Dutch)

Kranenborg N (1982) Sports participation and injuries. Toeg Soc Gen 60:224–227 (in Dutch)

Lindblad BE, Hoy K, Terkelsen CJ, Helleland HE (1991) The socioeconomic consequences of sports injuries in Randers, Denmark. Scand J Med Sci Sports 1:221–224

Lindenfeld TN, Noyes FR, Marshall MT (1988) Components of injury reporting systems. Am J Sports Med 16:69–80

McLain LG, Reynolds S (1989) Sports injuries in high school. Pediatrics 84:446–450

Meeusen R, Borms J (1992) Gymnastics injuries. Sports Med 13:337–356

Meeuwisse WH, Fowler PJ (1988) Frequency and predictability of sports injuries in intercollegiate athletes. Can J Sports Sci 13:35–42

National Sports Insurance Fund for Athletes (1996) Sports accidents 1983–1992. CONI SPORTASS, Rome

Nielsen AB, Yde J (1989) Epidemiology and traumatology of injuries in soccer. Am J Sports Med 17:803–807

Noyes FR, Lindenfeld TN, Marshall MT (1988) What determines an athletic injury (definition)? Who determines an injury (occurrence)? Am J Sports Med 16:65–68

Powell KE, Kohl HW, Caspersen CJ, Blair SM (1986) An epidemiological perspective on the causes of running injuries. Phys Sports Med 14:100–114

Sandelin J, Santavirta S, Lattila R, Sarna S (1987) Sports injuries in a large urban population: occurrence and epidemiological aspects. Int J Sports Med 8:61–66

Schootman M, Powell JW, Albright JP (1944) Statistics in sports injury reasearch. In: De Lee JC, Drez D (ed) Orthopaedic sports medicine. Saunders, Philadelphia, p 160

Sorensen CH, Sonne-Holm S (1980) Social costs of sports injuries. Br J Sports Med 14:24–25

Sperryn PN (1983) Sport and medicine. Butterworths, London, p ix

Steinbruck von K, Cotta H (1983) Epidemiology of sports injuries. Dtsch Z Sportmed 83:173–186 (in German)

Tolpin HG, Vinger PF, Tolpin DW (1981) Economic considerations. Int Ophthalmol Clin 21:179–201

Van Galen W, Diederiks J (1990) An extensive analysis of sports injuries in The Netherlands. De Vrieseborch, Haarlem (in Dutch)

Van Mechelen W, Hlobil H, Kemper HCG (1992) Incidence, severity, aetiology and prevention of sports injuries. A review of concepts. Sports Med 14:82–99

Van Vulpen A (1989) Sport for all: sport injuries and their prevention. Council of Europe. Nederlands Instituut voor Sport en Gezondheid, Papendal, NetherlandsVinger PF (1981) Principles of protection. Int Ophthalmol Clin 21:149–161

Wallace RB, Clark WR (1988) The numerator, denominator and the population at risk. Am J Sports Med 16:55–56

Walter SD, Sutton JR, McIntosh JM, Connolly C (1985) The aetiology of sports injuries: a review of methodologies. Sports Med 2:47–58

Weightman D, Browne RC (1974) Injuries in rugby and association football. Br J Sports Med 8:183

Williams JGP (1976) Injury in sport. In: Williams JGP, Sperryn PN (eds) Sport medicine. Arnold, London, p 245

2 Clinical Problems in Injured Athletes

C. Fabbriciani[1], A. Schiavone Panni[2], L. Lucania[3], and G. Milano[4]

CONTENTS

[1]C. Fabbriciani, MD, Department of Orthopaedics, University of Sassari, Via S. Godenzo 175, 00189 Rome, Italy
[2]A. Schiavone Panni, MD, Department of Orthopaedics, Catholic University, L.go A. Gemelli 8, 00168 Rome, Italy
[3]L. Lucania, MD, Department of Orthopaedics, Catholic University, L.go A. Gemelli 8, 00168 Rome, Italy
[4]G. Milano, MD, Department of Orthopaedics, Catholic University, L.go A. Gemelli 8, 00168 Rome, Italy

2.1 Glenohumeral Instability

Shoulder instability, sometimes associated with pain, is frequently observed in athletes. In specific terms, the high degree of stress withstood by the glenohumeral joint in throwing sports and swimming and direct as well as indirect shoulder traumas in contact sports can facilitate the onset of an unstable shoulder.

Shoulder instability may be classified according to cause, degree, frequency and direction of the instability, as well as the patient's control capability (Table 2.1). The most frequent cause of instability is an anterior traumatic dislocation of the shoulder (Rowe 1956), which in most cases is due to an indirect trauma with the shoulder in the external rotation position and abduction or extension (Matsen et al. 1990). Recurrent dislocation or subluxation after the first episode of anterior traumatic dislocation has been described in the literature with a frequency varying between 66% and 100% (Rowe 1980; Henry and Genund 1982; Simonet and Cofield 1984; Hovelius 1987; Wheeler et al. 1989; Marans et al. 1992). The incidence is especially high in subjects under 20 years of age and in athletes.

2.1.1 Physical Examination of Anterior Shoulder Instability

The diagnosis of shoulder instability may be simple in the presence of a previous acute or recurrent traumatic anterior dislocation history. In some patients, recurrent dislocation may also occur without any significant traumas. Such individuals are normally characterized by generalized ligamentous laxity. The diagnosis is more difficult in the presence of a recurrent subluxation. The patient does not report true dislocation episodes, but mainly pain, often complained of posteriorly, and sometimes a clicking sensation when making certain movements. In athletes,

Table 2.1. Classification of shoulder anterior instability

Cause	Traumatic
	Acute
	Repetitive
	Atraumatic
Degree	Dislocation
	Subluxation
Frequency	Acute
	Recurrent
Direction	Anterior
	Posterior
	Inferior
	Multidirectional
Patient control	Involuntary
	Voluntary

especially throwers, the pain is more intense during the cocking and acceleration phases of the throw (ROWE and ZARINS 1981). The initial symptoms may be caused by a traumatic event with the arm in external rotation combined with abduction and/or extension. In other cases, there is no macrotraumatic history. In these patients, the repetitiveness of the athletic performance leads to an "overuse" of capsuloligamentous and tendinous structures of the shoulder, and the cumulative effect of the microtrauma, in the long term, causes instability, often associated with subacromial impingement with damage to the rotator cuff (JOBE and KVITNE 1989; JOBE and GLOUSMAN 1991). JOBE (1991) and WALCH et al. (1992) have shown that throwers affected by anterior instability may also exhibit a posterosuperior impingement of the rotator cuff and glenoid labrum against the greater tuberosity during the abduction and extrarotation movements.

The clinical examination of the glenohumeral joint must begin with an inspection of the shoulder, which may reveal the presence of asymmetry or muscle atrophy. The passive and active range of motion must be evaluated in both shoulders. Clinical tests specific for instability must then be performed.

The *sulcus test* is carried out with the patient in the standing position. With the shoulder muscles in a relaxed position, the examiner performs a downward traction on the patient's wrist. In the presence of an inferior laxity, the humeral head will be subjected to downward subluxation, and a space below the acromion will become evident.

The *posterior apprehension test* is performed with the patient in a supine position and the shoulder not on the table. The limb is flexed at 90° and intrarotated; a posterior directed force is then ap-

plied to the flexed elbow. The onset of apprehension in the patient is indicative of posterior instability.

The *anterior apprehension test* is carried out with the patient in a supine position and the arm hanging over the side of the table. The limb is abducted at 90° and then slowly subjected to extrarotation. The onset of pain and apprehension in the patient is indicative of anterior instability. The symptoms may fade if the examiner places his hand on the patient's shoulder and exercises a posterior directed force (relocation test).

The *load and shift test* is performed with the patient in a supine position, with the arm abducted at 90°. The examiner places pressure on the flexed elbow with one hand and with the other exercises an anterior and posterior pressure on the humeral head. In the case of laxity, a soft clunk will be felt when the head of the humerus subluxates anteriorly or posteriorly.

2.1.2
Pathology of Anterior Shoulder Instability

Numerous studies have underlined the important role played by the anterior glenoid labrum in posttraumatic anterior shoulder instability (BANKART 1923; BOST and INMAN 1942; MOSELEY and OVERGAARD 1962). Recently, BAKER et al. (1990) have described a classification of lesions after an initial episode of traumatic anterior shoulder dislocation on the basis of their arthroscopic observations (Table 2.2).

In chronic anterior instability, the essential lesion is the laxity of the inferior glenohumeral ligament complex (IGHLC). In many cases, such a lesion is due to an avulsion of the glenoid labrum (Bankart lesion). In other cases, the labrum appears to be intact and the lesion consists in a tear of the glenohumeral ligaments, which remain loose after healing. NEVIASER (1992) described a lesion characterized by an avulsion of the anterior labrum and of the periosteal sleeve from the neck of the glenoid (ALPSA lesion). In such cases, the labrum is medially reinserted, and the synovial tends to fill the space above, simulating the labrum. Moreover, a small loose pocket is formed between the glenoid and the capsule, which makes the IGHLC incompetent. In some cases, WOLF (1992) observed glenohumeral ligament avulsion at the humeral insertion (HAGL lesion). Often, it is possible to observe osteochondral lesions of the posterior surface of the humeral head, the so-called Hill-Sachs lesions, which may elicit the

Table 2.2. Classification of acute anterior dislocation pathology[a]

Class	Clinical findings (under anesthesia)	Hemarthrosis	Pathology
I	Stable	<10 ml	Capsular stretch injury
II	Anterior subluxation	10–15 ml	Mild, partial detachment of glenoid labrum and IGHLC
III	Gross anterior instability	>15 ml	Complete capsular and labral detachment

IGHLC, inferior glenohumeral ligament complex.
[a] From BAKER et al. 1990.

Table 2.3. Classification of SLAP lesions[a]

Type	Pathology
I	Fraying and degeneration of the superior labrum with normal biceps tendon anchor
II	Possible fraying of the superior labrum with pathologic detachment of the labrum and biceps anchor from the superior glenoid
III	Bucket-handle tear of the superior labrum which may displace into the glenohumeral joint; the biceps anchor remains intact
IV	Bucket-handle tear of the superior labrum which extends into the biceps tendon; the remainder of the biceps anchor is well attached
Complex	A combination of two or more types

SLAP, superior labrum anterior to posterior.
[a] From SNYDER et al. 1990.

formation of loose bodies, frequently located in the subscapularis recess. The glenoid surface, too, may present chondral and osteochondral lesions, which sometimes are the result of a fracture avulsion of the anterior glenoid labrum (osseous Bankart lesion). The glenoid labrum may present flap, bucket-handle or degenerative lesions. ANDREWS et al. (1985) have described the presence of a lesion of the antero-superior labrum in throwers. Such lesions are secondary to an excessive traction of the long head of the biceps, and in 10% of the cases they are associated with biceps tendon and rotator cuff lesions.

Recently, SNYDER et al. (1990) described a superior labrum anterior to posterior (SLAP) lesion involving the insertion of the tendon of the long head of the biceps. Such lesions are often due to a traction and compression trauma (excessive traction on the bicipital anchor during the deceleration phase of the throw or a fall on the outstretched arm), and are often associated with anterior instability. SNYDER et al. (1990) have described four types of SLAP lesion, according to the arthroscopic appearance (Table 2.3).

2.1.3
Posterior Instability

Posterior instability may be characterized by an acute traumatic dislocation or by a recurrent subluxation. The latter may be involuntary (on a microtraumatic basis), traumatic-voluntary or atraumatic-voluntary.

The acute traumatic posterior dislocation in most cases is due to an indirect shoulder trauma with the limb in intrarotation, adduction and flexion, or to a strong contraction of intrarotator muscles (i.e., seizures, electroshock).

Involuntary recurrent posterior subluxation is the most frequent form of posterior instability and mainly affects throwers, swimmers, and archers, who develop significant posterior forces during sporting activities. In these patients, the main symptom is pain, which is more intense in the deceleration phase of the throw and may be clinically elicited by putting the limb into flexion, adduction and intrarotation. The load and shift test shows posterior laxity. However, most of these subjects do not complain of instability, and in many cases the apprehension test may also be negative. Often, a generalized ligamentous laxity is reported.

Intraarticular lesions in a posterior acute traumatic dislocation are characterized by a tear of the capsule or of the posterior labrum (posterior Bankart lesion), and often by an impact fracture of the anterior side of the humeral head (reverse Hill-

Sachs lesion). In involuntary recurring subluxation, on the other hand, the pathology is less evident. Often, the posterior Bankart lesion is absent, and only small degenerative lesions of the posterior labrum are observed (HAWKINS and BELLE 1989). At the level of the posterior glenoid, it is possible to observe signs of chondral damage, calcifications or erosions of the bone margin (BOWEN et al. 1991).

2.1.4
Multidirectional Instability

Multidirectional instability is mainly characterized by inferior instability, associated with an anterior and/or posterior instability (NEER 1990). Many of these patients suffer from a bilateral symptomatology, and in 20% of cases they also present subacromial impingement symptoms (ALTCHECK et al. 1991). In about 50% of cases, there is a generalized ligamentous laxity. The pathogenesis of multidirectional instability often occurs without trauma and is associated with a redundant inferior capsule, with a virtually complete absence of the medial glenohumeral ligament (MGHL) and of the IGHLC (NEER and FOSTER 1980). In other cases, the onset of the symptoms may be associated with a traumatic event. This type of instability is more frequent in athletes, in whom a "loose shoulder" is subjected more to microtraumas and presents a higher traumatic dislocation risk. In these patients, multidirectional instability is often associated with a Bankart lesion.

2.2
Rotator Cuff Pathology

Rotator cuff pathology in athletes is a problem that has aroused special interest over the past few years. Numerous clinical studies have shown that the incidence of rotator cuff disease is especially high (50%–80%) in tennis players, swimmers, throwers and all overhead athletes (BENNETT 1959; KENNEDY et al. 1978; RICHARDSON et al. 1980; HILL 1983; LEHMAN 1988; CIULLO and STEVENS 1989).

2.2.1
Etiopathogenesis

The etiology of rotator cuff lesions is still rather controversial. CODMAN (1934) was the first to describe cuff lesions, asserting the hypothesis of degenerative tendon lesions. In 1972, NEER and MARBERRY described the so-called impingement syndrome, observing that 95% of rotator cuff lesions are due to friction against the anteroinferior surface of the acromion. However, recent clinical and cadaver studies have shown that impingement may be characterized by a multifactorial etiology (OZAKI et al. 1988; UHTHOFF et al. 1988; OGATA and UHTHOFF 1990). In athletes, especially, impingement is a phenomenon secondary to eccentric muscle overload or to an associated glenohumeral instability. Indeed, the eccentric overload due to overuse during the practice of overhead sports may cause damage to the tendon fibers. Likewise, anterior or multidirectional instability may cause a functional overload of the rotator cuff to keep the humeral head centered, resulting in tendon damage. Over time, such phenomena may reduce the competence of the supraspinatus, bringing about a prevalence of the deltoid muscle, which then tends to displace the humeral head upwards, with the consequent onset of secondary impingement and further damage to the cuff and the long head of the biceps.

2.2.2
Physical Examination of Rotator Cuff Lesions

In assessing the painful shoulder of an athlete, the sport practiced must be considered, in addition to the level of participation, the type of motion that causes the pain and the training methods. In the case of a traumatic event, efforts should be made to identify the traumatic mechanism. In patients who perform symmetric sports (i.e. swimming and gymnastics), the bilateral nature of the symptoms must always be investigated. It is also important to identify the site of the pain – and try to rule out other diseases that may simulate an impingement syndrome – as well as the degree of pain, so as to formulate an adequate treatment approach.

The tenderness is frequently localized on the greater tuberosity (insertion of the supraspinatus) and in the bicipital groove in the case of tendinitis of the long head of the biceps. Tenderness of the acromioclavicular joint is indicative of the joint's involvement in impingement disorders. There are also specific maneuvers capable of eliciting pain in the case of an impingement syndrome. The pain is due to the contact between the supraspinatus and the anterior part of the undersurface of the acromion and the coracoacromial ligament. These maneuvers are the *impingement sign* (passive abduction of the limb on the scapular plane, with the humerus in intrarotation and the scapula stabilized by the hand of the examiner), the *Hawkins test* (the arm is abducted in the scapular plane up to the horizontal plane, then subjected to intrarotation and adduction), and the *Yocum test* (the arm is adducted by forcing the hand on the contralateral shoulder, after which a flexion against resistance is performed).

The *Neer test*, also known as the *impingement test*, is a clinical test of significant diagnostic value. It comprises an infiltration of about 7–10 ml of local anesthetic into the subacromial space. The disappearance of pain after the performance of this test is indicative of a subacromial impingement pathology.

The passive and active range of motion of the joint can be evaluated by flexion in the scapular plane, abduction, intrarotation and extrarotation. The active range of motion of the joint may be limited both by the pain and the muscle weakness due to a lesion of the rotator cuff. Therefore, these measures, too, must be evaluated before and after the Neer test.

The evaluation of muscle force is important in the diagnosis of a rotator cuff lesion. A scale from 0 to 5 is used. The force of the supraspinatus is evaluated by means of the *Jobe test* (abduction in the scapular plane with the arm in intrarotation; Fig. 2.1). The infraspinatus is evaluated by inducing the patient to engage in extrarotation with his elbows in adduction. The involvement of the long head of the biceps is assessed by means of the *palm up test* (arm flexion against resistance with an extended elbow and a supinated forearm) and the *Yergason test* (supination of the forearm against resistance). In the presence of an impingement syndrome, a force deficiency may be due to the presence of pain. In this case, after the performance of Neer's test the muscle force of the affected shoulder will be the same as that of the contralateral shoulder. A deficit of muscle strength that is evident even after infiltrating the local anesthetic into the subacromial space is indicative of a full-thickness tear of one or more tendons of the rotator cuff.

2.2.3
Classifications of Rotator Cuff Lesions

NEER (1983) identified three different stages in impingement syndrome. *Stage 1* is characterized by an edema and hemorrhage of the subacromial bursa and the cuff, and it affects young patients under 25 years of age. *Stage 2* is characterized by a fibrosis and thickening of the subacromial bursa, associated with partial lesions of the rotator cuff, and it affects patients aged 25 to 40 years of age. *Stage 3* is characterized by a full-thickness lesion of the rotator cuff, often associated with lesions of the long head of the biceps tendon, and by bone changes related to the impingement at the level of the coracromial arch and the humeral greater tuberosity. It almost exclusively affects patients over 40. Rotator cuff lesions may be of different sizes and severity.

Partial cuff lesions usually involve the tendon of the supraspinatus. ELLMAN (1990) divided partial lesions into articular (A) and bursal (B) lesions, (Fig. 2.2) and assigned them to three grades according to the depth of the lesion (Table 2.4). Full-thickness lesions were classified by MATSEN (1993) on the basis of the extension of the lesions and the tendons involved: *stage 1*, complete supraspinatus lesion (<2 cm); *stage 2*, complete lesion of the supraspinatus and at least one part of the infraspinatus (2–4 cm); *stage 3*, complete lesion of the supraspinatus, the infraspinatus and the subscapularis (>4 cm); *stage 4*, cuff tear arthropathy. Recently, SNYDER (1993) proposed a classification of rotator cuff lesions based on surface, severity and the site of the lesion.

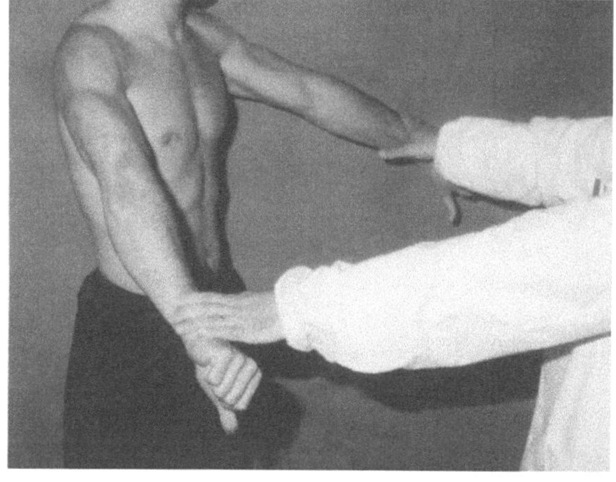

Fig. 2.1. Jobe's test: this test is carried out in standing position. The patient performs an abduction in the scapular plane against resistance with the arm in intrarotation. Jobe's test evaluates the muscular strength of the supraspinatus

Table 2.4. Classification of partial tears (after Ellman 1990)

Grade	Thickness
1	<1/4 (<3 mm)
2	<1/2 (3–6 mm)
3	>1/2 (>6 mm)

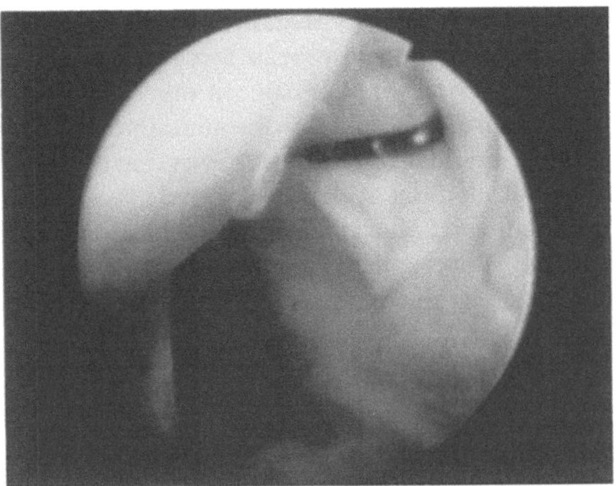

Fig. 2.2. Arthroscopic view of a Grade 2 articular-side partial tear of the rotator cuff according to Ellman's classification

2.3
Elbow Instability

Elbow instabilities can be classified according to the components of the elbow joint (ulnohumeral, radioulnar) involved, the direction and severity of instability and the presence of associated fractures.

The primary constraints to elbow instability are the medial collateral ligament (anterior band), the lateral collateral ligament (ulnar part) and an intact ulnohumeral joint. Secondary constraints include the radial head, the common extensor and flexor tendon origins and the anterior and posterior capsules.

2.3.1
Medial Elbow Instability (Ulnar Collateral Ligament Injury)

The anterior band of the ulnar collateral ligament is the primary structure resisting valgus stress at the elbow. The rupture of the ulnar collateral ligament often occurs in throwing athletes during the act of throwing. The athlete will complain of acute medial elbow pain accompanied by a "pop" felt or heard by the athlete. The "gravity stress test" can be useful in determining medial elbow instability, but frequently anesthesia is necessary to complete the gravity test because of the pain and muscle contracture. The test is carried out with the patient in a supine position, arm abducted at 90° with maximal external rotation

and the elbow flexed at 20°. In this way, the gravity of the force will open the medial compartment and laxity can be demonstrated by anteroposterior rays. Almost all patients with an acute ulnar collateral ligament injury have a history of pain and tenderness over the medial aspect of the elbow, a consequence of repeated high valgus stress.

2.3.2
Chronic Ulnar Collateral Ligament Insufficiency

The overuse syndrome in throwing athletes causes pathological processes within the ligament structure consisting of progressive destructive changes. This determines a slow deterioration in function of the elbow with pain and loss of control. The patient may also report pain or paresthesia radiating onto the ulnar aspect of the forearm, hand and fourth and fifth fingers. On clinical examination, valgus instability is always present. This is best examined with the patient seated and the hand and wrist held between the examiner's forearm and trunk. The patient's elbow is flexed by 25° to unlock the olecranon from its fossa, the humerus is externally rotated to lock the shoulder, and the medial aspect of the elbow receives a valgus stress. Local pain, tenderness and end-point laxity are revealed by this maneuver.

2.4
Wrist Instability

Wrist instability, frequently occurring in any type of sport and at all levels of activity, may be the consequence of a single traumatic event or of repeated microtraumas. The most frequent traumatic mechanism, however, is a trauma in hyperextension of the wrist. MAYFELD (1984) showed experimentally that ligament lesions generally begin on the radial margin of the carpus and radiate towards the ulnar margin as the intensity of the trauma increases.

2.4.1
Scapholunate Instability

The most frequent form of carpal instability is scapholunate dissociation or rotary subluxation of the scaphoid. There are three ligaments involved in scapholunate instability: the interosseous scapholunate ligament, the dorsal scapholunate ligament and the volar radioscapholunate ligament, which is the strongest and the most important of the three. In order for a dissociation to occur, at least two ligaments must be damaged, while subluxation may occur if only the volar radioscapholunate ligament is torn (LEWIS et al. 1970; TALEISNIK 1978).

Often, due to the faded symptoms, most of these lesions escape diagnosis (ISANI 1986). The clinical history of the subject generally includes a direct trauma with hyperextension, ulnar deviation and intercarpal wrist supination (MAYFIELD 1984; TALEISNIK 1985). The main symptoms are pain and swelling on the dorsoradial face of the wrist, especially at the level of the anatomical snuffbox. WATSON and HEMPTON (1980) proposed a clinical test for the diagnosis of scaphoulnar instability. By passively taking the wrist from ulnar to radial deviation and exerting volar pressure on the scaphoid tuberosity, the proximal pole of the scaphoid may be dislocated from the scaphoid fossa of the radius, thus causing pain. Instability that has been present for over 3 months is defined as chronic. The symptoms are characterized by the presence of intermittent pain which increases with wrist rotation or radial deviation.

2.4.2
Medial Instability

Medial or ulnar instability includes triquetrohamate or mediocarpal instability and triquetrolunate instability.

Triquetrohamate dissociation, the most common form of ulnar instability, is caused by ulnar arm lesion of the arcuate ligament (ALEXANDER and LICHTMAN 1984). These patients have a "clunk" that can be heard or palpated. It is reproduced by the ulnar deviation movements and wrist pronation. The clinical examination often reveals a typical tenderness over the triquetrum.

Triquetrolunate instability is less frequent. The exact etiopathogenetic mechanism is not well known. However, an isolated triquetrolunate lesion could be determined by hyperpronation of the hand on the forearm (TALEISNIK 1985) or by a trauma on the back of the hand in flexion, which determines the lesion of the radiotriquetrolunate ligament (WEBER 1980, 1984). Clinically, patients may have a painful wrist click. Local tenderness may be identified over the triquetrolunate joint.

2.5
Knee Instability

2.5.1
Ligamentous Injuries

Knee ligament injuries are more frequent in athletes who practice contact sports such as rugby, soccer and basketball.

Knee stability is determined both by the presence of passive ligament structures and active muscle-tendineous structures. Passive stability of the knee depends on the joint surfaces and on the cruciate ligaments as well as the collateral ligaments. The active stability depends on the musculotendineous structures, of which the main ones are the quadriceps muscle, the femoral biceps, the tensor fascia lata muscle, the hamstring muscles, the popliteus muscle and the gastrocnemius muscles.

2.5.1.1
Mechanism of Injury

The mechanisms that most frequently cause an anterior cruciate ligament (ACL) lesion are the following:

1. Pure hyperextension: In this case, the quadriceps contraction causes maximum stretching of the anterior cruciate ligament, which may break at the level of the intercondylar notch.
2. Hyperextension with internal rotation: This is the most frequent cause of an isolated ACL lesion. The internal rotation and the quadriceps contraction cause maximum stretching of the anterior cruciate ligament, which usually breaks at the middle third. This is the most frequent lesion mechanism in basketball in the landing phase, after a rebounding jump (SILBEY and FU 1994).
3. Valgus and external rotation: This is one of the most common mechanisms, as is often observed in skiing, football and soccer (SILBEY and FU 1994). The ACL lesion occurs after the medial collateral ligament injury. It may also be associated with a medial meniscus lesion (O'Donoghue's triad).

Varus and internal rotation injuries are less frequent.

Posterior cruciate ligament (PCL) lesions may be caused by:

1. Direct injury of the anterior tibial surface with flexed knee. This mechanism is typical of high-speed injuries such as those in motor sports.

2. Single-foot support hyperextension. This is very rare but extremely severe. The PCL is in maximum tension as of 25° of recurvatum. This is why the posteromedial and posterolateral corners break first, followed by PCL injury with posterior tibial subluxation.

There are also pure valgus or varus injury mechanisms without a rotation component:

The pure valgus mechanism is caused by a lateral direct injury and is the most frequent mechanism. It determines internal collateral ligament lesion and, depending on the severity of the trauma, an injury of the posteromedial corner, the ACL and the PCL.

The pure varus mechanism is caused by a medial direct injury and frequently determines lateral collateral ligament lesions. The posterolateral corner is almost always involved, with a different degree of lesion severity as the severity of the trauma.

2.5.1.2
Classification of Instability

Instability may be divided into direct or rotatory instability, according to the abnormal tibial movement on the femoral condyle. According to HUGHSTON's classification (1976a and b), there may be four main types of direct instability: medial, lateral, anterior and posterior. By definition, all rotating components are excluded from these forms of instability.

There are three types of rotatory instability: anteromedial, anterolateral and posterolateral. In anteromedial rotatory instability, there is a transient subluxation of the medial tibial plateau on the femur forwards and externally, due to a lesion of the medial structures. In the most severe forms, this is accompanied by a posterior cruciate ligament lesion. In anterolateral rotatory instability, however, there is an excessive anterior and internal rotating translation of the external tibial plateau on the femur. Typically, it is related to an anterior cruciate ligament and lateral capsuloligamentous injury. Posterolateral rotatory instability is characterized by a tibial posterior subluxation and is determined by a posterolateral structure lesion. In chronic lesions, there may be a combination of the different forms of rotatory instability. The most common association is that between anteromedial and anterolateral instability.

2.5.1.3
Physical Examination

2.5.1.3.1
COLLATERAL LIGAMENTS

Collateral ligament injuries may be divided into three grades, according to anatomic, functional and clinical criteria. In grade I, the ligament is anatomically integral, presenting no functional instability. Clinically, a moderate pain runs along the length of the ligament. Varus or valgus tests reveal an opening of the affected compartment no greater than 5 mm compared to the contralateral side. In grade II there is a partial interruption of the ligament with moderate instability. Clinically, pain is present in the proximity of the collateral ligament. Varus or valgus tests reveal an opening of the joint of 5–10 mm compared to the controlateral side. In grade III there is complete ligament rupture. Varus or valgus tests show a joint opening of more than 10 mm.

Lateral laxity tests comprise inducing valgus and varus lateral movements, with a flexed knee at 30° and in extension. Indeed, the extension tests are performed to evaluate the collateral ligaments, together with the posteromedial and posterolateral structures. Instability in extension may be indicative of a PCL lesion. The 30° flexion test makes it possible to evaluate collateral ligaments individually. In fact, in this position the posterior capsule and posteromedial and posterolateral corner structures are not stretched.

2.5.1.3.2
ANTERIOR CRUCIATE LIGAMENT

The anterior drawer sign may be elicited at 60° and 90° of knee flexion. The anterior drawer is elicited in three rotation positions: 30° of internal rotation (Slocum test), neutral position, and 15° of external rotation. The external and internal rotation positions allow for a better definition of the possible presence of associated lesions. The anterior drawer in external rotation evaluates the posteromedial corner, while the anterior drawer in internal rotation evaluates the posterior cruciate ligament and posteroexternal corner. The Lachman test is performed at 30° flexion and is the most reliable for the diagnosis of anterior cruciate ligament lesions. Indeed, the drawer test at 60°–90° of knee flexion sometimes cannot be performed due to the presence of an intraarticular swelling which constrains flexion, or due to hamstring contracture. In extension, the hamstrings' opposite force is annulled. The contact surface between the femoral condyle and the tibial plateau is relatively flat, favoring gliding.

There are also dynamic tests which evidence the high mobility of the lateral compartment, with an anterolateral click due to the anterior subluxation of the lateral tibial plateau. The most widely used dynamic tests are the Hughston jerk test, the pivot-shift test (GALWAY 1972), the MacIntosh test (GALWAY and MACINTOSH 1980), and the Losee test (LOSEE et al. 1978; LOSEE 1988). When these tests are positive, they are pathognomonic of an ACL lesion. However, they are often difficult to perform, especially in acute lesions but also in chronic lesions, as the patient has difficulty releasing the muscles.

2.5.1.3.3
POSTERIOR CRUCIATE LIGAMENT
The posterior drawer must be performed at 90° of knee flexion. It may be executed with the foot in neutral rotation (direct posterior drawer), in which case it is the expression of an isolated PCL lesion. In external rotation (external rotational posterior drawer), it is the expression of a PCL lesion associated with an injury of posterolateral structures. In internal rotation (internal rotational posterior drawer), it is the expression of a PCL injury associated with a lesion of posteromedial structures. The recurvatum test makes it possible to evaluate the possible presence of a retroposition's of the tibial tuberosity of the side involved. Hughston's external rotation recurvatum test makes it possible to evidence the recurvatum as well as the presence of a varus and an external rotation. It is the expression of rotatory posterolateral instability. Dynamic tests also exist for PCL lesion diagnosis, such as the reversed pivot-shift. They reveal the hypermobility of the external compartment, as evidenced by the external tibial plateau posterior subluxation.

2.5.2
Patellofemoral Instability

The term patellar instability refers to different clinical pictures of the patellofemoral joint, which range from subluxation to dislocation. Patellofemoral instability is most frequently observed in women who practice certain types of sports, especially ballet (LIEBLER 1974), gymnastics (WEISS 1994) and jumping and running in athletics (WHITMAN et al. 1981).

2.5.2.1
Etiopathogenesis

The patella, in its articular range, is guided and controlled by the quadriceps. The vastus lateralis exerts a superior and lateral traction on the patella. The vastus medialis, especially the vastus medialis obliquus (VMO), exerts a medial traction that counters the action of the more powerful vastus lateralis, for the more distal and horizontal insertion. The rectus femoris and the vastus intermedius, on the other hand, exert a superior traction along the femoral axis. The VMO is likely to be the critical muscle for the correct balance of the patella, and a VMO weakness may be the primary cause of patellofemoral instability. The active stabilizers of the patellofemoral joint also include the pes anserinus muscles, which, by determining tibial intrarotation, keep the tibial tuberosity aligned with the patella. Passive stabilizers, on the other hand, include the lateral and medial retinaculum and the shape of the patella and the trochlear groove. The position of the tibial tuberosity is equally important in determining patellar mediolateral stability. The relationship between the direction of the traction exerted by the quadriceps and the patellar tendon insertion on the tibial tuberosity is expressed by the Q angle. The value of the Q angle is given by the complementary angle between the line that goes to the midpatella from the anterosuperior iliac spine, which ideally represents the force quadriceps line, and the line that connects the midpatella with the tibial tuberosity. Normally, the Q angle ranges from 8° to 14° in males and 11° to 20° in females (AGLIETTI et al. 1983). Any Q angle increase will determine an increase in the lateral force vector that acts on the patella, and consequently causes a tendency towards patellar instability. The Q angle is greater in subjects with an increased femoral antiversion, an increased tibial extrarotation or with a valgus knee. Equally, a retraction of the lateral retinaculum may increase lateral traction forces on the patella, thus favoring instability.

2.5.2.2
Clinical Forms

In chronic subluxation, the patella is more lateral than in its normal position, at least in the first part of its range in the trochlear groove (MERCHANT 1994). Subluxation is often associated with a patellar tilt. Only occasionally, in patients with generalized hyperlaxity, subluxation is not associated with a tilt. The most severe form of patellofemoral instability is recurrent patellar dislocation, in which the patient presents numerous recurring instability episodes (MERCHANT 1994). It is especially important to distinguish between subluxation or dislocation and an isolated lateral tilt on the axial plane. FULKERSON and CAUTILLI (1993) classified patellofemoral malalignment according to three types. Type I is characterized by subluxation alone, type II by subluxation and a tilt, and type III by the tilt alone, without subluxation.

2.5.2.3
Physical Examination

The most frequent symptoms are pain, cracking and effusion during sporting activities in which there are increased patellofemoral contact forces. The pain is typically anterior, but it may be vague with an insidious onset. Mechanical symptoms may sometimes be present, such as locking. The pain is exacerbated by prolonged flexion of the knee, uphill running or climbing of stairs. The downward compression of the patella causes the patient to engage in an isometric contraction of the quadriceps, thus eliciting pain. The symptom related to instability is giving way with acute pain, which rapidly fades. Generally, patients suffering from patellar instability present a positive apprehension sign, which is elicited by moving the patella laterally. Patellar hypermobility may be measured by subluxating the patella medially and laterally and evaluating the magnitude of the shift. Moreover, most patients with patellar instability often experience bilateral symptoms.

2.6
Ankle Instability

Ankle sprains are the most frequent injuries in sport (GLICK et al. 1976; BALDUINI and TETZLAFF 1982; LASSITER et al. 1989). In a case series of 4673 patients treated for sports injuries, MAEHLUM and DALJORD (1984) reported an incidence rate as high as 16%. GARRICK (1977), moreover, observed that ankle sprains account for 45% of lesions in basketball, and 31% of lesions in soccer. The age group affected most frequently is that under 35 years, especially the range between 15 and 19 years (NILSSON 1982).

2.6.1
Etiopathogenesis

The most common lesion mechanism is a twisting injury in plantar flexion and inversion, which in over 90% of cases determines a lesion of the lateral ligament complex (BALDUINI and TETZLAFF 1982). This is due to the fact that when the foot is plantar-flexed, the narrower part of the talus is engaged in the tibiofibular mortise and the joint is mechanically less stable (INGLIS et al. 1976). The first ligament to be damaged is the anterior talofibular ligament (DIAS 1979). An isolated lesion of this ligament, even without the concomitant lesion of the calcaneofibular ligament, may cause residual instability (BROSTROM 1966). Moreover, an anterior talofibular ligament lesion, which is a thickening of the anterior joint capsule, represents a capsular lesion. As a result, even if there is no clinical instability, such a lesion may represent a spine irritating to the joint during sports activity, and may cause chronic pain (ANDREWS et al. 1984). The second ligament to be injured in an inversion trauma is the calcaneofibular ligament. However, in order for a lesion to occur, the talofibular ligament does not have to be completely ruptured. An isolated calcaneofibular ligament lesion may occur in the rare cases in which an inversion injury takes place with the foot in dorsiflexion. After a twisting injury in plantar flexion and inversion, there is an isolated lesion of the anterior talofibular ligament in 66% of cases, and a calcaneofibular ligament combined lesion in another 20% of cases (BROSTROM 1966). The isolated posterior talofibular ligament lesion, on the other hand, is very rare (BROSTROM 1966; BALDUINI and TETZLAFF 1982).

2.6.2
Physical Examination

The Standard Nomenclature of Athletic Injuries (1966) classified ankle ligament lesions into three grades. Grade I, mild, and is characterized by a sprain of the ligaments without an obvious macroscopic lesion, mild periarticular swelling and pain, no functional deficiency and no joint mechanical instability. In grade II, moderate, there is a partial lesion of the ligaments, with moderate pain, periarticular swelling and tenderness on palpation of the damaged structures. Functional deficiency is also recorded, with a modest joint instability. Grade III, severe, is characterized by a complete lesion of the ligaments with severe periarticular hemorrhagic swelling, severe functional impotence and joint instability. Another classification divides sprains into: grade I, defined as a partial or complete anterior talofibular ligament lesion; grade II, characterized by a lesion of both the anterior talofibular ligament and the calcaneofibular ligament; and grade III, characterized by a lesion of all three ligaments (LEACH 1983). Clinical tests for lateral ankle instability are the anterior drawer sign and the lateral talar tilt. The anterior drawer sign evaluates the anterior movement of the talus with respect to the tibia. When performing the test, the foot must be placed in slight dorsiflexion. The test must always be correlated to the healthy contralateral side. A positive anterior drawer test indicates a lesion of the anterior talofibular ligament. The lateral talar tilt evaluates the integrity of the calcaneofibular ligament. It is performed with a passive supination of the tibiotarsal joint with the foot in dorsiflexion. An increase in the tilt indicates an isolated lesion of the calcaneofibular ligament or a lesion associated with an anterior talofibular ligament lesion.

A medial sprain of the tibiotarsal joint, on the other hand, is caused by an eversion injury (STAPLES 1960). However, medial instability caused by a twisting injury is a rather rare event. Indeed, a deltoid ligament lesion is usually preceded by a fracture of the medial malleolus.

A syndesmotic or "high" ankle sprain may occur as an isolated lesion, or in conjunction with a lateral ankle sprain. A syndesmotic lesion accounts for about 10% of all tibiotarsal lesions, and it is more common in collision sports such as ice hockey, soccer and football (JAIVIN and FERKEL 1994). The most common mechanism determining the injury is an external rotation injury with the foot in forced dorsiflexion. The squeeze test may be used as a diagnostic test. It is performed by compressing the fibula to the tibia at the third middle of the calf. The test is positive when the compression determines pain in the area of the interosseous membrane and syndesmotic ligaments. Another diagnostic test is the external rotation test. It is performed by applying stress in external rotation on the foot, with the knee flexed at 90° and the ankle in a neutral position (BOYTIM et al. 1991). The test is positive if it elicits pain at the level of anterior and posterior tibiofibular ligaments and on the interosseous membrane.

Following an ankle sprain, the most common and serious residual disability is functional instability, that is, recurring twisting episodes and a feeling of giving way. Indeed, a ligament laxity may persist to such an extent that even minor injury will be sufficient to cause a serious lesion. EKSTRAND and TROPP (1990) reported a 50% rate of recurrence in soccer players with a history of ankle sprain. However, the exact etiopathogenetic mechanism responsible for chronic instability is still not well known. The numerous possible causes that have been suggested include mechanical instability (FREEMAN 1965; FREEMAN et al. 1965; TROPP 1985), peroneal muscle weakness (TROPP 1985), and a lesion of proprioceptive systems, which may determine a feeling of giving way in an otherwise stable joint, or a subtalar instability (ZWIPP and TSCHERNE 1984).

2.7
Ankle Impingement

2.7.1
Soft Tissue Impingement

Most ankle sprains heal definitively. However, in an investigation performed on basketball players, it was observed that 50% of the subjects presented residual symptoms after an ankle sprain, and that in 15% of such cases, the symptoms were such that they jeopardized the sports activity (SMITH and REISCHL 1986).

As early as 1950, WOLIN et al. described nine patients who, following an ankle inversion sprain, presented chronic pain and a mild swelling of the anterolateral side of the ankle. Arthrotomy revealed a mass of hyalinized connective tissue originating from the anterior talofibular ligament. Due to its resemblance to the meniscus of the knee, the authors gave the name "meniscoid" to this lesion. They believed that the trapping of this hyalinized tissue between the talus and the peroneal malleolus was responsible for the painful symptoms.

2.7.1.1
Etiopathogenesis

Soft tissue impingement is usually located in the anterolateral compartment of the ankle. It is caused by repeated injuries in plantar flexion and inversion of the ankle. FERKEL and FISCHER (1989) maintain that an anterolateral impingement is caused by a lesion of the anterior talofibular and anteroinferior tibiofibular ligaments. In these cases, the lesion is not so severe as to entail chronic instability. However, it does cause the formation of scar tissue and the onset of reactive hypertrophic synovitis, which is responsible for chronic pain. GUHL (1988) suggested that an impingement syndrome should be suspected also in fractures without displacement of the fibular malleolus followed by persistent pain. MEISLIN et al. (1993) have indeed reported that in a case series of 29 patients, 5 had suffered from a previous bimalleolar fracture. It is likely that in these cases, there is a lesion of the anteroinferior tibiofibular ligament, with a hypertrophic reactive synovitis of the tibiotalar joint. The meniscoid lesion probably represents a more advanced form of synovial impingement syndrome (FERKEL et al. 1991; Fig. 2.3). To date, there are no convergent opinions on the pathogenesis of the meniscoid lesion. WOLIN et al. (1950), who described the lesion first, suggested that the injury might cause an inflammatory exudate of the synovial membrane coating the damaged ligament. Its incomplete reabsorption may be responsible for the persistence of chronically inflamed scar tissue shaped by the compression between the talus and the fibular malleolus during normal joint movements. Other authors have maintained that the meniscoid tissue is comprised of damaged fibers of the capsule and lateral ligaments and of inflamed synovial tissue, which is interposed between the fibular malleolus and the talus (McGINTY et al. 1984; ANDREWS et al. 1984; McCARROL et al. 1987; SCHONHOLTZ 1987). However, the exact incidence of a meniscoid lesion in soft tissue impingement syndrome of the ankle is unknown. CHEN (1985) believes that the "meniscoid" tissue is connected with the anterior talofibular ligament and projects out onto the joint space between the talus and the lateral malleolus. He holds that the tissue is always present following an

ankle sprain. FERKEL et al. (1991) have reported a meniscoid lesion only in 4 (13%) out of 31 patients with lateral chronic pain. According to different authors, the term "meniscoid lesion" must therefore be abandoned, and this disorder must be considered as part of the wider context of the soft tissue impingement syndrome (FERKEL and FISCHER 1989; MARTIN et al. 1989b; MEISLIN et al. 1993).

2.7.1.2
Clinical Examination

The main symptom is chronic lateral and/or anterolateral pain. The pain is accentuated by load, with possible instability episodes, on an antalgic basis, and a consequently decreased sports performance. Especially running, if characterized by frequent and sudden changes in direction, will increase pain associated with clicking and instability. The manual compression of the fibular malleolus against the talus will also cause pain. Periarticular swelling is also frequently observed, especially after some strain.

2.7.2
Bone Impingement

One possible cause of chronic pain in the tibiotarsal region may be the presence of an anterior osteophyte in the tibia which projects out onto the tibiotalar joint (Fig. 2.4). Often, an osteophyte is also present in the neck of the talus. The dorsiflexion of the foot thus

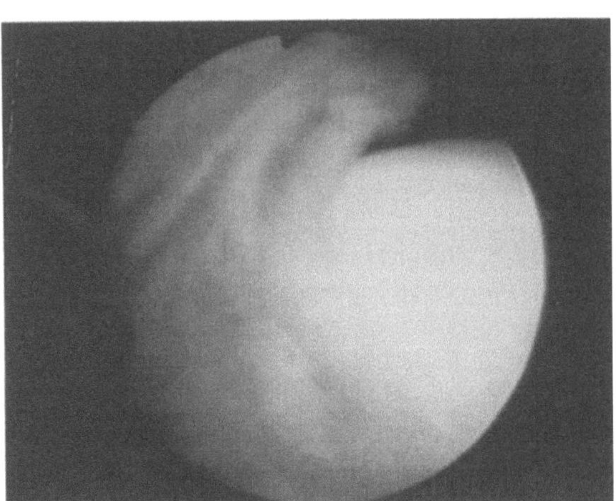

Fig. 2.3. Arthroscopic view of meniscoid lesion in the anterolateral gutter of the ankle

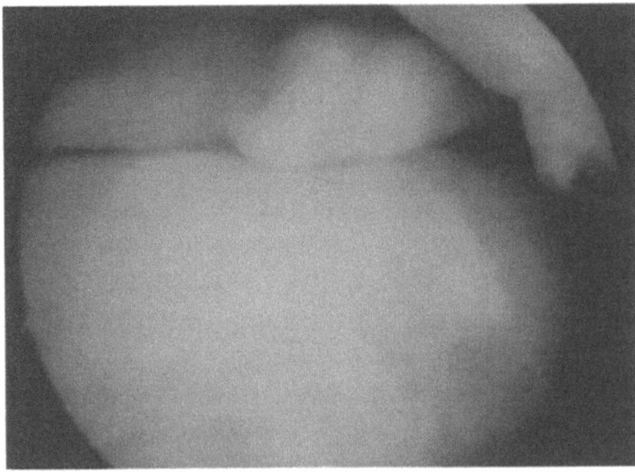

Fig. 2.4. Arthroscopic aspect of anterior osteophyte of the tibia protruding into the tibiotalar joint

determines an impingement of the osteophyte with the talus, with a consequently painful and restrained movement. This alteration was first described by MORRIS (1943), who defined it as "athlete's ankle". MCMURRAY (1950) then referred to this disorder as "footballer's ankle". Numerous other authors later described this alteration in athletes involved in sporting activities that require repetitive and forceful dorsiflexion movements of the ankle (O'DONOGHUE 1957; BRODELIUS 1960; PARKES et al. 1980; HARDAKER et al. 1985; MARTIN et al. 1989a; PARISIEN 1991).

2.7.2.1
Etiopathogenesis

Rather than being caused by a single injury, anterior impingement is due to repetitive microinjuries resulting from continuous inversion traumas and/or the constant repetition of sport activities that require a forceful dorsiflexion of the foot (OGILVIE-HARRIS et al. 1993). This explains the high incidence of this alteration in dancers, high jumpers, sprinters and skiers, who all subject their ankles to extreme dorsiflexion (KLEIGER 1982). A 59% anterior osteophyte incidence was reported in dancers (STOLLER et al. 1984), while in soccer players the frequency ranges from 45% to 60% (O'DONOGHUE 1957; MASSADA 1991). In addition to the microinjuries due to the forced dorsiflexion of the foot, in soccer players the formation of the osteophyte may also be due to the microtraumas caused by the impact of the ball with the neck of the foot. Frequent association with a narrowing of the articular space and degenerative midtarsal joint changes suggests that the anterior osteophyte may be the sign of an early degenerative process (MCDOUGALL 1955; O'DONOGHUE 1957; BRODELIUS 1960). Indeed, the presence of an osteophyte may be observed on the anterior margin of the tibia or on the neck of the talus, but also on the medial margin of the talus, on the anterior margin of the medial malleolus and on the lateral malleolus (PARISIEN 1991). Moreover, a posterior bone impingement has been described, especially in dancers. In fact, when a dancer dances on his toes, the tibiotarsal joint withstands an estimated load of 20 g/cm^2 (ENDE and WICKSTROM 1982), and the posterior tubercle of the talus is compressed between the posterior tibial margin and the posterior facet of the calcaneous (KLEIGER 1982). Forced plantar flexion may cause hypertrophy of the posterior tubercle of the talus, the formation of heterotopic ossifications,

and also a detachment of the os trigonum (KLEIGER 1982).

2.7.2.2
Physical Examination

Patients with bone impingement typically report chronic pain, painful restriction of mobility and sometimes periarticular swelling, especially in relation to the sports activity. These symptoms initially regress with rest. The clinical examination evidences pain upon pressure at the level of the anterior articular rima of the tibiotarsal joint. The passive dorsiflexion of the ankle is also painful.

2.8
Entrapment Neuropathies

2.8.1
Suprascapular Nerve

The potential sites of entrapment for the suprascapular nerve include the suprascapular notch, the superior-transverse scapular ligament, the inferior-transverse scapular ligament (KASPI et al. 1988) and the spinoglenoid notch at the lateral border of the scapular spine. The nerve lesion may be caused by repeated forced movements of the shoulder, as occur in baseball (RINGEL et al. 1990), in fencing (AIELLO et al. 1982), in weight lifting (AGRE et al. 1986) and in volleyball (FERRETTI et al. 1987). It may also be caused by a direct injury to the suprascapular region or by an anterior shoulder dislocation (GOODMAN 1983; HASHIMOTO et al. 1983). The main symptom is pain in the postero-lateral region of the shoulder, which increases as the shoulder is flexed. Clinical examination reveals weakness or atrophy of the supraspinatus and infraspinatus muscles or only of the infraspinatus. The pain may be reproduced or accentuated in scapular plane abduction or neck rotation toward the contralateral shoulder.

2.8.2
Ulnar Nerve

Ulnar nerve neuropathy at the elbow can be caused by repetitive elbow flexo-extension, a thickened or calcified ulnar ligament, loose bodies in the cubital tunnel, degenerative changes of the medial olecranon fossa, medial trochlear osteophytosis, or widening of the coronoid fossa and the olecranon (KING et al. 1969). It may also be due to a severe flexion-valgus deformity (JOBE and FANTON 1985), an accessory anconeus muscle (HIRASAWA et al. 1979), nerve hypermobility, or compressions inside the cubital canal. Ulnar nerve neuropathies are especially frequent in baseball (GODSHALL and HANSEN 1971; DEL PIZZO et al. 1977; INDELICATO et al. 1979; HANG 1981; WOJTYS et al. 1986), weight lifting (REGAN and MORREY 1994), tennis (McCUE 1982) and gymnastics (CHILDRESS 1956, 1975).

An ulnar nerve neuropathy in throwers may also be caused by an ischemic nerve lesion. Indeed, forced flexion of the elbow with wrist extension and shoulder abduction, as in the initial phase of throwing, may sprain the nerve or determine excessive compression by the aponeurosis of the flexor carpi ulnaris. This will result in greater intraneural pressure (PECHAN and JULIS 1975). The most frequent symptoms are medial pain of the elbow, which may be proximally or distally radiated and may be accompanied by hand paresthesias. Athletes suffering from nerve subluxation may also report a painful clicking, especially in rapid flexion-extension movements, with the onset of acute pain that radiates onto the forearm and hand (JOBE and FANTON 1985).

Ulnar nerve neuropathies of the wrist in Guyon's canal may be determined by an acute injury with fracture of the hamate (CARTER et al. 1977), the distal extremity of the radius (HOWARD 1986) or the pisiform. They may also be caused by repeated microinjuries to the hypothenar region which bring about chronic synovitis or degenerative changes of the pisopyramidal joint (SMAIL 1975; HELAL 1978). More rarely, they can be caused by thrombosis of the ulnar artery (KAPLAN and ZEIDE 1972) or by the presence of an anomalous muscle. The sports in which this syndrome is most frequently observed are cycling (handlebar palsy; ECKMAN et al. 1975; NOTH et al. 1980; PALMER et al. 1983), baseball, weight lifting, gymnastics, tennis and martial arts. The ulnar nerve inside the canal undergoes a bifurcation and forms two branches: the superficial branch, which is sensitive, and the deep branch, which is motor. The symptoms therefore vary according to the location of the lesion. A compression in the proximity of the bifurcation of the nerve will create both motor and sensitive symptoms. By contrast, a distal compression at the bifurcation will cause only motor or sensitive symptoms, depending on whether the deep motor or superficial sensitive branch is involved.

2.8.3
Median Nerve

Compression of the median nerve may occur in the distal part of the humerus at the level of Struthers' ligament, in the proximal forearm (pronator teres syndrome), at the level of the mid forearm (anterior interosseous syndrome) or in the wrist.

In some subjects, a bony spur, the supracondylar process, may be observed about 5 cm proximally of the medial epicondyle. Struthers' ligament (STRUTHERS 1854) runs from this process to the medial epicondyle. The symptoms are often vague and include pain in the elbow, weakness of pronation, fingers and wrist flexion and thumb abduction, and paresthesias in the median nerve region. If the symptoms are exacerbated by flexion of the elbow against resistance at 120°-135°, compression of the nerve at Struthers' ligament must be suspected.

The pronator teres syndrome is characterized by the compression of the nerve inside the pronator teres muscle due to a hypertrophy of the muscle itself, or due to the presence of a fibrous band at the insertion of the flexor digitorum superficialis muscle. It may also be attributed to the presence of a fibrous lacertus (HARTZ et al. 1981). This syndrome was observed in sports that require repetitive and forceful forearm pronation and elbow flexo-extension and gripping, as in baseball (KHURANA et al. 1975; BARNES and TULLOS 1987), tennis, gymnastics, weight lifting and other contact sports, and also observed following a direct injury to the proximal forearm. The symptoms include anterior pain in the forearm and paresthesias. If the symptoms are aggravated by the forearm's resistance to pronation, generally combined with the flexion of the wrist (to release the flexor digitorum superficialis muscle), compression of the two heads of the pronator teres is to be suspected (SOLNITZKY 1960; EVERSMANN 1988).

Anterior interosseous syndrome is an exclusively motor syndrome due to the chronic compression of the anterior interosseous nerve by the tendon of the deep head of the pronator quadratus (KILOH and NEVIN 1952; HILL et al. 1985). The sports that cause this syndrome most frequently are weight lifting and gymnastics, which require repeated forced pronosupination movements of the forearm and flexion of the elbow, associated with gripping. It may also be determined by direct acute forearm injury (BUTTERS and SINGER 1994). The symptoms are vague, and the onset is often insidious. The symptomatology is characterized by pain in the proximal volar region of the forearm, which generally increases with activity, loss of dexterity and reduced gripping capacity. No sensitivity disorders are reported, and the thenar eminance muscles are spared (BUCHTHAL et al. 1974). Objective examination reveals a loss of force in the deep flexor muscle of the fingers, and in the long flexor of the thumb, with a typical forceps attitude between the thumb and index. A hyperextension of the distal interphalangeal joints of the index is also observed, along with a hyperextension of the interphalangeal joints of the thumb (EVERSMANN 1988). Moreover, a pronator quadratus deficiency may also determine a deficiency in forearm pronation with a flexed elbow.

The carpal tunnel syndrome is frequently associated with sports activities which entail repeated flexion or gripping movements such as cycling, baseball and tennis (LAYFER and JONES 1977). Compression is more often caused by tenosynovitis of the flexor muscles. It may also be determined by a direct injury of the volar margin of the wrist (MATCH 1978). The symptoms include pain, which may radiate to the forearm, elbow and shoulder, and paresthesias in the median nerve distribution area (LAYFER and JONES 1977). Paresthesias and pain seem to occur prevalently at night.

2.8.4
Radial Nerve

Radial nerve neuropathy, at different levels, has been reported in numerous sporting activities that entail repetitive forearm rotation movements, as occur in rowing, swimming, tennis, golf, weight lifting and sports involving throwing (ROLES and MAUDSLEY 1972; POSNER 1990). The traumatic mechanisms may be a direct injury or a stretch and compression both by the lateral head of the triceps and a fibrous arch starting at the triceps (LOTEM et al. 1971; MITSUNAGA and NAKANO 1988). Lesions in the proximity of the nerve bifurcation into the posterior interosseous branch and in the superficial branch are defined as "high". The triceps may also be involved, depending upon the level of the lesion. The main symptoms are pain and paresthesias.

The posterior interosseous syndrome is characterized by the compression of the posterior interosseous nerve between the two heads of the supinator muscle at the level of Frohse's arch. No sensitivity disorders have been reported. The motor deficiency mainly involves the extension of the wrist and fingers. The main symptom is pain, typically

setting in at night (WERNER 1979) and located on the lateral margin of the forearm right beneath the elbow (LISTER et al. 1979; RITTS et al. 1987).

The repeated pronation movements of the forearm, combined with the flexion of the wrist, increase the intensity of pain. A decrease in the gripping force may also be observed, as a result of the pain caused by the extension of the wrist.

A compression of the superficial branch of the radial nerve may occur in the distal part of the forearm. Indeed, repetitive pronosupination and ulnar deviation movements may determine a stretch of the nerve, probably at the site where the nerve leaves the brachioradial muscle and extends subcutaneously.

2.9
Overuse Syndromes

Overuse syndromes are caused by repetitive microstrains on an anatomical structure for a prolonged period of time, without an adequate recovery phase allowing the structure to adapt to the stimulus. The common pathogenetic mechanism is therefore the persistence of repetitive microinjuries affecting a tissue (bone, muscle, tendon) whose repair capacity is inhibited by the persistence of the injury. The most common overuse syndromes are the iliotibial band syndrome, jumper's knee and stress fractures.

2.9.1
Iliotibial Band Friction Syndrome

The iliotibial band friction sydrome (ITBFS) is especially frequent in athletes practicing middle-distance and long-distance racing and in marathon runners, with an incidence ranging from 52% to 83% in different reports (NOBLE 1980; PINSHAW et al. 1984; MEIER 1986; BRUNET-GUEDY 1990). However, this syndrome may also affect athletes who practice other sports such as cycling (MIDDLETON 1990), skiing (ORAVA 1978) and soccer (LOHNES et al. 1994).

2.9.1.1
Etiopathogenesis

ITBFS is caused by the repetitive friction between the iliotibial band and the lateral femoral condyle during knee flexion-extension. This friction determines a chronic inflammatory response of the iliotibial band, the underlying bursa and the periostium of the lateral femoral epicondyle. There are both intrinsic and extrinsic factors that may foster the syndrome's onset. The intrinsic factors include the presence of a prominent femoral condyle (JONES and JAMES 1987), a highly taut iliotibial band, a varus knee (NOBLE 1980) that causes an increase in the tension forces on the lateral compartment, or an excessive pronation of the forefoot during walking (JONES and JAMES 1987). Such pronation is often associated with intrarotation of the tibia and determines an anteromedial translation of the distal insertion of the band, entailing greater tension of the latter and increased friction involving the femoral epicondyle (TAUNTON 1981). The extrinsic causes are errors in training entailing excessive stress on the lateral compartment, running downhill or on rough ground (RENNE 1975; MCNICHOL et al. 1981; BRUNET-GUEDY 1990), and sudden increases in speed during running (MIDDLETON 1990).

2.9.1.2
Physical Examination

The main symptom of ITBFS is pain, which increases with sports activity and is localized in the femoral epicondyle, some 2 cm above the articular rima, which can radiate along the fascia lata and onto Gerdy's tubercle. Objective examination reveals normal range of motion with slight pain during flexion between 0° and 90° (MIDDLETON 1990). Clinical tests have been described for the diagnosis of this pathology. In the Renne test, the patient, in single-foot support, is required to perform a flexion of the knee. The test is positive if pain is elicited at 30° to 40° flexion. The Noble test envisages palpation of the lateral epicondyle with the knee flexed at 90°, bringing the knee into extension. If the test causes pain at 30° flexion, it is positive.

2.9.2
Jumper's Knee

"Jumper's knee" is a syndrome involving the osteo-tendinous junction of the quadriceps and patellar tendon on the level of the lower or upper pole of the patella or the tibial tuberosity. The most frequent localization at any rate is the one involving the lower pole of the patella (FERRETTI 1986).

2.9.2.1
Etiopathogenesis

Jumper's knee affects athletes who perform both repetitive activities involving continuous tension peaks, such as running, and activities requiring sudden and maximal muscle-tendon engagement, such as volleyball or basketball (KARLSSON et al. 1991). In particular, in volleyball the incidence was reported at 40% among professional athletes (FERRETTI et al. 1985). This high frequency is due to the great number and variety of jumps that a volleyball player is forced to make. Indeed, jumping requires eccentric muscle work, so an overload is produced due to extension against resistance of the muscle-tendon unit with violent stress on the osteotendinous junction (PAVONE and MOFFATT 1985; BENNETT and STAUBER 1986; MOLNAR and FOX 1993). In the etiology of jumper's knee, the braking action of the quadriceps upon landing after a jump also seems to be important. Indeed, in this phase there is sudden strain on both the bone and muscle junction of the tendon (landing knee; BRUNET-GUEDY 1990). The factors that can affect the onset and evolution are divided into extrinsic and intrinsic. Extrinsic factors include the frequency and type of training and sports competition as well as the type of surface of the playing ground. Indeed, a higher incidence was observed in athletes who train on hard floors because the stress withstood by the tendinous structures is absorbed only by the elasticity of the tendinous tissue, not by the playing surface (FERRETTI et al. 1985). Intrinsic factors include alterations of the extensor apparatus, both in front and laterally.

2.9.2.2
Physical Examination

The main symptom of jumper's knee is pain localized in the patellar tendon junction on the lower pole of the patella, along the course of the tendon or on the tibial tuberosity (FERRETTI et al. 1983). The onset of pain is often insidious. Swelling and a peritendinous edema can be present. Pain can be elicited through palpation of the tendon with the knee flexed, the quadriceps contracted under resistance and passive maneuvers of maximum stretching of the quadriceps (Ely Test). BLAZINA et al. (1973) classified the athletes affected by "jumper's knee" according to four stages of pain. In stage 1, pain is reported only after sports activity. In stage 2, pain is present at the beginning of sports activity, disappears after adequate warming up, and then re-appears when fatigue sets in. In stage 3, pain is present both at rest and during physical exercise. In stage 4, there is complete rupture of the patellar tendon. Associated findings may be a hypermobile patella, chondromalacia patellae, patellar malalign-ment and hamstring contracture (BLAZINA et al. 1973). The quadriceps atrophy often present must be considered as a side effect of tendinous alteration (MARTENS et al. 1982).

2.9.3
Stress Fractures

Stress fractures represent roughly 10% of all sport pathologies (McBRYDE 1985; MATHESON et al. 1987). They are more frequent in running and, indeed, 69% of all stress fractures are reported in runners (HULKKO and ORAVA 1987). Although the lower limbs are more often involved (WITWOET 1990), in particular the tibia (34%), the fibula (24%), metatarsals (18%), femur (14%), and pelvis (6%) (McBRYDE 1985; MATHESON et al. 1987) may also be affected. Stress fractures are particularly fre-quent in male athletes in their 20s and 30s (MARKEY 1987).

2.9.3.1
Etiopathogenesis

Bone is a dynamic structure that reshapes in re-sponse to stress. Lack of adjustment to repetitive stress determines an increase in osteoclastic activity not offset by an adequate osteoblastic activity, until the repeated microstrain on the bone finally exceeds its reparative capacity (JOHNSON et al. 1963). Stress fractures can be defined as an interruption of the bone characterized by interruption of the cortical bone with inconstant involvement of the cancellous bone, caused by repetitive and cyclical loads involv-ing an otherwise healthy bone (CECILIANI 1989). In fact, a stress fracture is not associated with reduced bone density. Repeated microtraumas therefore de-termine an interruption in the bone with the subse-quent formation of osteoid tissue which is less resistant to stress and tends to refracture due to the persistence of stress.

2.9.3.2
Physical Examination

The main symptom of a symptomatic stress fracture is local pain, of insidious onset, which exacerbates with activity. Initially, the symptoms appear only af-ter physical activity. However, if stress continues, pain appears during sports activity and decreases with rest. The clinical history of the patient often reveals a recent change in the training programme, such as an increase in the intensity or distance cov-ered or a change in the running or training surface (FREDERICSON et al. 1995). Clinical examination re-veals the presence of pain that exacerbates with palpation and pressure on the bone segment, associ-ated with a perilesional edema (JAMES et al. 1987; McBRYDE 1985). Moreover, pain can be induced by mobilizing the joint adjacent to the bone segment involved.

References

Aglietti P, Insall JH, Cerulli G (1983) Patellar pain and incon-gruence. I. Measurements of incongruence. Clin Orthop 122:217–224
Agre JC, Ash N, Cameron C, House J (1986) Suprascapular neuropathy after intensive progressive exercise: case re-port. Arch Phys Med Rehabil 68:236–238
Aiello I, Serra G, Traina C, Tugnoli V (1982) Entrapment of the suprascapular nerve at the spinoglenoid notch. Ann Neurol 12:314–316
Alexander CE, Lichtman DM (1984) Ulnar carpal instabilities. Orthop Clin North Am 15:307–320
Altchek DW, Warren RF, Skyhar MJ, Ortiz G (1991) T-Plasty modification of the Bankart procedure for multidirectional instability of the anterior and inferior types. J Bone Joint Surg [Am] 73:105–112
Andrews JR, Drez DJ, McGinty JB (1984) Symposium: Arthroscopy of joints other than the knee. Contemp Orthop 9:71–100
Andrews JR, Carson WG, McLeod WD (1985) Glenoid labrum tears related to the long head of the biceps. Am J Sports Med 13:337–341
Baker CL, Uribe JW, Whitman C (1990) Arthroscopic evalua-tion of acute initial anterior shoulder dislocations. Am J Sports Med 18:25–28
Balduini FC, Tetzlaff J (1982) Historical perspectives on inju-ries of the ligaments of the ankle. Clin Sports Med 1:3–12
Bankart AS (1923) Recurrent or habitual dislocation of the shoulder joint. Br J Surg 2:1132–1133
Barnes DA, Tullos HS (1987) An analysis of 100 symptomatic baseball players. Am J Sports Med 6:62–67
Bennett GE (1959) Elbow and shoulder lesions of baseball players. Am J Surg 98:484–492
Bennett JG, Stauber WT (1986) Evaluation and treatment of anterior knee pain using eccentric exercise. Med Sci Sports Exerc 18:526–530
Blazina M, Kerlan R, Jobe FW, Carter VS, Carlson CJ (1973) Jumper's knee. Orthop Clin North Am 4:665–678

Bost FC, Inman VT (1942) The pathological changes in recurrent dislocation of the shoulder. J Bone Joint Surg [Am] 24:595–613

Bowen MK, Warren RF, Altchek DW, O'Brien SJ (1991) Posterior subluxation of the glenohumeral joint treated by posterior stabilization. Orthop Trans 15:764

Boytim MJ, Fischer DA, Neumann L (1991) Syndesmotic ankle sprains. Am J Sports Med 19:294–298

Brodelius A (1960) Osteoarthritis of the talar joints in footballers and ballet dancers. Acta Orthop Scand 30:309–314

Brostrom L (1966) Sprained ankles: VI. Surgical treatment of "chronic" ligament ruptures. Acta Chir Scand 132:537–550

Brunet-Guedy E (1990) Les tendinites du genou. Lesions traumatiques des tendons chez le sportif. Saillant Masson, Catonnè, pp 100–108

Buchthal F, Rosenfalck A, Trojaborg W (1974) Electrophysiological findings in entrapment of the median nerve to wrist and elbow. J Neurol Neurosurg Psychiatry 37:340

Butters KP, Singer KM (1994) Nerve lesions of the arm and elbow. In: De Lee JC, Drez D (eds) Orthopaedic sports medicine. Principles and practice. Saunders, Philadelphia, pp 802–811

Carter PR, Eaton RG, Lottler SW (1977) Ununited fracture of the hook of the hamate. J Bone Joint Surg [Am] 59:583–588

Ceciliani L (1989) Le fratture da durata. Atti 5° Convegno Nazionale "Attualità in traumatologia dello sport", pp 193–209

Chen YC (1985) Arthroscopy of the ankle joint. In: Watanabe M (ed) Arthroscopy of small joints. Igaku-Shoin, Tokyo, p 116

Childress HM (1956) Recurrent ulnar nerve dislocations at the elbow. J Bone Joint Surg [Am] 35:978

Childress HM (1975) Recurrent ulnar nerve dislocations at the elbow. Clin Orthop 180:168–173

Ciullo JV, Stevens GG (1989) The prevention and treatment of injuries to the shoulder in swimming. Sports Med 7:82–204

Codman EA (1934) The shoulder. Todd, Boston, pp 1–261

Del Pizzo W, Jobe FW, Norwood L (1977) Ulnar nerve entrapment syndrome in baseball players. Am J Sports Med 5:182–185

Dias LS (1979) The lateral ankle sprain. An experimental study. J Trauma 19:266–269

Eckman PB, Perlstein G, Altrocchi PH (1975) Ulnar neuropathy in bicycle riders. Arch Neurol 32:130–131

Ekstrand J, Tropp H (1990) The incidence of ankle sprains in soccer. Foot Ankle 11:41–44

Ellman H (1990) Diagnosis and treatment of incomplete rotator cuff tears. Clin Orthop 254:64–74

Ende LS, Wickstrom J (1982) Ballet injuries. Phys Sportsmed 10:101–118

Eversmann WW (1988) Entrapment and compression neuropathies In: Green DP (ed) Operative hand surgery, vol 2. Churchill Livingstone, New York, pp 1423–1478

Ferkel RD, Fischer SP (1989) Progress in ankle arthroscopy. Clin Orthop 240:210–220

Ferkel RD, Karzel RP, Del Pizzo W, Friedman MJ, Fischer SP (1991) Arthroscopic treatment of anterolateral impingement of the ankle. Am J Sports Med 19:440–446

Ferretti A (1986) Epidemiology of jumper's knee. Sports Med 3:289–295

Ferretti A, Ippolito E, Puddu G (1983) Jumper's knee. Am J Sports Med 11:58–62

Ferretti A, Puddu G, Mariani PP, Neri M (1985) The natural history of jumper's knee: patellar or quadriceps tendinitis. Int Orthop 8:239–242

Ferretti A, Cerullo, Russo G (1987) Suprascapular neurophathy in volleyball players. J Bone Joint Surg [Am] 69:260–263

Fredericson M, Bergman G, Hoffman K, Dillingham M (1995) Tibial stress reaction in runners. Am J Sports Med 23:472–481

Freeman MAR (1965) Treatment of ruptures of the lateral ligament of the ankle. J Bone Joint Surg [Br] 47:661–668

Freeman MAR, Dean MRE, Hanham IWF (1965) The etiology and prevention of functional instability of the foot. J Bone Joint Surg [Br] 47:678–685

Fulkerson JP, Cautilli RA (1993) Chronic patellar instability: subluxation and dislocation. In: Fox JM, Del Pizzo W (eds) The patellofemoral joint. McGraw-Hill, New York, pp 135–147

Galway R (1972) Pivot-shift syndrome. J Bone Joint Surg [Br] 54:558

Galway R, MacIntosh DL (1980) The lateral pivot shift: symptom and sign of anterior cruciate ligament insufficiency. Clin Orthop 147:45–50

Garrick JM (1977) The frequency of injury, mechanism of injury, and epidemiology of ankle sprains. Am J Sports Med 5:241–242

Glick JM, Gordon RB, Nishimoto D (1976) The prevention and treatment of ankle injuries. Am J Sports Med 4:136–141

Godshall RW, Hansen CA (1971) Traumatic ulnar neuropathy in adolescent baseball pitchers. J Bone Joint Surg [Am] 53:359–361

Goodman GE (1983) Unusual nerve injuries in recreational sports. Am J Sports Med 2:224–227

Guhl JF (1988) Ankle arthroscopy: pathology and surgical techniques. Slack, Thorofare

Hang YS (1981) Tardy ulnar neuritis in a Little League baseball player. Am J Sports Med 9:244–246

Hardaker WT, Margello S, Goldner JL (1985) Foot and ankle injuries in theatrical dancers. Foot Ankle 6:59–69

Hartz CR, Linscheid RL, Gramse RR (1981) The pronator teres syndrome: compressive neuropathy of the median nerve. J Bone Joint Surg [Am] 63:885–890

Hashimoto K, Oda K, Kuroda Y (1983) Case of suprascapular nerve palsy manifesting as selected atrophy of the infraspinatus muscle. Clin Neurol 23:970–973

Hawkins RJ, Belle RM (1989) Posterior instability of the shoulder. AAOS Instr Course Lect 38:211–216

Helal B (1978) Racquet player's pisiform. Hand 10:87–90

Henry JH, Genund JA (1982) Natural history of glenohumeral dislocation revisited. Am J Sports Med 10:135–137

Hill JA (1983) Epidemiologic perspective on shoulder injuries. Clin Sports Med 2:241–245

Hill NA, Howard FM, Huffer BR (1985) The incomplete anterior interosseous nerve syndrome. J Hand Surg 10:4–16

Hirasawa Y, Sawamaura H, Sakakida K (1979) Entrapment neuropathy due to bilateral epitrochleoanconeus muscles: a case report. J Hand Surg 4:181–184

Hovelius L (1987) Anterior dislocation of the shoulder in teenagers and young adults: five year prognosis. J Bone Joint Surg [Am] 69:393–399

Howard FM (1986) Controversies in nerve entrapment syndromes in the forearm and wrist. Orthop Clin North Am 17:375–381

Hughston JC, Andrews JR, Cross MJ (1976a) Classification of knee ligament instabilities. I. The medial compartment and cruciate ligaments. J Bone Joint Surg [Am] 58:159–172

Hughston JC, Andrews JR, Cross MJ (1976b) Classification of knee ligament instabilities. II. The lateral compartment. J Bone Joint Surg [Am] 58:173–179

Hulkko A, Orava S (1987) Stress fractures in athletes. J Sports Med 8:221–226

Indelicato PA, Jobe FW, Kerlan RK (1979) Correctable elbow lesions in professional baseball players: a review of 25 cases. Am J Sports Med 7:72–75

Inglis AE, Scott WN, Sculco TP (1976) Ruptures of the tendon Achilles: an objective assessment of surgical and nonsurgical treatment. J Bone Joint Surg [Am] 58:990–993

Isani A (1986) Small joint injuries requiring surgical treatment. Orthop Clin North Am 24:360–367

Jaivin JS, Ferkel RD (1994) Ankle and foot injuries. In: Fu FH, Stone DA (eds) Sports injuries. Williams and Wilkins, Baltimore, pp 977–1000

James SL, Bates BT, Osterning LR (1987) Injuries to runners. Am J Sports Med 6:40–50

Jobe CM (1991) Evidence linking posterior superior labral impingement and shoulder instability. American Shoulder and Elbow Surgeons Closed Meeting, Seattle

Jobe FW, Fanton GS (1985) Nerve injuries. In: Morrey BF (ed) The elbow and its disorders. Saunders, Philadelphia, pp 497–501

Jobe FW, Glousman RE (1991) Rotator cuff dysfunction and associated glenohumeral instability in the throwing athlete. In: Paulos LE, Tibone JE (eds) Operative techniques in shoulder surgery. Aspen, Gaithersburg, p 85

Jobe FW, Kvitne RS (1989) Shoulder pain in the overhead or throwing athlete: the relationship of anterior instability and rotator cuff impingement. Orthop Rev 18:963–975

Johnson LC, Stradford HT, Geits RW (1963) Histogenesis of stress fractures. J Bone Joint Surg [Am] 45:1542

Jones DC, James SL (1987) Overuse injuries of the lower extremity: shin splints, iliotibial band friction syndrome, and exertional compartment syndromes. Clin Sports Med 6:273–284

Kaplan EB, Zeide NS (1972) Aneurysm of the ulnar artery: case report. Bull Hosp Joint Dis 33:197–199

Karlsson J, Lundin O, Lossing IW, Peterson L (1991) Partial rupture of the patellar ligament. Results after operative treatment. Am J Sports Med 19:403–408

Kaspi A, Yanai J, Pick CG, Mann G (1988) Entrapment of the distal suprascapular nerve. An anatomical study. Orthopaedics 12:273–275

Kennedy JC, Hawkins RJ, Krissoff WB (1978) Orthopaedic manifestations of swimming. Am J Sports Med 6:309–322

Khurana RK, Schlagenhauff RE, Zwirecki RJ (1975) The pronator syndrome (a case report and reappraisal). Neurology 23:46–48

Kiloh LG, Nevin S (1952) Isolated neuritis of the anterior interosseous nerve. Br Med J 1:850

King JW, Bielsford HJ, Tullos HS (1969) Analysis of the pitching arm of the professional baseball pitcher. Clin Orthop 67:116–122

Kleiger B (1982) Anterior tibiotalar impingement syndromes in dancers. Foot Ankle 3:69–73

Lassiter TE, Malone TR, Garret WE (1989) Injury to the lateral ligaments of the ankle. Orthop Clin North Am 20:629–640

Layfer LE, Jones JB (1977) Hand paresthesias after racquetball. Ill Med J 152:190–191

Leach RE (1983) Acute ankle sprains: vigorous treatment for best results. J Musculoskel Med 1:68

Lehman RC (1988) Shoulder pain in the competitive tennis player. Clin Sports Med 7:309–327

Lewis OJ, Hamshere RJ, Bucknill TM (1970) The anatomy of wrist joint. J Anat 106:539

Liebler WA (1974) Treatment of patellar lesions for instability, a perplexing problem. Orthop Rev 6:25–37

Lister GD, Belsole RB, Kleinert HE (1979) The radial tunnel syndrome. J Hand Surg 4:52–59

Lohnes JH, Garrett WE, Monto RR (1994) Soccer. In: Fu FH, Stone DA (eds) Sports injuries. Williams and Wilkins, Baltimore, pp 603–624

Losee RE (1988) The pivot shift. In: Feagin JA (ed) The crucial ligament. Churchill Livingstone, New York, pp 301–316

Losee RE, Johnson TR, Southwick WO (1978) Anterior subluxation of the lateral tibial plateau. A diagnostic test and operative repair. J Bone Joint Surg [Am] 60:1015–1030

Lotem M, Fried A, Levy M (1971) Radial palsy following muscular effort: a nerve compression syndrome related to a fibrous arch of the lateral head of the triceps. J Bone Joint Surg [Br] 53: 500–506

Maehlum S, Daljord OA (1984) Football injuries in Oslo: a one year study. Br J Sports Med 18:186–190

Marans HJ, Angel KR, Schemitsch EH, Wedge JH (1992) Fate of traumatic anterior shoulder dislocations in children. Annual Meeting of the American Academy of Orthopaedic Surgeons, Washington

Markey KL (1987) Stress fractures. Clin Sports Med 6:405–425

Martens M, Wouters P, Burssens A, Mulier JC (1982) Patellar tendinitis: pathology and results of treatment. Acta Orthop Scand 53:445–450

Martin D, Baker C, Curl W (1989a) Operative ankle arthroscopy: long-term follow-up. Am J Sports Med 17:16–23

Martin D, Curl W, Baker C (1989b) Arthroscopic treatment of chronic synovitis of the ankle. Arthroscopy 5:110–114

Massada JL (1991) Ankle overuse injuries in soccer players. J Sports Med Phys Fitness 31:447–451

Match RM (1978) Laceration of the median nerve from skiing. Am J Sports Med 6:22–25

Matheson GO, Clement DB, McKenzie DC (1987) Stress fractures in athletes: a study of 320 cases. Am J Sports Med 15:46–58

Matsen FA (1993) Pathogenesis and clinical evolution of rotator cuff disease. In: Ellmman H, Gartsmann GM (eds) Arthroscopic shoulder surgery and related procedures. Lea & Febiger, Philadelphia, p 98

Matsen FA, Thomas SC, Rockwood CA (1990) Glenohumeral instability. In: Rockwood CA, Matsen FA (eds) The shoulder, vol 1. Saunders, Philadephia, pp 526–529

Mayfield JK (1984) Patterns of injury to carpal ligaments. A spectrum. Clin Orthop 187:36–42

McBryde AM (1985) Stress fractures in runners. Clin Sports Med 4:737–752

McCarrol JR, Schrader JW, Shelbourne KD, Retting AC, Bisesi MA (1987) Meniscoid lesions of the ankle in soccer players. Am J Sports Med 15:255–257

McCue FC (1982) The elbow, wrist and hand In: Curland D (ed) The injured athlete. Lippincott, Philadelphia, pp 295–329

McDougall A (1955) Footballer's ankle. Lancet 2:1219–1220

McGinty JB, Andrews JR, Drez DJ, Ewing JW, Johnson LL (1984) Symposium: arthroscopy of joints other than knee. Contemp Orthop 9:71–100

McMurray TP (1950) Footballer's ankle. J Bone Joint Surg [Br] 32:68–69

McNichol K, Taunton JE, Clemente DB (1981) Iliotibial tract friction syndrome in athletes. Can J Appl Sport Sci 6:76–80

Meier JL (1986) Douleur du compartiment externe du genou chez le sportif. J Traumatol Sport 3:7–12

Meislin RJ, Roe DJ, Parisien JS, Springer S (1993) Arthroscopic treatment of synovial impingement of the ankle. Am J Sports Med 21:186–189

Merchant AC (1994) Clinical classification of patellofemoral disorders. Sports Med Arthroscopy Rev 2:211–219

Middleton P (1990) Syndrome de la bandellette ileo-tibiale. In: Rodineau J, Simon L (eds) Microtraumatologie du sport. (Collection de pathologie locomotrice, vol 13) Masson, Pasis, pp 250–253

Mitsunaga MM, Nakano K (1988) High radial nerve palsy following strenuous muscular activity. Clin Orthop 234:39–42

Molnar TJ, Fox F (1993) Overuse injuries of the knee in basketball. Clin Sports Med 12:349–362

Morris LH (1943) Athlete's ankle. J Bone Joint Surg 25:220

Moseley HJ, Overgaard B (1962) The anterior capsular mechanism in recurrent anterior dislocation of the shoulder: morphological and clinical study with special reference to the glenoid labrum and glenohumeral ligaments. J Bone Joint Surg [Br] 44:913–927

Neer CS (1983) Impingement lesions. Clin Orthop 173:70–77

Neer CS (1990) Shoulder reconstruction. Saunders, Philadelphia, pp 273–362

Neer CS, Foster CR (1980) Inferior capsular shift for involuntary and multidirectional instability of the shoulder. J Bone Joint Surg [Am] 62:897–908

Neer CS, Marberry TA (1972) Anterior acromioplasty for the chronic impingement syndrome in the shoulder. J Bone Jonit Surg [Am]: 41–50

Neviaser T (1992) ALPSA lesions. Arthroscopy Association of North America Annual Meeting, Instructional Course, Boston

Nilsson S (1982) Sprains of the lateral ankle ligaments. Part I. Epidemiological and clinical considerations. J Oslo City Hosp 32:3–29

Noble CA (1980) Iliotibial band friction syndrome in runners. Am J Sports Med 8:232–234

Noth J, Dietz V, Mauritz KH (1980) Cyclist's palsy. J Neurol Sci 46:111–116

O'Donoghue DH (1957) Impingement exostoses of the talus and tibia. J Bone Joint Surg [Am] 39:835

Ogata S, Uhthoff HK (1990) Acromial enthesopathy and rotator cuff tear. A radiologic and histologic postmortem investigation of the coracoacromial arch. Clin Orthop 254:39–48

Ogilvie-Harris DJ, Mahomed N, Demaziere A (1993) Anterior impingement of the ankle treated by arthroscopic removal of bony spurs. J Bone Joint Surg [Br] 75:437–440

Orava S (1978) Ileotibial tract friction syndrome in athletes. Br J Sports Med 12:69–73

Ozaki J, Fujimoto S, Nakagawa Y, Masuhara K, Tamai S (1988) Tears of the rotator cuff of the shoulder associated with pathological changes in the acromion. J Bone Joint Surg [Am] 70:1224–1230

Palmer AK, Levinsohn EM, Kurma GR (1983) Arthrography of the wrist. J Hand Surg 8:15–23

Parisien JS (1991) Arthroscopic surgery in osteocartilaginous lesions of the ankle. In: McGinty JB (ed) Operative arthroscopy. Raven, New York, pp 739–741

Parkes JC, Hamilton WG, Patterson AH, Rawles JG (1980) The anterior impingement syndrome of the ankle. J Trauma 20:895–898

Pavone E, Moffatt M (1985) Isometric torque of the quadriceps femoris after concentric, eccentric and isometric training. Arch Phys Med Rehabil 66:168–170

Pechan J, Julis I (1975) The pressure measurement in the ulnar nerve: a contribution to the pathophysiology of the cubital tunnel syndrome. J Biomech 8:75–79

Pinshaw R, Atlas V, Noakes TD (1984) The nature and response to therapy of 196 consecutive injuries seen at a runner's clinic. S Afr Med J 65:291–298

Posner MA (1990) Compressive neuropathies of the median and radial nerves at the elbow. Clin Sports Med 9:343–363

Regan WD, Morrey BF (1994) Entrapment neuropathies about the elbow. In: De Lee JC, Drez D (eds) 'Orthopaedic sports medicine. Principles and practice. Saunders, Philadelphia, pp 844–859

Renne JW (1975) The iliotibial band friction syndrome. J Bone Joint Surg [Am] 57:1110–1111

Richardson AB, Jobe FW, Collins HF (1980) The shoulder in competitive swimming. Am J Sports Med 87:159–163

Ringel SP, Treihaft M, Carry M, Fisher R, Jacobs P (1990) Suprascapular neuropathy in pitchers. Am J Sports Med 18:80–86

Ritts ED, Wood MB, Linscheid RL (1987) Radial tunnel syndrome: a ten year surgical experience. Clin Orthop 279:201–205

Roles NC, Maudsley RH (1972) Radial tunnel syndrome: resistant tennis elbow as a nerve entrapment. J Bone Joint Surg [Br] 54:499–508

Rowe CR (1956) Prognosis in dislocations of the shoulder. J Bone Joint Surg [Am] 38: 957–977

Rowe CR (1980) Acute and recurrent anterior dislocations of the shoulder. Orthop Clin North Am 11:253–270

Rowe CR, Zarins B (1981) Recurrent transient subluxation of the shoulder. J Bone Joint Surg [Am] 63:863–872

Schonholtz GJ (1987) Arthroscopic surgery of the shoulder, elbow and ankle. Thomas, Springfield

Silbey MB, Fu FH (1994) Knee injuries. In: Fu FH, Stone DA (eds) Sports injuries.Williams and Wilkins, Baltimore, pp 949–976

Simonet WT, Cofield RH (1984) Prognosis in anterior shoulder dislocation. Am J Sports Med 12:19–24

Smail DF (1975) Handlebar palsy. N Engl J Med 292:322

Smith RW, Reischl SF (1986) Treatment of ankle sprains in young athletes. Am J Sports Med 14:465–471

Snyder SJ (1993) Evaluation and treatment of the rotator cuff. Orthop Clin North Am 24:173–192

Snyder SJ, Karzel RP, Del Pizzo W (1990) SLAP lesions of the shoulder. Arthroscopy 6:274–279

Solnitzky O (1960) Pronator syndrome: compression neuropathy of the median nerve at the level of pronator teres muscle. Georgetown Med Bull 13:232–238

Staples OS (1960) Injuries to the medial ligaments of the ankle. J Bone Joint Surg [Am] 42:1287–1307

Stoller SM, Hekmat F, Kleiger B (1984) A comparative study of the frequency of anterior impingement exostoses of the ankle in dancers and nondancers. Foot Ankle 4:201

Struthers J (1854) On some points in the abnormal anatomy of the arm. Br Forensic Med Surg Rev 14:170

Subcommittee on Classification of Sports Injuries, American Medical Association, Committee on the Medical Aspects of Sports (1966) Standard nomenclature of athletic injuries. American Medical Association, Chicago

Taleisnik J (1978) Wrist: anatomy, function, and injury. AAOS Instr Course Lect 27:61–87

Taleisnik J (1985) The wrist. Churchill Livingstone, New York

Taunton JE (1981) Iliotibial band friction syndrome in athletes. Can J Appl Sports Sci 76–80

Tropp H (1985) Functional instability of the ankle joint. Medical dissertation. Linkoping University, Sweden, pp 1–92

Uhthoff HK, Hammond DI, Sarkar K, Hooper GJ, Papoff WJ (1988) The role of the coracoacromial ligament in the impingement syndrome: a clinical, radiological and histological study. Int Orthop 12:97–104

Walch G, Boileau P, Noel E, Donell ST (1992) Impingement of the deep surface of the supraspinatus tendon on the posteriosuperior glenoid rim: an arthroscopic study. J Shoulder Elbow Surg 1:238

Watson HK, Hempton RF (1980) Limited wrist arthrodesis: the triscaphoid joint. J Hand Surg 5:320–327

Weber ER (1980) Biomechanical implications of scaphoid wrist fractures. Clin Orthop 149:83–89

Weber ER (1984) Concepts governing the rotational shift of the intercalated segment of the carpus. Orthop Clin North Am 15:193–207

Weiss JR (1994) Gymnastics In: Fu FH, Stone DA (eds) Sports injuries. Williams and Wilkins, Baltimore, pp 383–396

Werner CO (1979) Lateral elbow pain and posterior interosseous nerve entrapment. Acta Orthop Scand Suppl 174:1–62

Wheeler JH, Ryan JB, Arciero RA, Molinari RN (1989) Arthroscopic versus nonoperative treatment of acute shoulder dislocations in young athletes. Arthroscopy 5:213–217

Whitman PA, Melvin M, Nicholas JA (1981) Common problems seen in a sport injury clinic. Physician Sports Med 9:105–110

Witwoet J (1990) Microtraumatismes sportifs du genou: mecanisme, consequences cliniques et radiologiques. In: Rodineau J, Simon L (eds) Microtraumatologie du sport. (Collection de pathologie locomotrice, vol 13) Masson, Paris, pp 74–77

Wojtys EM, Smith PA, Hankin FM (1986) A cause of ulnar neuropathy in a baseball pitcher. A case report. Am J Sports Med 14:422–424

Wolf E (1992) Arthroscopic management of shoulder instability. Arthroscopy Association of North America Annual Meeting. Instructional Course, Boston, p 201

Wolin I, Glassman F, Sideman S (1950) Internal derangement of the talofibular component of the ankle. Surg Gynecol Obstet 91:193–200

Zwipp H, Tscherne H (1984) Zur Behandlung der chronischen Rotationsinstabilität im hinteren unteren Sprunggelenk. Unfallheilkunde 87:196–200

3 The Role of MR Imaging in Sports Injuries of the Muscles

M. T. McNamara[1] and A. Greco[2]

CONTENTS

3.1
Introduction

Magnetic resonance (MR) imaging has clearly documented its utility as an important imaging modality for the study of soft tissue (BERQUIST and EHMAN 1987; EHMAN and BERQUIST 1986; FLECKENSTEIN et al. 1989a, 1991a; DESMET et al. 1990; FLECKENSTEIN and SHELLOCK 1991; GRECO et al. 1991; BERQUIST et al. 1985; HANNA et al. 1991; BIONDETTI and EHMAN 1992). It has demonstrated excellent results for depicting normal anatomy and a wide variety of soft tissue lesions. This is due largely to the inherent capability of MR pulse sequences which are designed to take advantage of alterations of soft tissue composition, in order to produce a predictable modification of the signal pattern relative to normal tissue. Such changes in image contrast can be produced without need for administration of paramagnetic contrast media (PCM), although certain lesions may also be best visualized with greater sensitivity and/or specificity using intravenous PCM.

By far the most frequent indication for MR imaging of soft tissue lesions at our institution is the

evaluation of skeletal muscle pathology (BERQUIST and EHMAN 1987; EHMAN and BERQUIST 1986; FLECKENSTEIN et al. 1989a, 1991b; DESMET et al. 1990; FLECKENSTEIN and SHELLOCK 1991; GRECO et al. 1991; DEUTSCH and MINK 1989; MOON et al. 1983; SCOTT et al. 1984; SPEER et al. 1993; HIROSHI et al. 1994; FISCHER et al. 1986; WHITEHOUSE 1992). Diseases of muscles include acute trauma, both direct and associated with overuse or strain, inflammation, fibrosis, infection, and neoplasm, as well as other infrequent lesions.

Prior to the development of MR, clinicians relied on plain radiographs, computed tomography (CT), sonography, and scintigraphy for the routine evaluation of musculoskel et al lesions (BERQUIST 1985a,b; BOWERMAN 1977; MIDDLETON et al. 1985; ALLARD et al. 1992; GARRETT et al. 1989; MATIN 1988; MATIN et al. 1983; SHIRKODA et al. 1983; TERMOTE et al. 1980; VALK 1983). While each of these techniques has demonstrated utility in diagnosing muscle diseases, it is MR that provides the greatest sensitivity and specificity for revealing muscle pathology (BERQUIST and EHMAN 1987; EHMAN and BERQUIST 1986; FLECKENSTEIN et al. 1989a, 1991b; DESMET et al. 1990; FLECKENSTEIN and SHELLOCK 1991; GRECO et al. 1991; DEUTSCH and MINK 1989; MOON et al. 1983; SCOTT et al. 1984; SPEER et al. 1993; HIROSHI et al. 1994; FISCHER et al. 1986; WHITEHOUSE 1992; DOOMS et al. 1985).

3.2
Technical Considerations

Contrast between normal tissue and pathologic lesions on MR is derived from differences in relaxivity of the various tissues under the influence of magnetic fields, both fixed and switching, and radiofrequency pulse sequences produced by the MR system in order to make the MR image. Each tissue, organ, or cell type may often have a characteristic range of T1 and T2 relaxation time values at a given field strength. Human skeletal muscle has a relatively

[1] M.T. McNamara, MD, Department of Magnetic Resonance Imaging, Princess Grace Hospital, P.D.B. 489, 98000 Monte Carlo, Monaco
[2] A. Greco, MD, Department of Magnetic Resonance Imaging, Princess Grace Hospital, P.D.B. 489, 98000 Monte Carlo, Monaco

short T2 relaxation time (FISHER et al. 1986; BERNARDINO et al. 1989; KUNO et al. 1988; POLAK et al. 1988), and therefore even insignificant changes in the composition of muscle may result in profound alterations in the signal intensity on certain MR images. Concomitant changes in T1 also occur, but from a practical imaging point of view, these changes are usually less significant and less useful than T2 alterations.

Since it is the change in T2 that predominates on MR images, most of this chapter focuses on depiction of muscle injuries using sequences that take advantage of this phenomenon. Acute muscle trauma produces a combination of muscle edema and hemorrhage, the degree of which varies according to the cause of injury. Invariably, a prolongation of muscle T2 relaxation time occurs with acute muscle injury such as strain or contusion (EHMAN and BERQUIST 1986; GRECO et al. 1991).

On long-TR, long-TE spin echo T2-weighted images, such lesions appear as regions of higher signal intensity than the unaffected normal muscle tissue, which is of intermediate to low intensity. Gradient echo T2*-weighted images have relatively low sensitivity for detection of sports injuries of skeletal muscle and are therefore not recommended to diagnose such lesions.

The short-tau-inversion-recovery (STIR) sequence is another powerful MR imaging sequence for detecting muscle pathology (DWYER et al. 1988; BYDDER and YOUNG 1985). Unlike the T2-weighted sequence, which depicts MR signal changes related to changes in tissue T2 relaxation rate, the STIR sequence reveals any prolongation of both T1 and T2 times EHMAN and BERQUIST 1986; BERQUIST et al. 1985; FLECKENSTEIN et al. 1988; FISHER et al. 1990). As on T2-weighted images, most acute traumatic muscle lesions appear hyperintense on STIR images. Normal muscle tissue has intermediate and fairly homogeneous signal intensity, due in part to the fact that the contribution of fat to the MR signal is reduced by the STIR sequence.

Despite the apparent superiority of the STIR sequence over the T2-weighted sequence, there are some drawbacks to STIR imaging. Image acquisition time is long, and a two-signal average (i.e., two excitations) image with medium resolution (192 × 256 pixels, for example) will exceed 10 min in duration. Another problem is the limited number of image sections per sequence. In order to cover a sufficient volume of tissue, it therefore becomes necessary to increase slice thickness to at least 10 mm. When

higher signal-to-noise ratio is sought, it may be necessary to use two-signal averages, which may necessitate the use of low image resolution (128 × 256 pixels) in order to keep the imaging time reasonably low.

More recently, STIR imaging has been made available using a fast STIR technique in which image acquisition time is reduced (FLECKENSTEIN et al. 1989b, 1991c). This technique permits a greater number of image sections per acquisition and the reduced scanning time allows higher spatial resolution without requiring excessively long acquisition time. Imaging time may be an important factor in imaging sports injuries with MR. If the study is performed shortly after the injury occurs and the patient is in pain, it may be difficult for him or her to remain absolutely immobile for a prolonged period of time, particularly for a long STIR sequence. The resulting patient-related noise may render an image uninterpretable, even if patient motion is of limited duration during the long acquisition.

It is also possible to significantly reduce the contribution of fat to tissue signal intensity on spin echo images. This may be accomplished with spectral radiofrequency fat presaturation (HIROSHI et al. 1994; HERNANDEZ et al. 1992). As on STIR images, fat presaturation T2-weighted images offer greater homogeneity of skeletal muscle signal intensity, thus making the long T2 components of edema and hemorrhage more obvious. This is particularly important in small peripheral muscle lesions, such as musculofascial muscle strains, where the high signal intensity of the muscle strain occurs in close proximity to perimuscular fatty tissue. Distinguishing between the strain and fat can be virtually impossible on routine T2-weighted images without fat presaturation.

An additional consideration in the choice between the STIR and fat-saturated T2-weighted sequence is the field strength of the MR system. High field strength offers heightened separation of the fat and water peaks, and therefore this sequence is often utilized for general musculoskeletal work in general at high field strength. At low to intermediate field strength, however, there is less fat/water peak separation, and therefore fat presaturation is less efficient. Suppression of fat signal is not field-dependent in STIR imaging, however, and is therefore potentially more valuable in this range of field strength. Our system operates at 1.5 T (General Electric Signa), but nevertheless we routinely employ the STIR sequence because we are routinely called upon to diagnose small muscle strains in athletes and it may be difficult to distinguish between muscle edema or hemorrhage and normal blood vessels, which tend to be hyperintense on fat-saturated T2-weighted images.

Fat presaturation may also be utilized on T2-weighted gradient echo images. Such images are rapidly acquired. Although they offer less sensitivity than other imaging techniques discussed in this chapter for detection of acute muscle injuries, we have employed T2*-weighted fat presaturation sequences to help provide precise anatomic localization of muscle strain and hemorrhage in the lower extremities of professional and high-level athletes. These athletes have a low percentage of body, fat, and intermuscular fat may be very sparse, thus making it difficult to define fascial cleavage planes between specific muscles. The greater susceptibility effects and/or chemical-shift effects depict the fascial plane as a readily defined hypointense linear structure. A short-TR, short-TE spin echo T1-weighted sequence offers an alternative imaging technique to aid in depiction of normal muscle anatomy, but in many cases it may be just as difficult to define fascial muscle planes as on spin echo T2-weighted images, again due to the paucity of intermuscular fat in well-conditioned athletes.

From a practical standpoint, the choice of the plane of section should be based on the region of the body being examined. Most sports-related muscle injuries involve the lower extremities. We have found the axial sequence to be best suited as the initial sequence because it minimizes the partial volume artifacts that tend to occur on coronal and sagittal sequences. Therefore, our protocol entails an initial axial STIR sequence centered on the site of pain. Ten-millimeter sections are routinely employed with a 2.5-mm gap between sections. Care should be taken to cover a large volume of muscle tissue in acute lower extremity muscle strain because intermuscular or perimuscular hemorrhage may migrate along fascial planes, resulting in more pain distal to the strain than at the site of muscle injury itself. This may result in false-negative studies because the imaged volume of tissue may not include the proximally situated muscle strain.

Following the initial transverse sequence, we use a longitudinal STIR sequence to provide a view of the strain or injury in a plane that parallels the lesion and/or the muscle anatomy. This view provides insight into the true longitudinal dimension of the injury. It also better depicts the site of the lesion,

allowing improved accuracy for detecting purely intramuscular injuries versus musculofascial strain or musculotendinous strain. In fact, it is important to acquire this sequence even if the axial images reveal no pathology, for the reason stated in the previous paragraph, because a normal-appearing axial sequence is not sufficient to rule out muscle pathology, particularly sports-related injuries. Some authors advocate the use of a vitamin E capsule taped to the skin at the site of pain as a marker to facilitate localization of the lesion.

As implied by their name, purely intramuscular strains are confined to the muscle, usually the muscle belly, without peripheral involvement and without extension to the proximal or distal portion of the muscle. Musculofascial lesions and musculotendinous muscle strains will be more specifically discussed in Sect. 3.3.1.

In choosing the plane of section for longitudinal section, the goal is to align the image acquisition parallel to the long axis of the involved muscle. For example, in the lower extremity, this entails the use of a coronal STIR sequence for adductor compartment thigh injuries and a sagittal STIR sequence for quadriceps (anterior thigh) and hamstring (posterior thigh) strains. Keep in mind that one of the major assets of MR imaging is the capability to orient image acquisition in oblique nonorthogonal planes of sections. A frequent application for oblique longitudinal imaging of muscle injuries occurs in the evaluation of the size and extent of soleus muscle or gastrocnemius muscle (calf) injuries, whereby we utilize an obliquely oriented STIR sequence following the initial axial transverse STIR sequence. The oblique sequence is oriented by traversing the hyperintense muscle strain seen on the axial images, with the section placed such that it obliquely traverses the "short axis" of the muscle, as seen on the axial. In this fashion, the radiologist can best appreciate the true extent of the muscle strain and can most readily determine the exact muscle involved because the fascial plane(s) between muscles will be oriented perpendicular to the plane of section and therefore will not be obscured by partial volume effects.

In specific cases, the choice of the second longitudinal sequence may depend on the appearance of the lesion on the initial axial sequence and possibly upon the clinical history of the athlete. Theoretically, both the STIR and the long-TR, long-TE spin echo sequence with fat presaturation should readily depict muscle injury. Muscle hematoma may result from significant muscle strain or, more frequently, from direct trauma to the muscle. Previously, it has been demonstrated that acute hematoma may exhibit signal patterns that reflect a short T2 component (RUBIN et al. 1987; UNGER et al. 1986), thus appearing hypointense to isointense relative to normal adjacent muscle tissue on spin echo T2-weighted images. However, since the T1 and T2 changes are additive on STIR images, hyperacute hematomas may also have a low signal intensity (Fig. 3.1). We prefer he STIR sequence in this instance because it provides good depiction of the hemorrhagic changes and of the muscle edema surrounding the blood collection. It is nevertheless necessary to stress that the STIR sequence is an extremely powerful tool for detecting muscle injury, but lacks in specificity in differentiating between simple fluid and hemorrhage.

Subacute to chronic hematomas have been shown to contain variable amounts of paramagnetic methemoglobin (DOOMS et al. 1985; RUBIN et al. 1987; UNGER et al. 1986). In selected cases, an additional axial or longitudinal short-TR, short-TE spin echo sequence may be useful to exhibit these characteristics (Fig. 3.2). The paramagnetic properties of methemoglobin cause it to appear hyperintense with this technique, which may permit separation of the various components of blood collection and

muscle tissue. This is particularly valid in our experience in the evaluation of hemorrhagic reinjury of muscle, in which the T1-weighted sequence may help separate acute hemorrhage from older blood, with older blood being hyperintense on the T1-weighted images due to the presence of methemoglobin. Mature chronic hematomas may also contain little to no visible methemoglobin, thus appearing hypointense to muscle on T1-weighted images. Both of these components are usually nonspecifically hyperintense on STIR or T2-weighted images (Figs. 3.3, 3.4).

In nearly all cases referred for the evaluation of muscle injury or trauma, the MR examination is performed with the patient in the supine position. This allows maximum patient comfort. As in MRI of any part of the body, patient comfort is important in order to optimize MR image quality by avoiding motion due to pain or discomfort resulting from improper positioning. In rare instances, it may not be possible for the patient to lie in the supine position due to buttock or back muscle injury or concomitant skeletal injury. In this case, the patient may have to be positioned in the prone or lateral decubitus position.

Optimum signal-to-noise ratio (SNR) and image quality may be obtained by using the proper receiver imaging coils. For most pelvic, hip and upper thigh

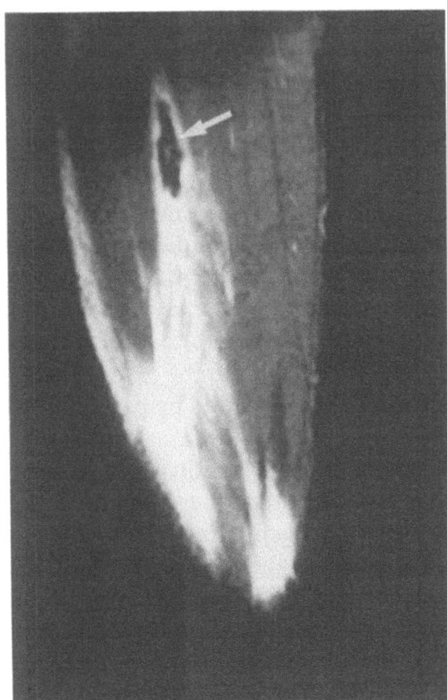

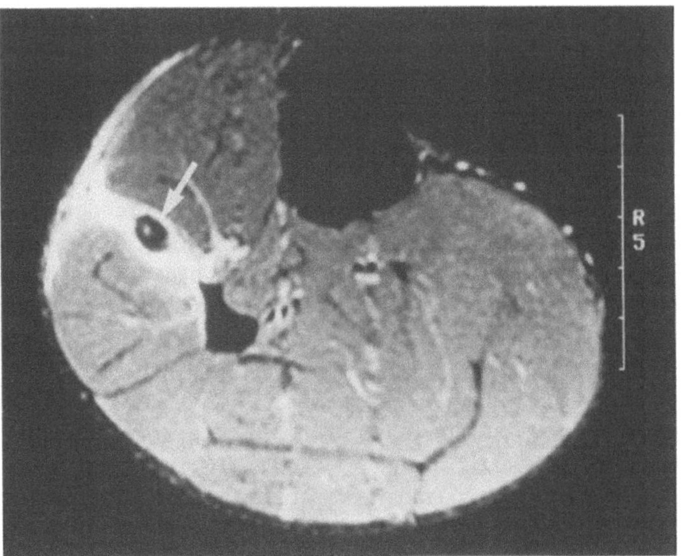

Fig. 3.1a,b. Acute muscle hematoma of an 18-year-old male soccer player with significant pain while running. a The sagittal fast STIR (3000/150/39) image and b the axial STIR (3200/160/40) image demonstrate a hypointense blood collection (*arrows*) between the peroneus muscles and the extensor digitorum longus muscle. *STIR*, short tan inversion recovery

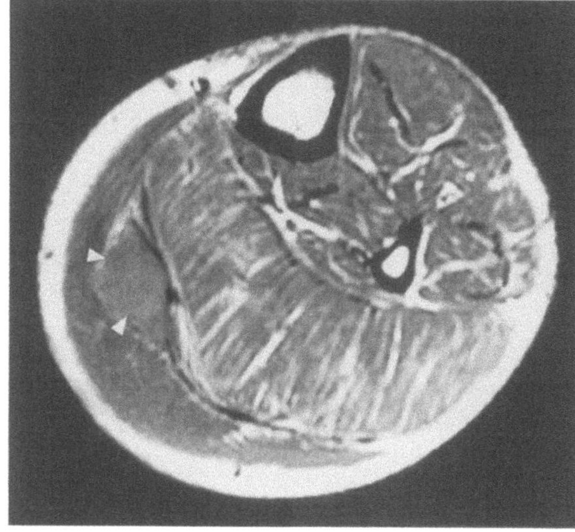
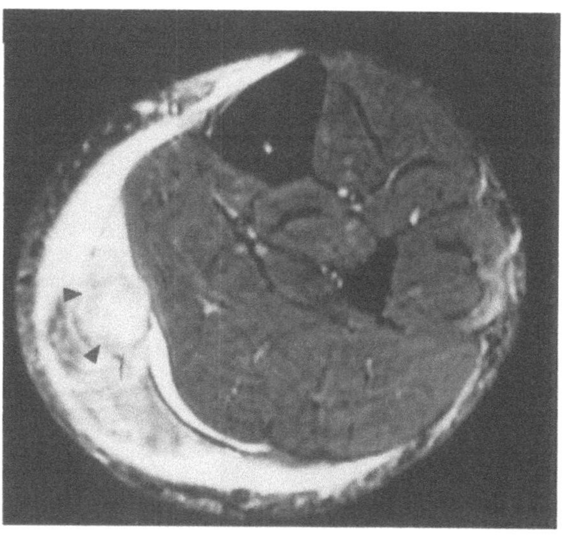

Fig. 3.2a,b. Subacute gastrocnemius muscle hematoma. This 43-year-old man experienced sudden onset of calf pain while playing tennis. The hematoma (*arrowheads*) is slightly hyperintense to the gastrocnemius muscle on the **a** axial T1-weighted sequence (420/12) and hyperintense on the **b** fast STIR (4400/150/42) image. Intermuscular and perimuscular blood is also hyperintense on the STIR image

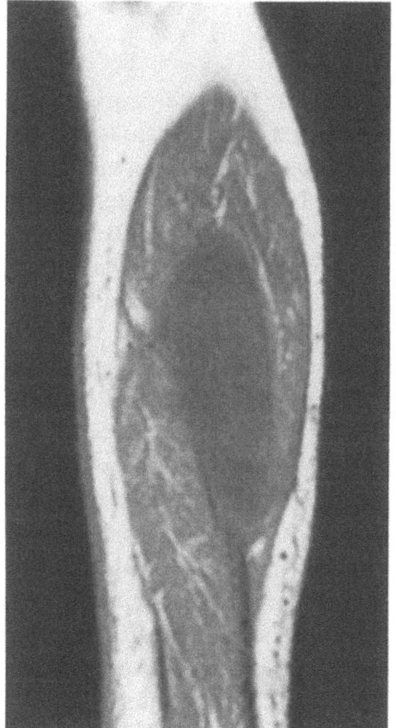
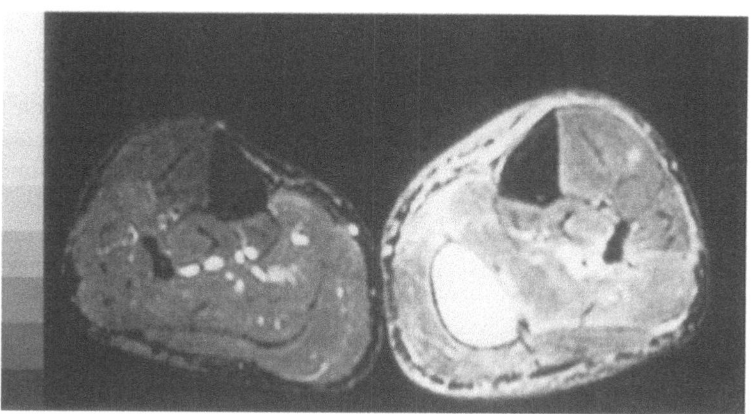

Fig. 3.3a,b. Chronic hematoma of a 43-year-old man with a 1-month history of left calf swelling and pain following direct trauma. Cyst-like chronic hematoma is situated between medial gastrocnemius and soleus muscles and is hypointense on **a** coronal T1-weighted (600/20) STIR and **b** markedly hyperintense on axial STIR (3200/160/30) image. Note increased signal in the surrounding musculature and within the soft tissues on axial STIR image

examinations, the body coil affords a large field of view (FOV), also allowing comparison between the two lower extremities or between the lesion and contralateral side of the body.

A flexible receive-only surface coil provides excellent SNR for the torso, pelvis, and lower extremities. It is also useful in small sizes for the upper extremities, including the elbow region. The extremity coil,

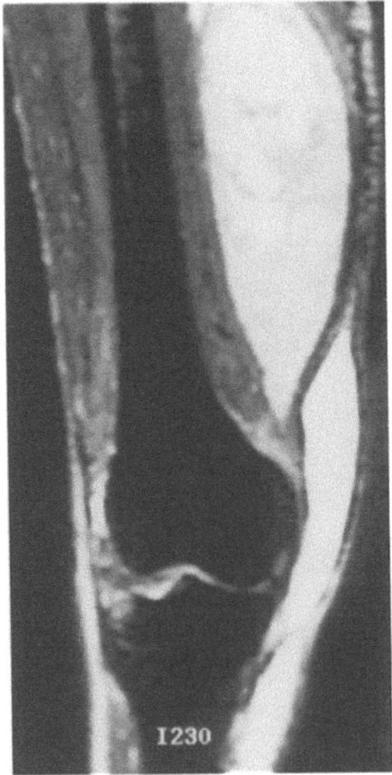

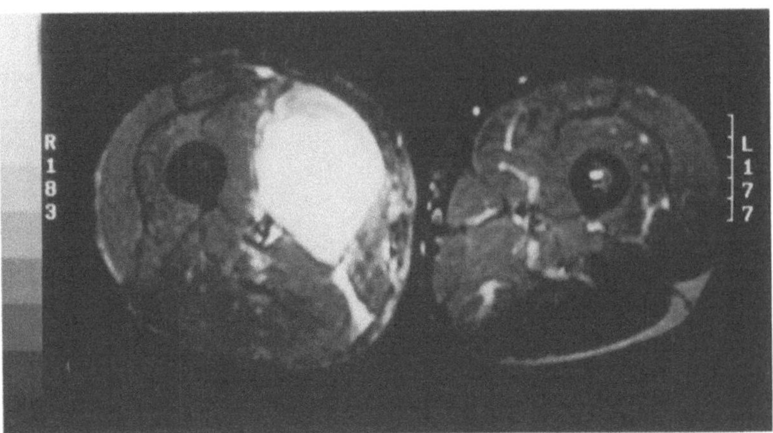

Fig. 3.4a,b. Subacute thigh hematoma of a 41-year-old male patient with a history of direct trauma; coronal (**a**) and axial (**b**) fast STIR (3000/150/39) images. Extensive right vastus medialis subacute hematoma is hyperintense with intermixed areas of relatively higher signal intensity. There is also a loculated subcutaneous fluid collection medial to the knee

which is routinely used for knee studies, is also useful for evaluation of calf injuries.

3.3
Pathology

3.3.1
Muscle Strain

Muscle strain or tear is an indirect traumatic injury produced by excessive stretching of the myotendinous unit. In most cases, it results from muscle contraction during forced lengthening of a muscle. The frequency of muscle strain is ever rising with the steadily increasing number of athletes participating in a wide variety of sporting activities (MUCKLE 1981; GARRETT 1986, 1988; JACKSON and FEAGIN 1973; ZARINS and CIULLO 1983). Thus, it is not surprising that the evaluation of muscle strain and musculotendinous injury is the major indication for MRI of the soft tissues at our institution. Certain muscle structures are more vulnerable to traumatic injury than others, including those that contain a high proportion of fast-twitch type II fibers (GARRETT 1986, 1988) and those that span more

than one joint. Included in these categories are the muscles we are most often asked to evaluate for acute muscle trauma, including the hamstring muscles (biceps femoris, semimembranosus, semitendinosus), the rectus femoris muscle, and the gastrocnemius muscle. Other muscles that are frequently affected by strain are the thigh adductor muscles and the soleus muscle.

It has been shown that the most frequent site of muscle strain is the myotendinous junction (GARRETT 1986, 1988). Most sports-related traumatic muscle injuries therefore occur at this site. The muscle-tendon unit, however, can be involved at a number of other sites, including the muscle belly, the tendon, the bone-tendon junction, within the bone, or within an unfused apophyseal growth plate. Muscle strains occur most frequently in the lower extremity, particularly in athletes. Our experience is based largely on acute and chronic muscle injury in soccer players. Such lesions typically involve the lower extremity muscles, with most lesions occurring at the myotendinous junction. It is not uncommon to observe multiple adjacent muscle strains, particularly in the upper thigh adductor muscles, the hamstring muscles and the calf, where the gastrocnemius and soleus are often concomitantly involved.

3.3.2
Characterization of Muscle Strain

Purely intramuscular strain typically involves the muscle belly. The intensity and morphology of the hyperintense signal corresponds to the severity of the injury. The mildest degree of muscle strain produces a focus of weakly to mildly hyperintense high signal intensity on STIR or fat-saturated T2-weighted images. This corresponds clinically to a first-degree muscle strain, in which there is low-grade muscle inflammation without tissue disruption. In this type of lesion, there is no loss of muscle strength or range of motion. This type of lesion is very homogeneous, without visibly perceptible areas of more intense signal within or adjacent to the injury (Figs. 3.5, 3.6).

A moderate muscle strain is characterized by partial muscle fiber tearing and results in some loss of muscle strength. This is also known as a second-degree strain. This type of strain will result in single or multiple foci of intramuscular hemorrhage, appearing as brighter areas of signal change over a background of mildly elevated signal intensity on STIR or fat-saturated T2-weighted images (Fig. 3.7). A majority of purely intramuscular lesions will take on this appearance in our experience. This type of lesion does not involve enough muscle fibers to alter the thickness of the muscle. Peripheral second-degree strains involve the musculofascial junction. The hallmark of this injury is a perifascial blood collection which appears uniformly hyperintense on

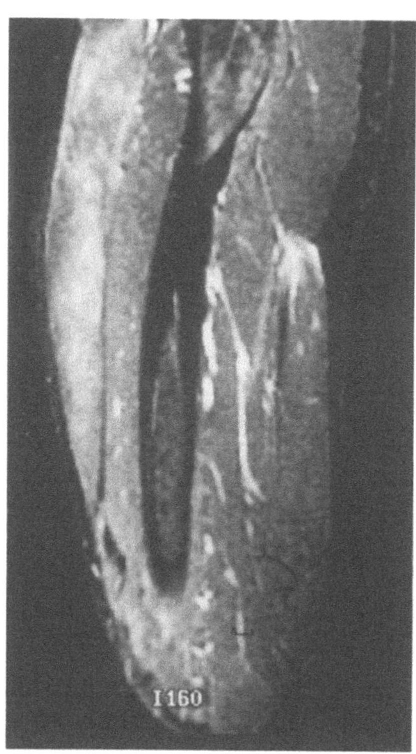

Fig. 3.6. First-degree muscle strain; pain following exertion in an 18-year-old soccer player. The rectus femoris muscle is diffusely hyperintense on the sagittal fast STIR (4000/140/39) image

STIR and T2-weighted images. This hemorrhage may track along intermuscular fascial planes for a significant distance from the site of muscle fiber disruption, and may be associated with discomfort.

Severe muscle strain, also known as third-degree strain, causes complete disruption of a portion of the muscle or of the muscle-tendon unit, causing significant muscle weakness. STIR or T2-weighted sequences demonstrate actual separation of muscle fibers or of the muscle-tendon unit, with hyperintense hemorrhagic fluid seen within the area of disruption. Perimuscular hematoma is invariably present to a certain degree (Fig. 3.8).

Frank tearing of a significant number of muscle fibers results in appreciable reduction in cross-sectional muscle. In the acute lesion of this type and in the absence of previous muscle injury at the same site, such tears often result from direct muscle trauma. In the most severe form of this type of injury, complete muscle tear with retraction of the muscle ends may be readily detected on longitudinal (sagittal or coronal) images.

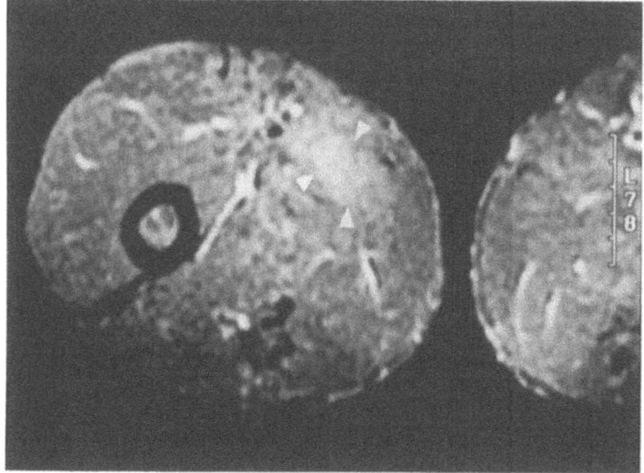

Fig. 3.5. First-degree muscle strain of an 18-year-old soccer player with mild pain following exertion. Strained adductor muscle displays hazy signal increase on axial fast STIR (3200/160/40) image (*arrowheads*)

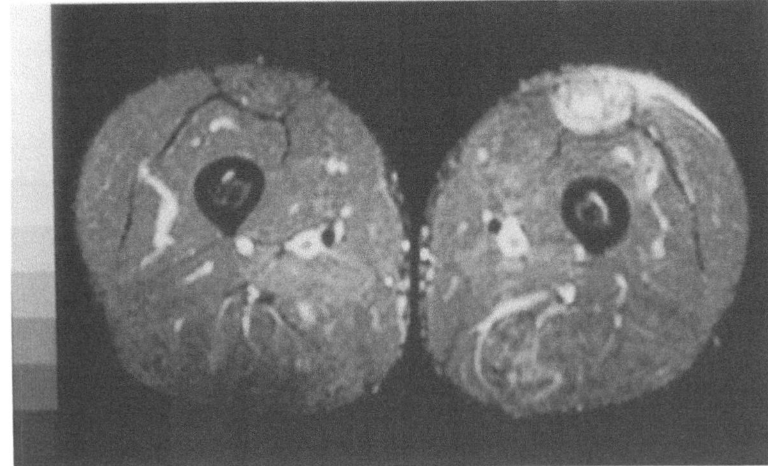

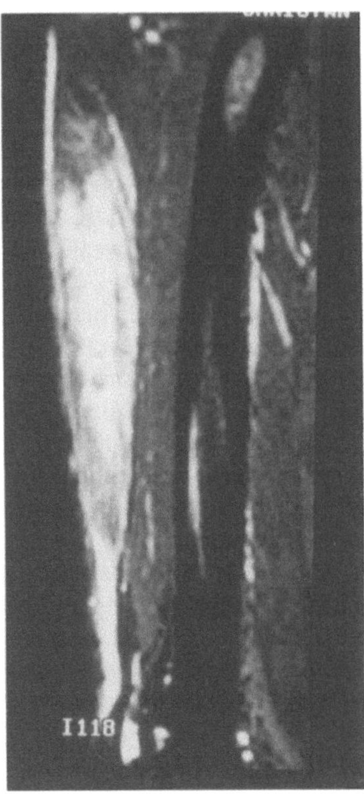

Fig. 3.7a,b. Second-degree muscle strain. This 18-year-old soccer player experienced sudden pain while kicking a ball. **a** Axial STIR (3200/160/30) and **b** sagittal fast STIR (3000/150/26) images of left rectus femoris tear. There is an intramuscular hemorrhagic signal (*arrow*) from grade II strain and an associated subcutaneous hemorrhagic signal (*long white arrow*). The sagittal image is essential to demonstrate the full longitudinal extent of this muscle strain

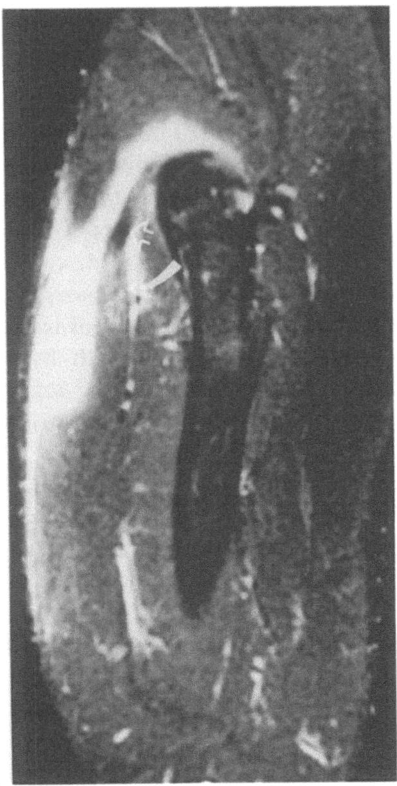

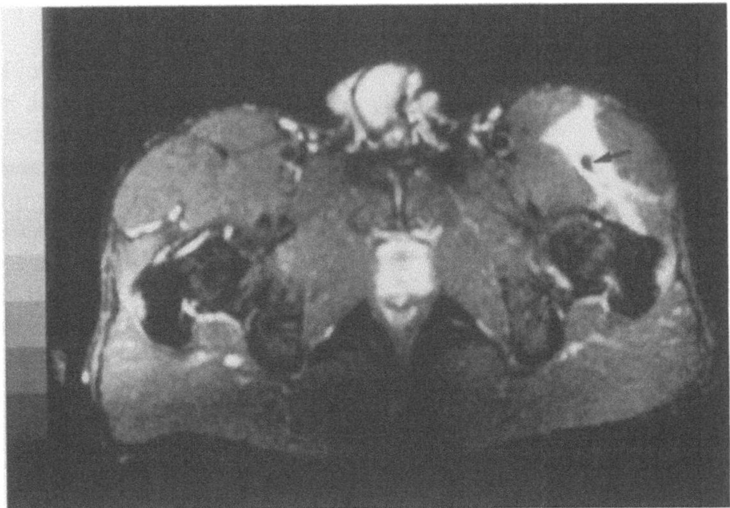

Fig. 3.8a,b. Myotendinous junction strain. This 35-year-old male professional basketball player injured his thigh while jumping. **b** The sagittal fast STIR (3000/150/39) image demonstrates high signal intensity of the proximal rectus femoris muscle at the level of the musculotendinous junction (*curved arrow*) and marked muscle thinning. The prominent low signal intensity and thickening of the tendon (*open arrow*) are due to fibrosis from a remote injury. Perimuscular blood is uniformly hyperintense. B The axial fast STIR (3200/160/40) image shows the tendon scar on the *left* (*arrow*) compared to the normal *right* rectus femoris tendon

3.3.3
Muscle Strain in Sports Medicine: Clinical Examples

As mentioned earlier, our experience is largely based on acute and chronic muscle strains in professional and amateur soccer players. These lesions involve virtually any muscle or combination of muscles of the lower extremity. A majority of lesions occur in the hamstring muscles, involving the semimembranosus and semitendinosus muscles and the long head of the biceps femoris muscles with relatively equal frequency. A vast majority of hamstring strains are moderate second-degree injuries. Most of these have a musculofascial involvement and thus will have a perifascial fluid collection which is readily identified on STIR or T2-weighted images due to its very hyperintense signal (Fig. 3.9). On the initial axial sequence, it is often the perifascial fluid that alerts us to the presence of a muscle strain, particularly when the intramuscular edema or hemorrhage associated with a moderate strain is small in size.

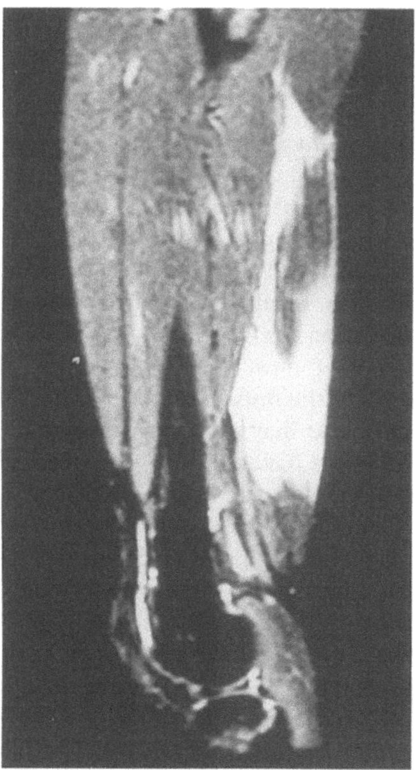

Fig. 3.9. Hamstring musculofascial strain. This 19-year-old soccer player felt sharp posterior thigh pain while training. The sagittal fast STIR (3000/150/39) image demonstrates significant hyperintense perifascial hemorrhage

Perifascial fluid may track completely around the muscle.

The role of MR in the follow-up of muscle strains may be quite important, particularly in professional and world-class athletes, where therapeutic decisions concerning the return to activity may weigh heavily on the outcome of the lesion and upon the performance of the athlete. Failure to correctly document complete muscle strain healing is particularly important with severe third-degree injuries because further complications may produce more weakness and disability due to exacerbation of the tear and due to the sequelae from the injury, including muscle fibrosis, foreshortening and detachment (Fig. 3.8).

Muscle injury may result from a certain repetitive activity or action, as opposed to a typical muscle strain which results from a single traumatic event. This occurs most often in response to athletic and occupational overuse and is therefore named muscle overuse syndrome (McKeag 1984; Stern 1990; Dennett and Fry 1988; Frymoyer and Mooney 1986; Ireland 1986; Lockwood 1989; Larsson et al. 1988; Simons 1975, 1976; •• 1987). The result is essentially the same as from a single event, namely, muscle strain or myotendinous injury. In sports medicine, one of the most common types of overuse syndrome occurs in tennis players, producing what is commonly known as "tennis leg." This usually involves the medial gastrocnemius myotendinous junction (Figs. 3.2, 3.10). The soleus muscle is less frequently involved.

Muscle overuse syndrome may also involve the epicondylar tendon insertions in tennis players, known as "tennis elbow." This may also affect golfers and carpenters (Fig. 3.11). Repetitive microtrauma produces pain over the radiohumeral joint due to tearing of the extensor tendon fibers at the lateral epicondyle. STIR or T2-weighted images demonstrate thickening and/or high signal intensity edema of the common extensor tendon, often with associated avulsive changes within the epicondyle. When avulsion is present, MR images usually demonstrate the presence of fluid.

3.3.4
Muscle Contusion

Direct trauma to muscle results in a combination of hemorrhage and edema. The degree of disruption of muscle fibers is proportional to the severity of the contusion. STIR and fat-saturated T2-weighted images demonstrate high signal intensity which may be

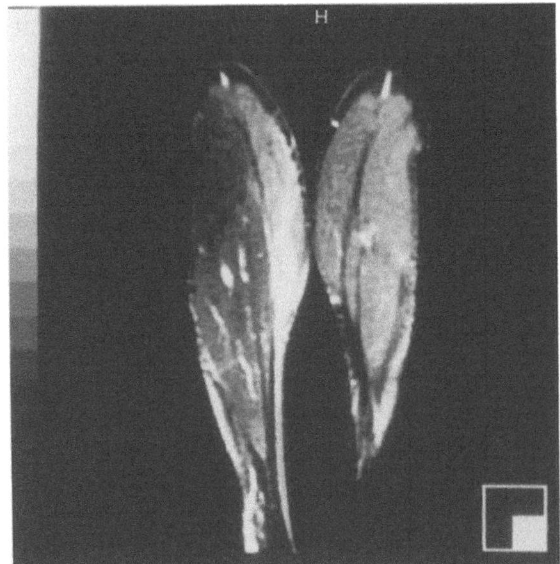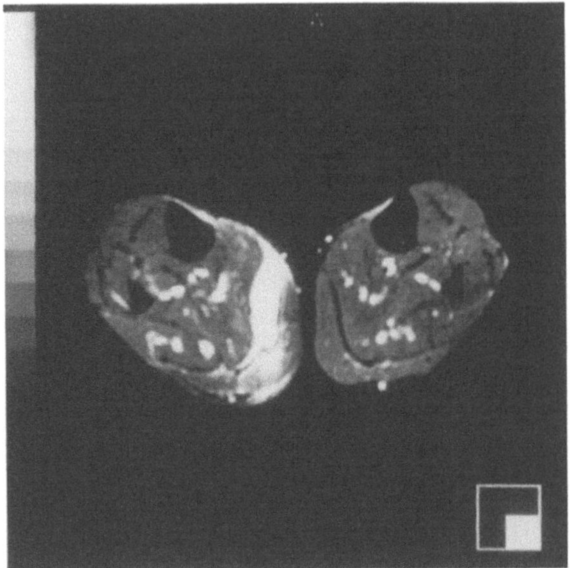

Fig. 3.10a,b. Tennis leg of a 56-year-old tennis player with a 10-day history of calf pain. Coronal (a) (2000/100/40) and axial (b) (2000/100/40) STIR images show distal myotendinous hyperintense muscle signal and perifascial blood

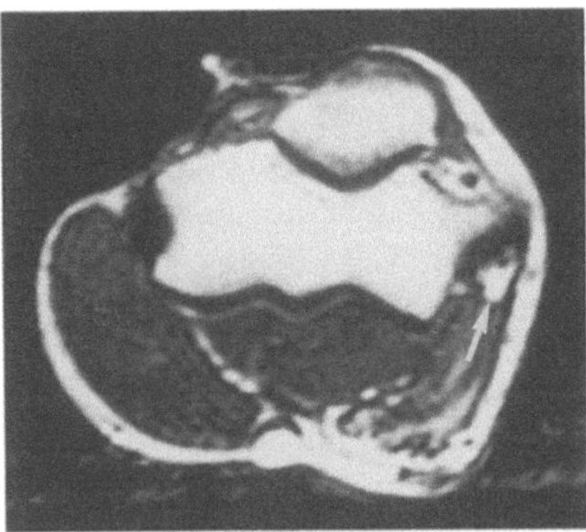

Fig. 3.11. Golf elbow. This 55-year-old male golfer has had lateral epicondylar pain of 4 months duration. The axial T2-weighted (2000/80) image shows high signal intensity at the insertion of the extensor tendon (*arrow*) in the lateral epicondyle

difficult to distinguish from muscle strain. Muscle contusion may involve the deep muscle structures with relative sparing of the superficial muscle. It also tends to produce more hematomas than simple muscle strain, although the presence of hematoma is certainly not a specific finding for either entity. The goal of MR is to determine the significance of muscle fiber disruption, particularly in the presence of a significant hematoma. The MR appearance may influence subsequent therapeutic decisions because in some cases the treating physician may elect to percutaneously drain the blood collection in order to pro-

mote apposition of the torn muscle fibers to facilitate healing.

3.3.4.1
Muscle Fibrosis

Muscle injury may result in fibroblast proliferation and subsequent muscle fibrosis (GRECO et al. 1991; WHYTE et al. 1989; SUNDARAM et al. 1987). Clinical second-degree muscle strain is usually not associated with significant scar formation. In most instances, third-degree muscle strain or significant contusion are precursors to muscle fibrosis, the amount of muscle scarring being related to the severity of the muscle injury. Many authors feel that muscle scar may predispose skeletal muscle to recurrent strain (GRECO et al. 1991; FLECKENSTEIN 1990). Muscle fibrosis has a hypointense signal intensity compared to normal skeletal muscle on all MR sequences (Fig. 3.12). Since scar tissue has a short T2 relaxation time (WHYTE et al. 1989; SUNDARAM et al. 1987), fibrosis is most easily appreciated on T2-weighted images and on STIR images. Fibrosis occurs in nearly all cases in close proximity to the myotendinous junction (Fig. 3.8). Immature fibrosis may initially appear as heterogeneous signal intensity, depending on the age of the injury and the phase of muscle healing. Since muscle fibrosis occurs most frequently at the myotendinous junction, it may be difficult to distinguish between

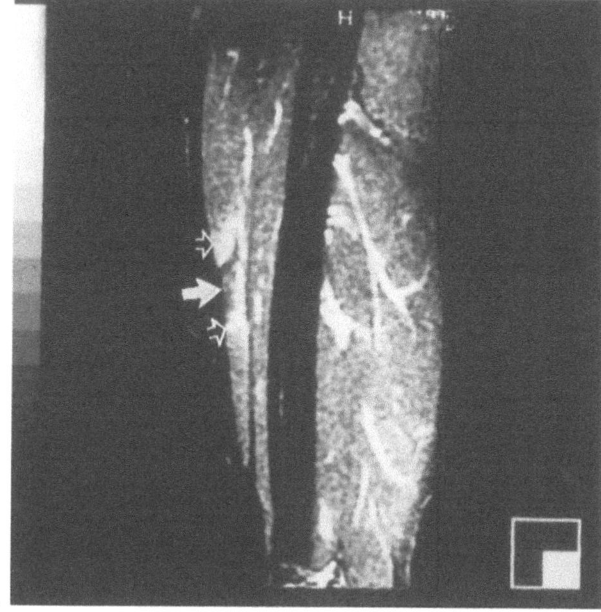

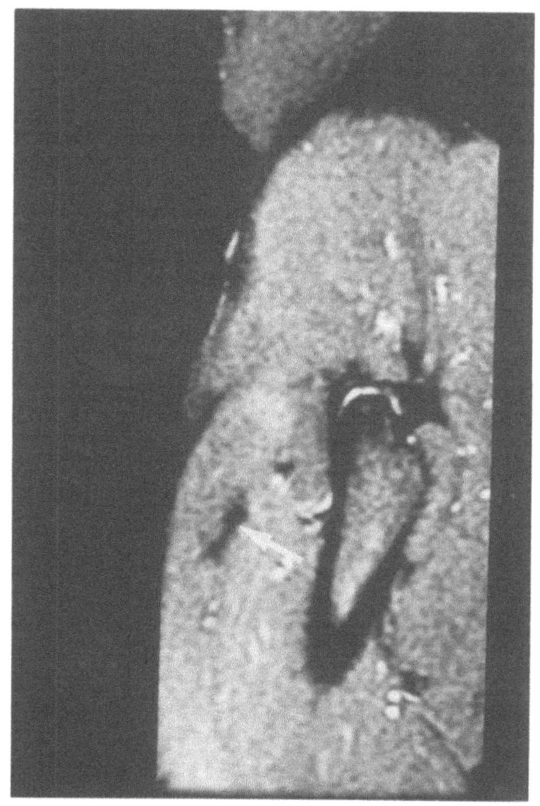

Fig. 3.12a,b. Muscle fibrosis. a A 28-year-old male soccer player with a history of repetitive anterior thigh muscle strains. The sagittal STIR (2000/100/40) image demonstrates low signal intensity muscle scar (*arrow*). The proximal and distal high signal intensity regions (*open arrows*) may repre-sent either incomplete healing or recurrent muscle strain. b A 25-year-old professional soccer player with remote anterior thigh muscle injury. Sagittal fast STIR (3000/150/26) image shows hypointense rectus femoris scar (*arrow*)

the normally hypointense tendon (FULLERTON et al. 1985; BELTRAN et al. 1987) and fibrosis. In this instance, a comparative axial transverse or coronal sequence displaying both extremities will demon-strate the thickening of the scarred tendon com-pared to the normal contralateral tendon (Fig. 3.8).

Since muscle fibrosis may predispose to recurrent muscle strain, MR is well suited for the evaluation of recurrent pain in proximity to a site of previous muscle strain or contusion. Hyperintense signal will be readily detected on STIR or fat-saturated T2-weighted sequences (Fig. 3.12).

3.3.4.2
Myositis Ossificans

Muscle injury may produce this uncommon sequela by a mechanism of unknown origin that consists of muscle swelling, pain, and loss of muscle function (JOHNSON 1948). The condition is benign and self-limiting (BOOTH and WESTERS ••). Myositis ossificans consists of a fibroblastic reaction that or-ganizes to produce peripheral new bone at 6–8 weeks of age (HUDSON 1987). Within 6 months, the lesion will mature into peripheral compact bone with a cen-tral core of lamellar bone (AMENDOLA et al. 1983; ZEANAH and HUDSON 1982).

In the early stage, MR STIR on T2-weighted im-ages demonstrates nonspecific high signal intensity (KRANSDORF et al. 1991). Peripheral hypointense curvilinear or irregular ossification may be seen in the subacute phase. Chronic mature myositis ossificans contains cortical bone and fibrotic tissue which appear hypointense on MR images, involving both the periphery and central portion of the lesion. If the lesion contains bone trabeculae with fatty bone marrow, hyperintense signal intensity will be noted on T1-weighted images.

3.3.4.3
Compartment Syndrome

This lesion is a result of muscle trauma or injury, whereby raised intracompartmental pressure is produced by edema and hemorrhage within fascial boundaries (RAETHER and LUTHER 1982; WHITESIDES et al. 1975). This may result in a 20% increase in muscle volume during exercise, which is due to increased capillary filtration that is not removed by normal mechanisms. In compartment syndrome, tissue pressures may increase to as much as 40–60 mmHg (WHITESIDES et al. 1975), thereby impairing capillary perfusion and oxygen supply, which causes pain, reduced function, and sensory deficits. In our experience, compartment syndrome occurs most commonly in the calf, but it has also been reported in the arm and thigh (FLECKENSTEIN and SHELLOCK 1991; RAETHER and LUTHER 1982; WHITESIDES et al. 1975; FLECKENSTEIN et al. 1989c; WOLFORT et al. 1973; BINKOVITZ et al. 1990; AMENDOLA et al. 1990).

On STIR and T2-weighted images of compartment syndrome, there is muscle swelling and diffuse high signal intensity (AMENDOLA et al. 1990). Note that this appearance is nonspecific and careful clinical correlation is required to make the diagnosis. A constant finding in these patients is pain brought on by exercise (AMENDOLA et al. 1990).

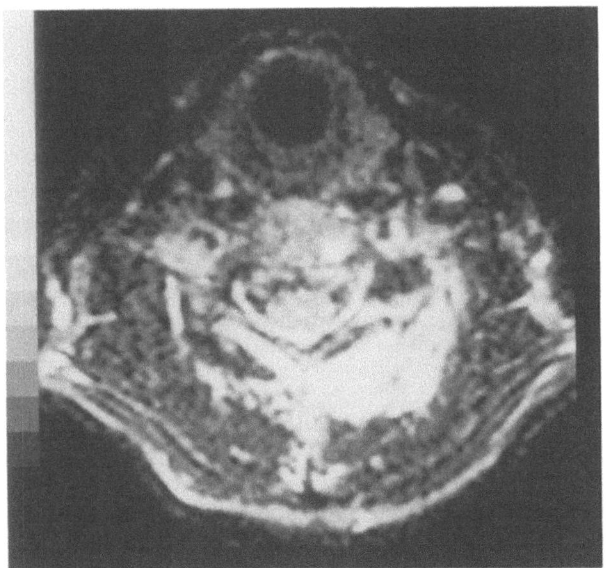

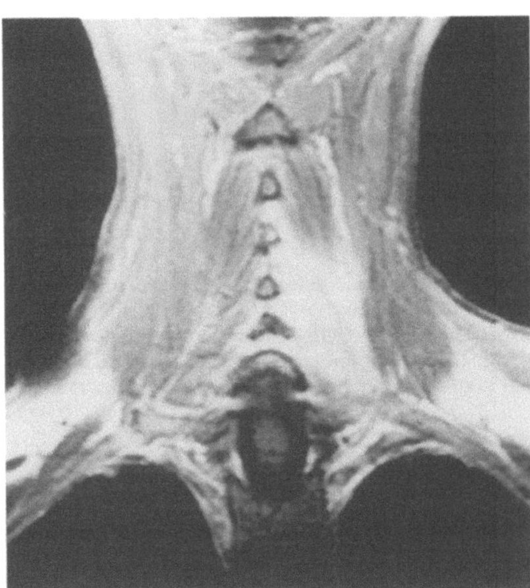

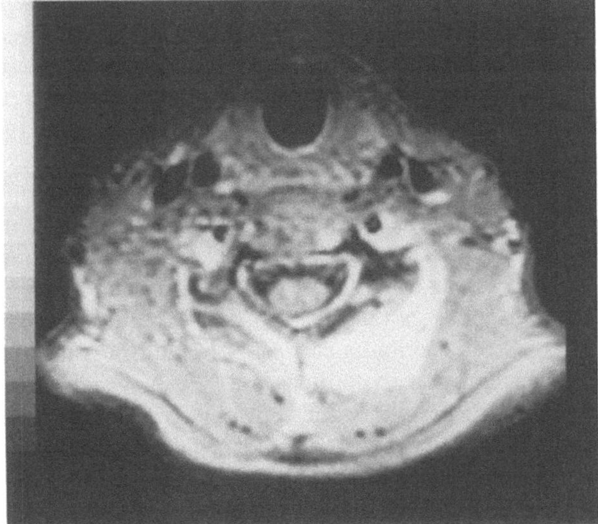

Fig. 3.13a–c. Presumed left posterior neck compartment infectious myositis in a 49-year-old woman with a 2-month history of left-sided neck pain. Axial (a) fat-saturated FSE (3000/96) T2-weighted and axial (b) and coronal (c) fat-saturated FSE (500/11) T1-weighted postcontrast images. There is extensive signal increase of left posterior deep musculature, with marked enhancement following gadolinium chelate intravenous injection. There is also focal hyperintensity, inflammatory or infectious in origin, in the left posterior C6 vertebral body. The lesion resolved following antibiotic therapy. *FSE*, fast spin echo

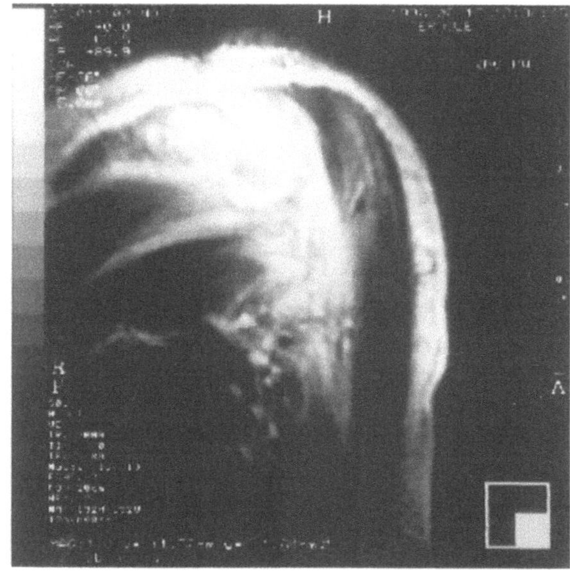

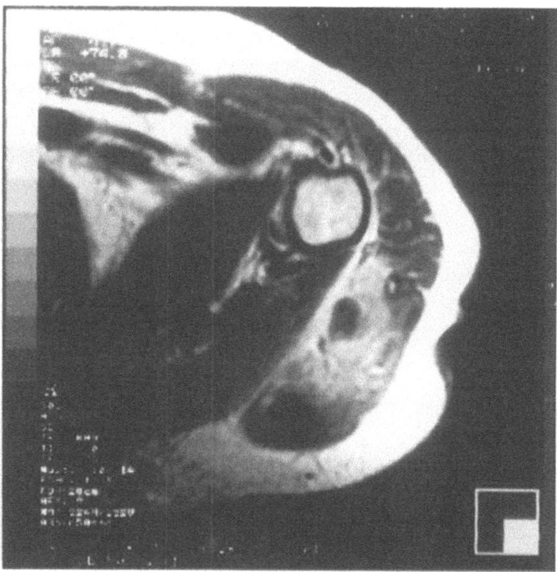

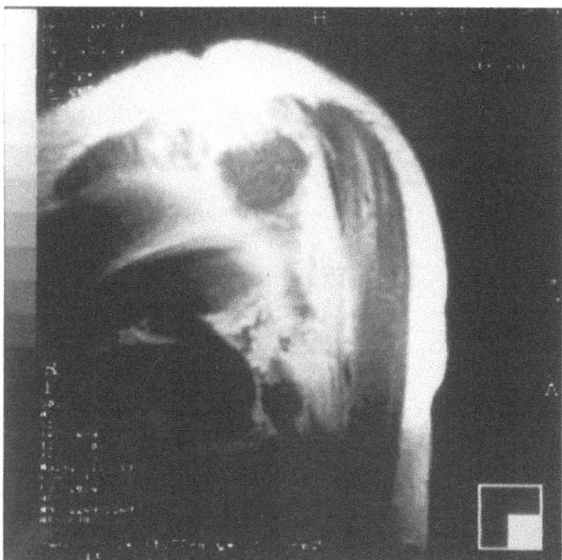

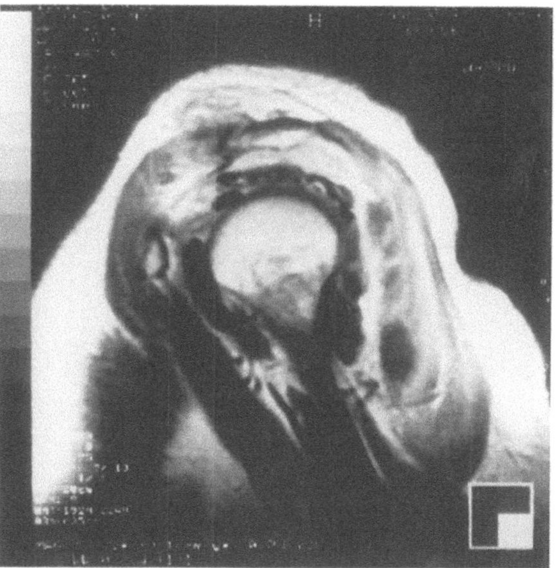

Fig. 3.14a–d. Infectious myositis in a 63-year-old woman with staphylococcus deltoid myositis abscess. Coronal T2-weighted (2000/80) spin-echo image (**a**) shows increased signal intensity involving posterior deltoid muscle. On coronal (**b**) (620/ 25), axial (**c**) (600/25) and sagittal (**d**) (560/25) T1-weighted images obtained following intravenous gadolinium chelate injection, there is diffuse muscle enhancement surrounding an area of no contrast uptake, consistent with an abscess

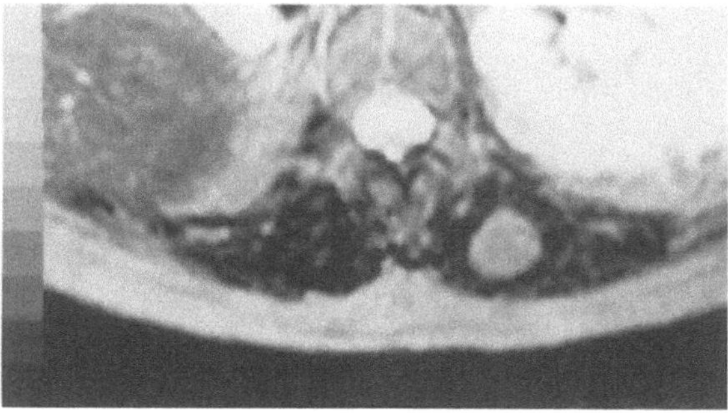

Fig. 3.15. Paraspinal muscle metastasis in a 45-year-old female patient with primary leiomyosarcoma. Metastatic lesion appears hyperintense on fat-saturated axial FSE (4000/104) T2-weighted image

Fig. 3.16. Obturator externus metastasis in a 49-year-old male patient with colon adenocarcinoma. Metastasis is hyperintense on fat-saturated FSE (4000/119) T2-weighted image

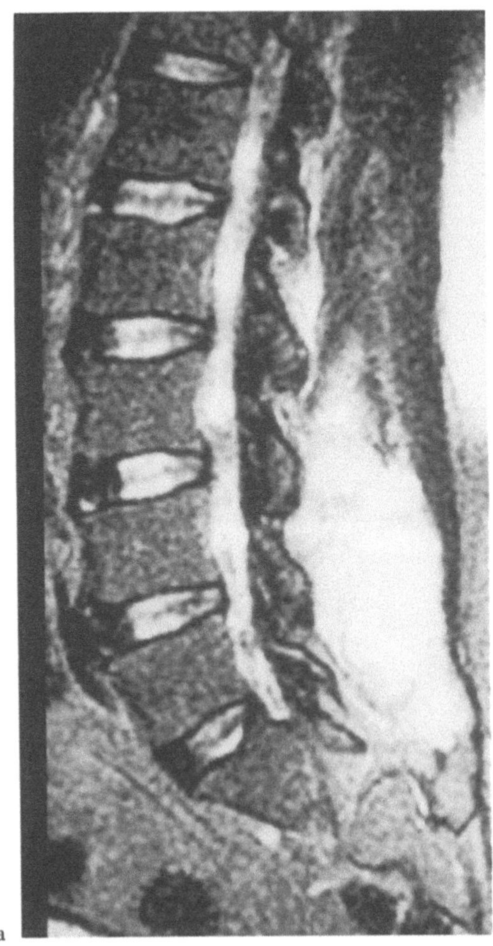

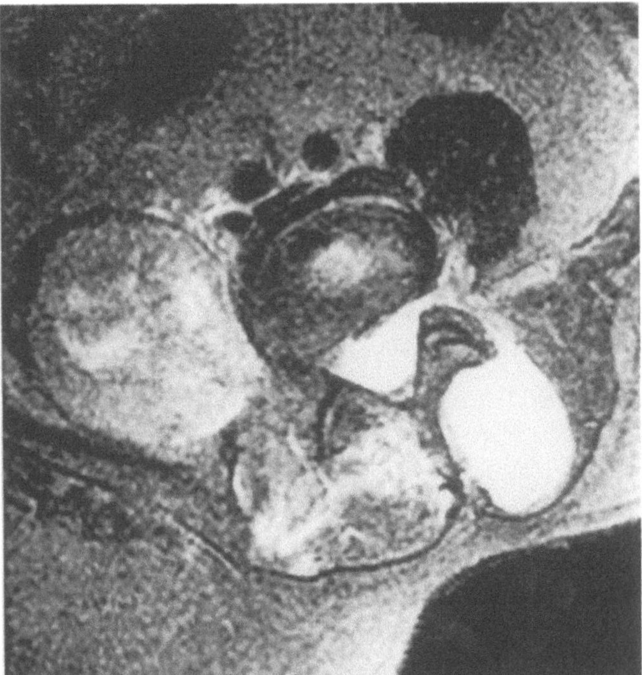

b

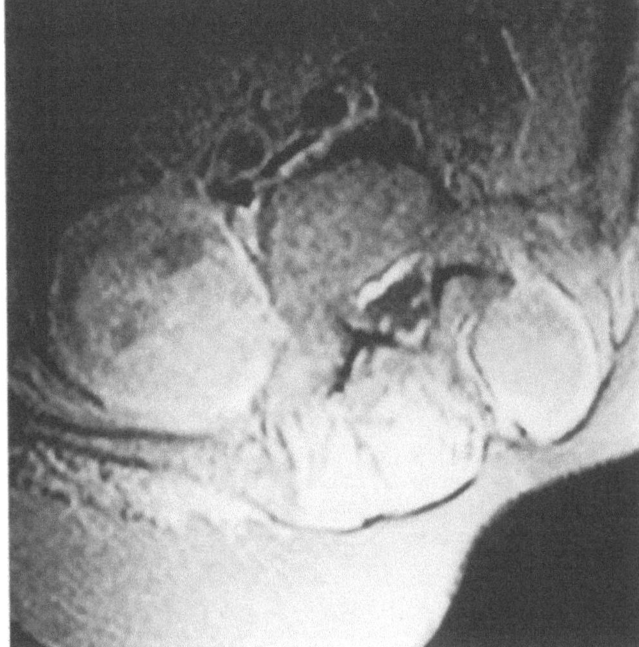

c

Fig. 3.17a–c. Non-Hodgkin lymphoma in a 48-year-old man. Sagittal (**a**) and axial (**b**) T2-weighted fat-saturated FSE (3500/90) and postcontrast axial fat-saturated FSE (500/11) T1-weighted images (**c**). Necrotic lymphomatous involvement of left posterior paraspinal and right psoas muscles is hyperintense. There is ring-like enhancement following intravenous gadolinium chelate administration. Also, note on T2-weighted images patchy areas of increased signal intensity involving right posterior paraspinal muscles

3.3.4.4
Calcific Myonecrosis

This relatively rare muscle lesion consists of fusiform mass-like swelling of a single muscle with associated peripheral nerve damage. Authors have suggested that myonecrosis may be caused by underlying compartment syndrome and ischemia (MALISANO and HUNTER 1992; VIAU et al. 1983). The calf is the most frequent site of occurrence, and concomitant fracture is also found. Injury to the peroneal nerve has also been suggested as a causative factor in calf calcific myonecrosis (JANZEN et al. 1993).

In calcific myonecrosis, there is central muscle liquefaction that is hyperintense on STIR and T2-

weighted images. There are plaquelike peripheral calcifications which are typically hypointense. Central calcifications such as those seen in myositis ossificans are not a feature of calcific myonecrosis.

3.3.4.5
Miscellaneous Conditions

Diseases unrelated to sports injury or trauma may produce nonspecific high signal intensity in skeletal muscle. Myositis (Fig. 3.13) and abscess may have clinical and MR features that help to differentiate them from other lesions such as neoplasm and hematoma (FLECKENSTEIN et al. 1991a; BERQUIST et al. 1985; HERNANDEZ et al. 1992; BERQUIST 1987). The abscess may be distinguishable from hyperintense surrounding muscle edema on STIR or T2-weighted images. The central portion of the abscess may have a liquid-like signal intensity. Intravenous administration of paramagnetic gadolinium chelate usually produces enhancement of both the central portion of the abscess and the surrounding soft tissue inflammation (Fig. 3.14). The liquid-like center of the abscess typically does not enhance.

Although they present infrequently with muscle pain, muscle neoplasms should be considered in the differential diagnosis of muscle swelling. A majority of the muscle tumors that we detect with MR are metastatic in origin. STIR or T2-weighted images will demonstrate a hyperintense, usually heterogeneous mass with variable amounts of hemorrhage, necrosis, and calcification. Most metastatic muscle tumors are fairly well circumscribed (Figs. 3.15, 3.16). It is generally accepted at this time that MR cannot reliably differentiate between benign and malignant muscle tumors (HANNA et al. 1991; BIONDETTI and EHMAN 1992; CRIM et al. 1992; BERQUIST et al. 1990; WETZEL and LEVINE 1990; MORTON et al. 1991; MURPHY et al. 1991). Even with gadolinium chelate enhancement, the pattern of enhancement does not increase either the diagnostic sensitivity or the specificity of MR compared to unenhanced STIR or T2-weighted images (Fig. 3.17).

3.4
Summary

MR imaging has inherent attributes which make it a very useful imaging modality for the depiction of the soft tissues, particularly the musculoskeletal system. It is very sensitive for the detection of a wide variety of pathologic alterations of the composition of skeletal muscle, including hemorrhage, edema, inflammation, infection, necrosis, calcification and fibrosis. At our institution, it has become the method of choice for the detection and characterization of nearly all muscle lesions, particularly those related to sports. By providing a rapid and accurate diagnosis, MR imaging permits the rapid initiation of treatment and may even reduce morbidity and postinjury sequelae, thus providing cost effectiveness when compared to other methods of diagnosis.

References

Allard JC, Bancroft J, Porter G (1992) Imaging of plantaris muscle rupture. Clin Imaging 16:55–58

Amendola MA, Glazer GM, Agha FP, Francis IR, Weatherbee L, Martel W (1983) Myositis ossificans circumscripta: computed tomographic diagnosis. Radiology 149:775–779

Amendola A, Rorabeck CH, Vellett D, Vezina W, Rutt B, Nott L (1990) The use of magnetic resonance imaging in exertional compartment syndromes. Am J Sports Med 18:29–34

Anonymous (1987) Repetition strain injury (editorial). Lancet 2:316

Anzel SH, Covey KW, Weiner AD, et al. (1959) Disruption of muscles and tendons: an analysis of 1,014 cases. Surgery 45:406–414

Baker BE (1984) Current concepts in diagnosis and treatment of musculotendinous injuries. Med Sci Sports Exerc 16:323–327

Beltran J, Noto AM, Herman LJ, Lubbers LM (1987) Tendons: high-field-strength, surface coil MR imaging. Radiology 162:735–740

Bernardino ME, Chaloupka JC, Malko JA, Chezmar JL, Nelson RC (1989) Are hepatic and muscle T2 values different at 0.5 and 1.5 tesla? Magn Reson Imaging 7:363–367

Berquist TH (1985a) Imaging of orthopedic trauma and surgery. Saunders, Philadelphia

Berquist TH (1985b) Imaging Techniques in the acutely injured patient. Urban and Schwarzenberg, Baltimore

Berquist TH (1987) Musculoskeletal infection. In: Berquist TH, Ehman RL, Richardson ML (eds) Magnetic resonance imaging of the musculoskeletal system. Raven, New York, pp 109–126

Berquist TH, Ehman RL (1987) Musculoskeletal trauma. In: Berquist TH, Ehman RL, Richardson ML (eds) Magnetic resonance imaging of the musculoskeletal system. Raven, New York, pp 127–163

Berquist TH, Brown ML, Fitzgerald RH Jr, May GR (1985) Magnetic resonance imaging: application in musculoskeletal infection. Magn Reson Imaging 3:219–230

Berquist TH, Ehman RL, King BF, Hodgman CG, Iistrup DM (1990) Value of MR imaging in differentiating benign from malignant soft-tissue masses: study of 95 lesions. AJR AM J Roentgenol 155:1251–1255

Binkovitz LA, Berquist TH, McLeod RA (1990) Masses of the hand and wrist: detection and characterization with MR imaging. AJR Am J Roentgenol 154:323–326

Biondetti PR, Ehman RL (1992) Soft-tissue sarcomas: use of textural patterns in skeletal muscle as a diagnostic feature in postoperative MR imaging. Radiology 183:845–848

Booth DW, Westers BM. The management of athletes with myositis ossificans traumatica. Can J Sport Sci 14:10–16

Bowerman JW (1977) Radiology of injury in sports. Appleton-Century-Crofts, New York

Bydder GM, Young IR (1985) MR imaging: clinical use of the inversion recovery sequence. J Comput Assist Tomogr 9:659–675

Cooney WP (1984) Sports injuries to the upper extremity. How to recognize and deal with some common problems. Postgrad Med 76:45–50

Crim JR, Seeger LL, Yao L, Chandnani V, Eckardt JJ (1992) Diagnosis of soft-tissue masses with MR imaging: can benign masses be differentiated from malignant ones? Radiology 185:581–586

Dennett X, Fry HJ (1988) Overuse syndrome: a muscle biopsy study. Lancet 1:905–908

DeSmet AA, Fisher DR, Heiner JP, Keene JS (1990) Magnetic resonance imaging of muscle tears. Skeletal Radiol 19:283–286

Deutsch AL, Mink JH (1989) Magnetic resonance imaging of musculoskeletal injuries. Radiol Clin North Am 27:983–1002

Dooms GC, Fisher MR, Hricak H, Higgins CB (1985) MR imaging of intramuscular hemorrhage. J Comput Assist Tomogr 9:908–913

Dwyer AJ, Frank JA, Sank VJ, Reinig JW, Hickey AM, Doppman JL (1988) Short-T1 inversion recovery pulse sequence: analysis and initial experience in cancer imaging. Radiology 168:827–836

Ehman RL, Berquist TH (1986) Magnetic resonance imaging of musculoskeletal trauma. Radio Clin North Am 24:291–319

Fisher MR, Dooms GC, Hricak H, et al. (1986) Magnetic resonance imaging of the normal and pathologic muscular system. Magn Reson Imaging 4:491–496

Fisher MJ, Meyer RA, Adams GR, Foley JM, Potchen EJ (1990) Direct relationship between proton T2 and exercise intensity in skeletal muscle MR images. Invest Radiol 25:480–485

Fleckenstein JL (1990) Skeletal muscle disorders: the emerging role of MR imaging. In: Kressel HY, Modic MT, Murphy WA (eds) Syllabus: a special course in MR 1990. Radiological Society of North America, Oak Brook, pp 197–206

Fleckenstein JL, Shellock FG (1991) Exertional muscle injuries magnetic resonance imaging evaluation. Top Magn Reson Imaging 3:50–70

Fleckenstein JL, Canby RC, Parkey RW, Peshock RM (1988) Acute effects of exercise on MR imaging of skeletal muscle in normal volunteers. AJR Am J Roentgenol 15:231–237

Fleckenstein JL, Weatherall PT, Parkey RW, Payne JA, Peshock RM (1989a) Sports related muscle injuries: evaluation with MR imaging. Radiology 172:793–798

Fleckenstein JL, Archer BT, Barker BA, Vaughan JT, Parkey RW, Peshock RM (1989b) Fast, short tau inversion recovery (FASTIR) imaging (abstr). Magn Reson Imaging 7:87

Fleckenstein JL, Bertocci LA, Nunnally RL, Parkey RW, Peshock RM (1989c) Exercise-enhanced MR imaging of variations in forearm muscle anatomy and use: importance in MR spectroscopy. AJR AM J Roentgenol 153:693–698

Fleckenstein JL, Burns DK, Murphy FK, Jayson HT, Bonte FJ (1991a) Differential diagnosis of bacterial myositis in AIDS: evaluation with MR imaging. Radiology 179:653–658

Fleckenstein JL, Weatherall PT, Bertocci LA, et al. (1991b) Locomotor system assessment by muscle magnetic resonance imaging. Magn Reson Q 7:79–103

Fleckenstein JL, Archer BT, Barker BA, Vaughan JT, Parkey RW, Peshock RM (1991c) Fast short-tau inversion-recovery imaging. Radiology 179:499–504

Frymoyer JW, Mooney V (1986) Occupational orthopaedics. J Bone Joint Surg [Am] 68:469–474

Fullerton GD, Cameron IL, Ord VA (1985) Orientation of tendons in the magnetic field and its effect on T2 relaxation times. Radiology 155:433–435

Garrett WE (1986) Basic science of musculotendinous injuries. In: Nicholas JA, Hershman EB (eds) The lower extremity and spine in sports medicine. Mosby, St Louis, pp 42–58

Garrett WE (1988) Injuries to the muscle tendon unit. Instr Course Lect 37:275–282

Garrett WE (1990) Muscle strain injuries: clinical and basic aspects. Med Sci Sports Exerc 22:436–443

Garrett WE, Rich FR, Nikolaou PK, et al. (1989) Computed tomography of hamstring muscle strains. Med Sci Sports Exerc 21:506–514

Glick JM (1980) Muscle strains: prevention and treatment. Physician Sports Med 8:73–77

Greco A, McNamara MT, Escher MB, Trifilio G, Parienti J (1991) Spin-echo and STIR MR imaging of sports-related muscle injuries at 1.5 T. J Comput Assist Tomogr 15:994–999

Hanna SL, Fletcher BD, Parham DM, Bugg MF (1991) Muscle edema in musculoskeletal tumors: MR imaging characteristics and clinical significance. J Magn Reson Imaging 1:441–449

Hernandez RJ, Keim DR, Chenevert TL, Sullivan DB, Aisen AM (1992) Fat-suppressed MR imaging of myositis. Radiology 182(1):217–219

Hiroshi Y, Anno I, Niitsu M, Takahashi H, Matsumoto K, Itai Y (1994) MRI of muscle strain injuries. J Comput Assist Tomogr 18:454–460

Hudson TM (1987) Radiologic-pathologic correlation of musculoskeletal lesions. Williams and Wilkins, Baltimore, pp 589–604

Ireland DC (1986) Repetitive strain injury. Aust Fam Physician 15:415–418

Jackson DW, Feagin JA (1973) Quadriceps contusions in young adults: relationship of severity of injury to treatment and prognosis. J Bone Joint Surg [Am] 55:95–105

Janzen DL, Connell DG, Vaisler BJ (1993) Calcific myonecrosis of the calf manifesting as an enlarging soft tissue mass: imaging features. AJR Am J Roentgenol 160:1072–1074

Johnson LC (1948) Histogenesis of myositis ossificans. Am J Pathol 24:681–682

Kibler WB (1990) Clinical aspects of muscle injury. Med Sci Sports Exerc 22:450–452

Kransdorf MJ, Meis JM, Jelinek JS (1991) Myositis ossificans: MR appearance with radiologic-pathologic correlation. AJR Am J Roentgenol 157:1243–1248

Kuno S-Y, Katsuta S, Inouye T, Anno I, Matsumoto K, Akisada M (1988) Relationship between relaxation times and muscle fiber composition. Radiology 169:567–568

Larsson SE, Bengtsson A, Bodegard L, Hendricksson KG, Larsson J (1988) Muscle changes in work-related chronic myalgia. Acta Orthop Scand 59:552–556

Lockwood AH (1989) Medical problems of musicians. N Engl J Med 320:221–227

Malisano LP, Hunter GA (1992) Liquefaction and calcification of a chronic compartment syndrome of the lower limb. J Orthop Trauma 6:245–247

Matin P (1988) Basic principles of nuclear medicine techniques for detection and evaluation of trauma and sports medicine injuries. Semin Nucl Med 18:90–112

Matin P, Lang G, Garretta R, et al. (1983) Scintigraphic evaluation of muscle damage following extreme exercise: concise communication. J Nucl Med 24:308–311

McKeag DB (1984) The concept of overuse: the primary care aspects of overuse syndromes in sports. Prim Care 11:43–59

Middleton WD, Edelstein G, Reinus WR, Melson GL, Totty WG, Murphy WA (1985) Sonographic detection of rotator cuff tears. AJR Am J Roentgenol 144:349–353

Moon KL, Genant HK, Helms CA, Chafetz NI, Crooks LE, Kaufman L (1983) Musculoskeletal applications of nuclear magnetic resonance. Radiology 147:161–171

Morton MJ, Berquist TH, McLeod RA, Unni KK, Sim FH (1991) Pictorial essay. MR imaging of synovial sarcoma. AJR Am J Roentgenol 156:337–340

Muckle DS (1981) Injuries in professional football. Br J Sports Med 15:77–79

Murphy WD, Hurst GC, Duerk JL, Feiglin DH, Christopher M, Bellon EM (1991) Atypical appearance of lipomatous tumors on MR images: high signal intensity with fat-suppression STIR sequences. J Magn Reson, Imaging 1:477–480

Noonan TJ, Garrett WEJ (1992) Injuries of the myotendinous junction. Clin Sports Med 11:783–806

O'Donoghue DH (1984) Principles in the management of specific injuries. In: O'Donoghue DH (ed) Treatment of injuries to athletes, 4th edn. Saunders, Philadelphia, pp 39–91

Orava S, Sorasto A, Aalto K, Kvist H (1984) Total rupture of the pectoralis major muscle in athletes. Int J Sports Med 5:272–274

Polak JF, Jolesz FA, Adams DF (1988) NMR of skeletal muscle differences in relaxation parameters related to extracellular/intracellular fluid spaces. Invest Radiol 23:107–111

Raether PM, Luther LD (1982) Recurrent compartment syndrome in the posterior thigh. Report of a case. Am J Sports Med 10:40–43

Rubin JI, Gomori JM, Grossman RI, Gefter WB, Kressel HY (1987) High-field MR imaging of extracranial hematomas. AJR Am J Roentgenol 248:813–817

Ryan AJ (1969) Quadriceps strain: rupture and charley horse. Med Sci Sports 1:106–111

Scott JA, Rosenthal DI, Brady T (1984) The evaluation of musculoskeletal disease with magnetic resonance imaging. Radiol Clin North Am 22:917–924

Shirkoda A, Mauro MA, Staab EV, Blatt PM (1983) Soft-tissue hemorrhage in hemophiliac patients: computed tomography and ultrasound study. Radiology 147:811–814

Simons D (1975) Muscle pain syndromes. I. Am J Phys Med 54:289–311

Simons D (1976) Muscle pain syndromes. II. Am J Phys Med 55:15–42

Speer KP, Lohnes H, Garrett WE (1993) Radiographic imaging of muscle strain injury. Am J Sports Med 21:89–95

Stern PJ (1990) Tendinitis, overuse syndromes, and tendon injuries. Hand Clin 6:467–476

Sundaram M, McGuire MH, Schajowicz F (1987) Soft-tissue masses: histologic basis for decreased signal (short T2) on T2-weighted MR images. AJR Am J Roentgenol 148:1247–1250

Termote J, Baert A, Crolla D, Palmers Y, Bulcke JA (1980) Computed tomography of the normal and pathologic muscular system. Radiology 137:439–444

Unger EC, Glazer HS, Lee JKT, et al. (1986) MRI of extracranial hematomas: preliminary observations. AJR Am J Roentgenol 146:403–407

Valk P (1983) Muscle localization of Tc-99m MDP after exertion. Clin Nucl Med 24:308–311

Viau MR, Pederson HE, Salciccioli GG, Manoli A (1983) Ectopic calcification as a late sequela of compartment syndrome. Clin Orthop 176:178–180

Wetzel LH, Levine E (1990) Soft-tissue tumors of the foot: value of MR imaging for specific diagnosis. AJR Am J Roentgenol 155:1025–1030

Whitehouse GH (1992) Magnetic resonance imaging in the diagnosis of muscle and tendon injuries. Imaging 4:95–105

Whitesides TE, Haney TC, Moremoto K (1975) Tissue pressure measurements as a determinator for need for fasciotomy. Clin Orthop 113:43–51

Whyte AM, Lufkin RB, Bredenkamp J, Hoover L (1989) Sternocleidomastoid fibrosis in congenital muscular torticollis: MR appearance. J Comput Assist Tomogr 13:163–166

Wolfort FG, Modelvang LC, Filtzer HS (1973) Anterior tibial compartment syndrome following muscle hernia repair. Arch Surg 106:97–99

Zarins B, Ciullo JV (1983) Acute muscle and tendon injuries in athletes. Clin Sports Med 2:167–182

Zeanah WR, Hudson TM (1982) Myositis ossificans: radiologic evaluation of two cases with diagnostic computed tomograms. Clin Orthop 168:187–192

4 Tendinous Disease

H. Imhof[1], M. Breitenseher[2], J. Haller[3], F. Kainberger[4], and S. Trattnig[5]

CONTENTS

4.1
Introduction

Tendinous diseases are very common, particularly in younger athletes. In previous times, diagnosis of tendinous injuries depended less on imaging and almost exclusively on clinical parameters (e.g., grade of maximum joint angulation).

Since the advent of sonography, computed tomography (CT) and especially magnetic resonance imaging (MRI), this situation has changed dramatically. Changes in size, structure and intactness of fibers are readily detected. This has led to new staging and therapy strategies in many different joint and tendon injuries. Healing of tendon injuries usually takes twice as long as bone injuries, so they are very often neglected, which may lead to chronic injuries. With the new imaging modalities, healing and nonhealing can be much more exactly differentiated.

[1]H. Imhof, MD, and [2]M. Breitenseher, MD, MR and Osteology; Universitätsklinik für Radiodiagnostik AKH, Ludwig-Boltzmann-Institut für radiologische-physikalische Tumordiagnostik, Währinger Gürtel 18–20, 1090 Vienna, Austria

[3]J. Haller, MD, Roentgeninstitut, Hanusch-Krankenhaus, Heinrich-Collinstrasse 30, Vienna, Austria

[4]F. Kainberger, MD, and [5]S. Trattnig, MR and Osteology; Universitätsklinik für Radiodiagnostik AKH, Ludwig-Boltzmann-Institut für radiologische-physikalische Tumordiagnostik, Währinger Gürtel 18–20, 1090 Vienna, Austria

4.2
Plain Film Radiography, Computed Tomography and Arthrography in Tendon Injury

4.2.1
Principles of Imaging

Radiographic diagnosis of a tendon injury can be difficult, although soft tissue swelling changes in tendon contour and bony displacement may be detected. Other techniques such as xerography, low-kV radiography and arthrography, possibly in combination with CT, can be helpful. Low-kV radiography offers increased contrast and resolution, and many subtle abnormalities of soft tissues which would otherwise not be seen may be clearly appreciated. A magnifying glass is required to analyze the radiographic detail in low-kV radiography, limiting the field of vision and facilitating a systematic analysis of these detailed radiographic images (Fischer 1988).

Certain abnormalities, such as complete rupture, are easy to recognize clinically, while others may produce nonspecific symptoms and signs, in which cases arthrography can be helpful. The latter abnormalities include partial tears, dislocation and post-traumatic tenosynovitis (Fig. 4.1).

CT combined with arthrography has been used to assess chondral defects in some joints. The technique is also valuable in the detection of osteochondral bodies in any articulation, but may not be useful in tendon injuries (Resnick 1988).

Contrast opacification of tendon sheath (tenography) or tendons (tendeography) may reveal abnormal patterns in patients with tendon tears.

Effusions related to fluid production within the sheath may produce distension, and villous hypertrophy of the synovial lining can lead to thickening and irregularity of the tendon sheath wall, visible as a nodular-corrugated pattern of the contrast material. Displacement of the sheaths may occur (Resnick 1988).

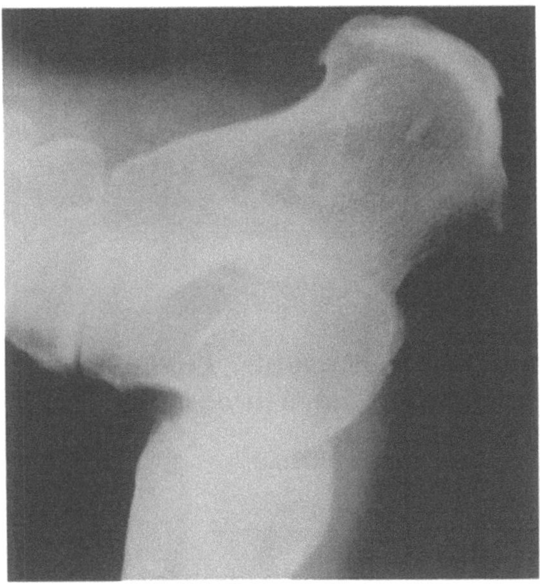

Fig. 4.1. Lateral radiograph of the foot with posttraumatic Achilles tendinitis. Thickening of the tendon and blurring of the anterior margin 3 weeks after soccer injury

Posttraumatic ossification of injured ligaments can be observed (Fig. 4.2). Abnormal stress on tendons may lead to characteristic avulsions of bony attachments. Avulsion injuries around the pelvis and the hips of young athletes occur in sprinters at the anterior superior iliac spine as a result of stress of the tensor fasciae femoris muscle or the sartorius muscle (Fig. 4.3).

Avulsion injuries of the apophysis of the ischial tuberosity (Fig. 4.4) owing to abrupt contraction of the hamstring muscles often occur in hurdlers, whereas avulsion of the apophysis of the iliac crest owing to severe contraction of the abdominal muscles can be seen in athletes with abrupt directional change during running (RESNICK 1988).

4.2.2
Clinical Application

4.2.2.1
Rotator Cuff

A decrease in the soft tissue mass between humerus and acromion causes the humeral head to become juxtaposed to the undersurface of the acromion. The fat that separates the rotator cuff from the adjacent subdeltoid bursa may vanish on conventional radiographs in internal rotation and indicate a rupture of the rotator cuff (Fig. 4.5a). These findings are incon-

stant, so it is important to consider additional radiographic manifestations that accompany rotator cuff injuries such as narrowing of the acromial humeral space, reversal of the normal inferior acromial convexity, cystic lesions and sclerosis to the acromion and humeral head. Most of these manifestations are seen more often in cases of chronic rotator cuff tears than in acute injury. Arthrography of the glenohumeral joint is better suited for discovering acute, complete or partial tears of the rotator cuff (Fig. 4.5b, c). A partial tear may involve the deep surface of the rotator cuff, the superficial surface, or the interior substance of the tendon. Tears within the substance of the cuff will generally escape arthrographic detection but may not require operative repair. Tears involving the superior surface of the cuff will also not be demonstrated on glenohumeral joint arthrography, although they may rarely be seen with direct subacromial bursography (SCHNEIDER et al. 1975).

Entrapment or rupture of the long head of the biceps tendon following trauma may be detected only after arthrography, possibly followed by computed tomography (Fig. 4.6).

4.2.2.2
Quadriceps and Patellar Tendon

Quadriceps tendon rupture most often involves elderly patients with degenerative changes of tendons. Tears may be partial or complete and usually involve an area 1–2 cm above the patellar tip. The central anterior portion of the tendon tears first and may then extend medially or laterally with continuing force.

Radiographic diagnosis is difficult using plain films only. Abnormalities are confined to the lateral view. Hemarthrosis and blurring of this usually sharply defined margin of the quadriceps tendon caused by adjacent hemorrhage are noted. A suprapatellar soft tissue mass with inner calcification provides an important diagnostic clue. The mass represents the retracted portion of the tendon. The calcification may be a consequence of prior degenerative changes in the tendon of newly avulsed fragments from the patella. Although the patella position should be low, this is not always apparent on radiographs obtained in supine position. Laxity of the patellar tendon may be demonstrable. Full-thickness tears can be confirmed after an injection of radiopaque material into the patellar pouch, demonstrat-

Fig. 4.2. A.p. radiograph of the shoulder: Coracoclavicular and acromioclavicular separation with subsequent ossification of the coracoclavicular ligament (*arrow*)

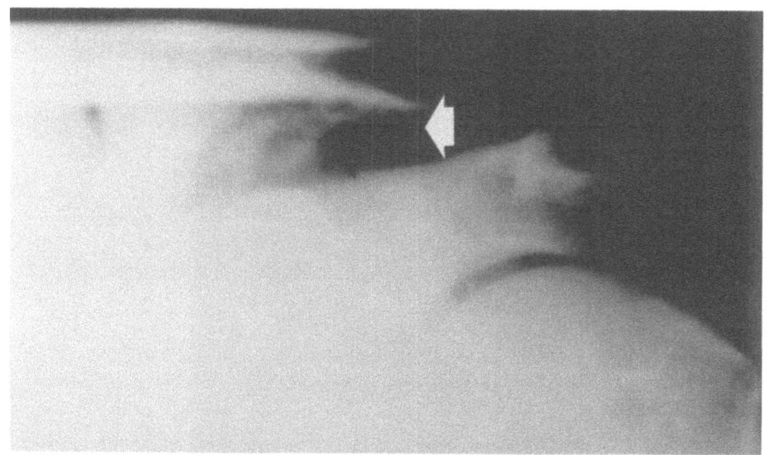

Fig. 4.3. A.p. radiograph of the pelvis: avulsion fracture (*arrow*) of the anterior-superior iliacal spine involving a young gymnast

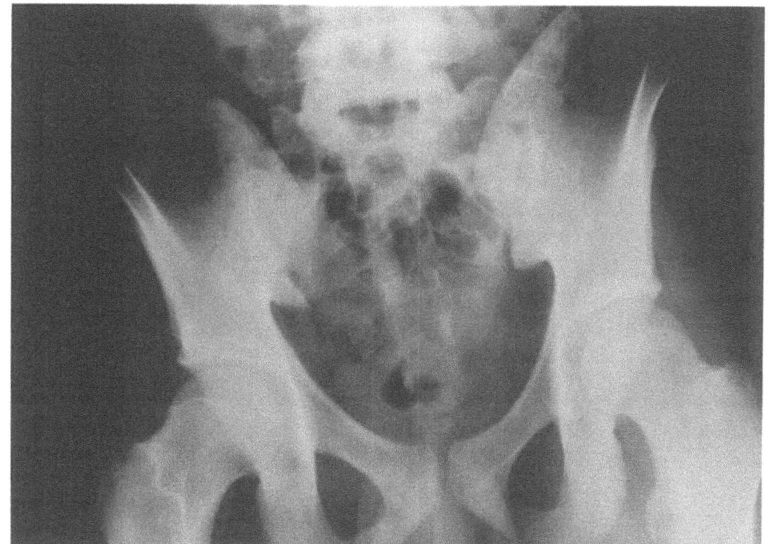

Fig. 4.4. A.p. radiograph of the pelvis: bilateral avulsion injury of the ischial tuberosity in a young competitive hurdler

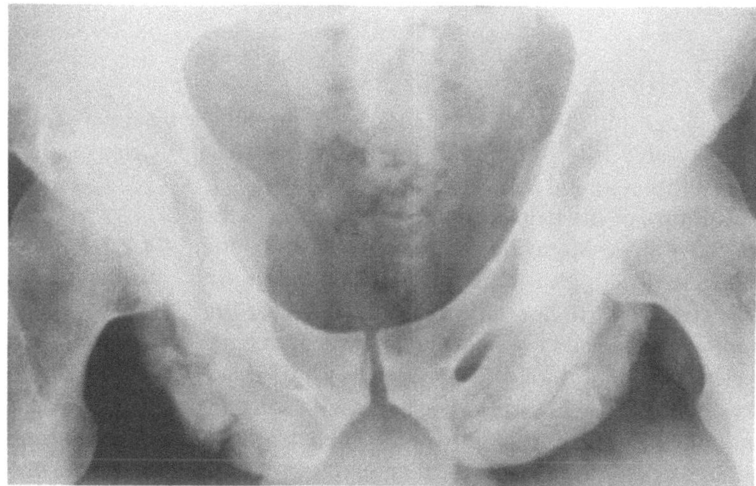

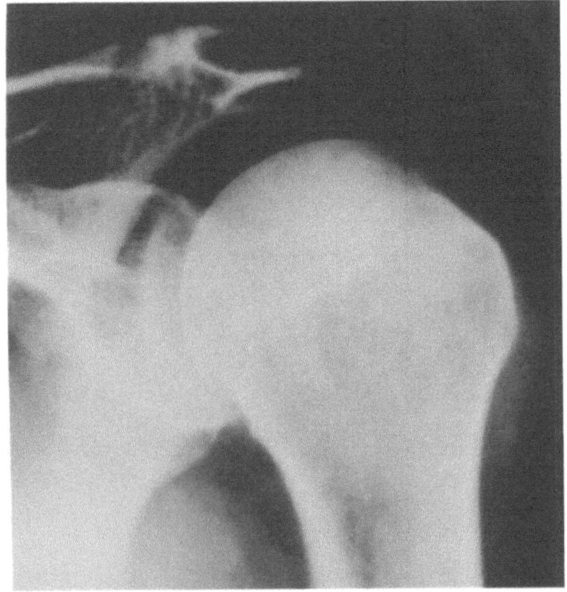

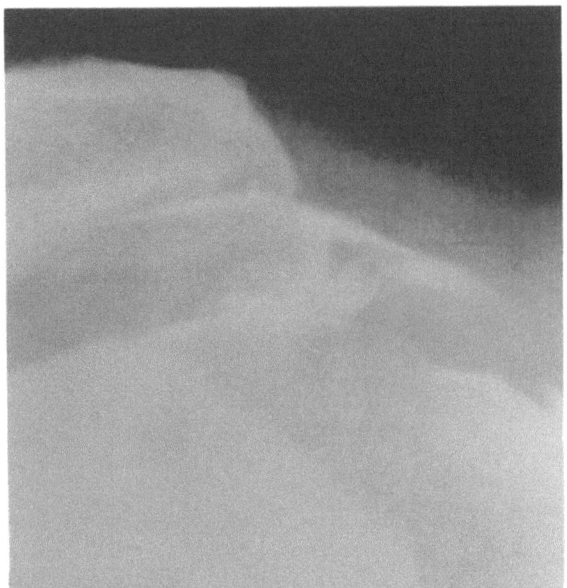

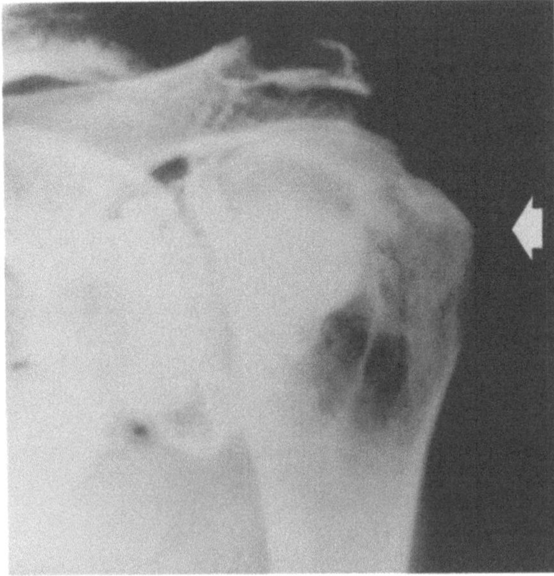

Fig. 4.5. **a** A.p. radiograph of the shoulder with internal rotation, demonstrating loss of fat pad underneath subdeltoid bursa. **b** Same patient after injection of contrast material into the glenohumeral joint. Full-thickness tear of the supraspinatus tendon with subsequent filling of the subacromial-subdeltoid bursa can be seen. **c** Shoulder arthrogramm in a young athletic patient following trauma. Air in subdeltoid bursa (*arrow*) indicating evidence of full-thickness tear of the rotator cuff

ing leakage into the soft tissues anterior to the patella and possibly into the prepatellar and infrapatellar bursae (JELASO and MORRIS 1975).

Rupture of the patellar tendon produces a deficit in active knee extension and usually affects young athletes. Swelling around the patella tendon with obliteration of its normally sharp adjacent fat lines and an abnormally high patella position are characteristic radiographic features (Fig. 4.7). For the assessment of patella position, lateral views are taken in mild flexion. The length of the patella tendon should be compared with the diagonal length of the patella and the ratio should not exceed 1.3:1 (INSALL and SALVATI 1976).

4.2.2.3
Peroneus Tendon

Contrast opacification of the peroneus tendon may provide useful information in patients with traumatic disorders. The normal peroneal tenogram outlines the common sheath of the peroneus longus and peroneus brevis muscles as well as the point of bifur-

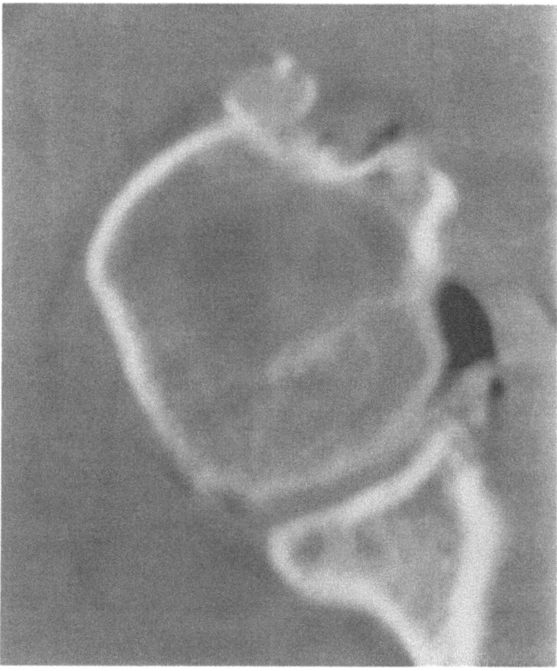

Fig. 4.6. CT-arthrogram of the shoulder after trauma demonstrating air in the glenohumeral joint and biceps tendon sheath. Bone fragments of the lateral wall of the bicipital groove and adhesions within the sheath are responsible for entrapment of the biceps tendon

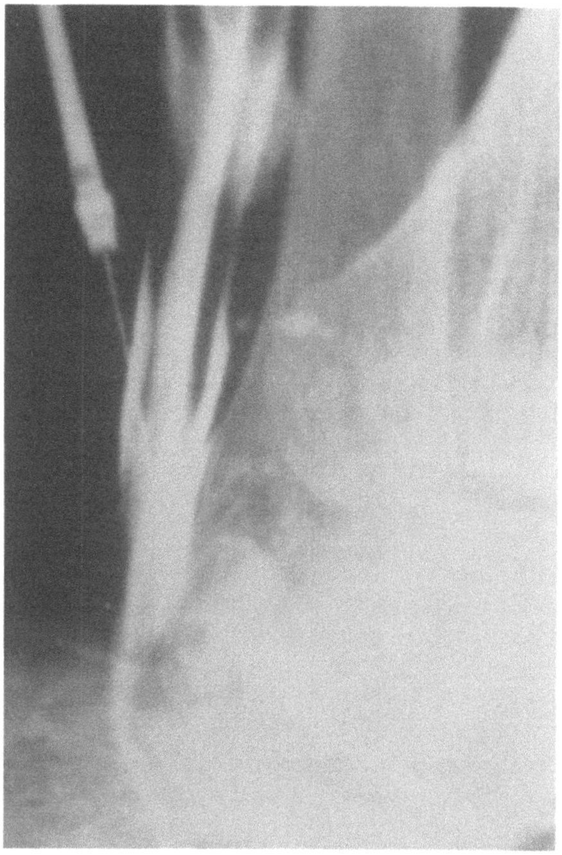

Fig. 4.8. Peroneal tenography: impingement of peroneal tendon sheaths caused by posttraumatic deformation of the calcaneus (*arrow*)

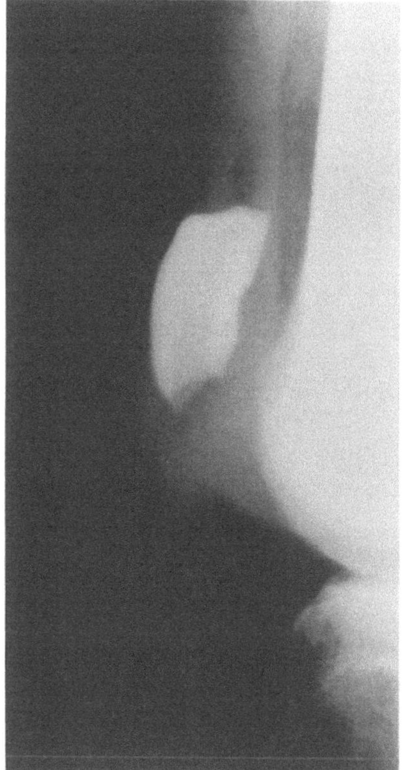

Fig. 4.7. Lateral radiograph of the knee joint showing marked soft tissue swelling and patella alta following rupture of the patella tendon

cation of this sheath into separate sheaths enclosing each tendon. The sheath appears smooth in outline and contains a radiolucent tendon without displacement. Painful disability following calcaneal fractures may result from posttraumatic stenosing tenosynovitis of the peroneal tendons. In most instances, peroneal dysfunction may be suspected on the basis of deformity and widening of the lateral aspect of the calcaneus. The source of pain may be more obscure. In these patients, peroneal tenography is useful and may show extrinsic compression, irregularity of the sheath, tendon displacement, obstruction of contrast flow or tendon rupture (Fig. 4.8).

Furthermore, lidocaine injection may help to localize the source of obscure pain (RESNICK and GOERGEN 1975).

4.2.2.4
Achilles Tendon

Normally the tendon is 4–9 mm thick, thinnest in its distal third and commonly increasing in thickness proximally. With proper positioning, the Achilles tendon has well-defined margins anteriorly and, if there is sufficient fatty tissue between it and the skin, posteriorly as well. Lesions related to overstrain of the Achilles tendon range from irritation of the paratenon to complete rupture, usually secondary to degenerative changes that reduce the strength of the tendon. The signs of paratendinitis are increased thickness and blurring of the anterior margin as a result of edema, which may extend considerably into the pre-Achilles fatty tissue.

The signs of incomplete rupture of the Achilles tendon depend on the interval between the causative event and the low-kV radiographic examination. A few hours after the event, the tendon is swollen due to intratendinous edema and bleeding with localized swelling at the site of incomplete rupture. The normally gently curved tendon may be straightened by the presence of edema in the pre-Achilles fatty tissue. Perifocal edema and bleeding as well as shredding of the severed ends of the Achilles tendon are likely to abolish its outline at the site of complete rupture. However, even when its contours are well outlined and tendon thickness is normal, an increase in the anterior curvature of the tendon reducing Toygar's angle to less than 150° indicates complete rupture (TOYGAR 1947).

4.3
Sonography

4.3.1
Principles of Imaging

With the development of high-frequency probes, the field of musculoskeletal sonography has improved and expanded rapidly. It is a direct, painless and relatively inexpensive examination. Dynamic imaging facilitates the display of the physiologic range of motion of the tendons. With the capability of ultrasound (US) to take images in various planes, the course, shape and thickness of tendons can be investigated thoroughly.

4.3.1.1
Anatomy

The sonographic appearance of all tendons reflects their fibrillar structure: collagen fibers are hypoechoic with intermingled hyperechoic loose connective tissue. Adaptation of the collagen fibres to mechanical load due to sporting activities has not only been demonstrated in experimental studies but also with ultrasonography (KAINBERGER et al. 1990; SOMMER 1987). The diameter of the Achilles tendon which normally measures 4–6 mm, is increased in runners to up to 7 mm (KAINBERGER et al. 1990).

Tendons may be encircled by synovial sheaths in areas of stress in major or minor joints. Normally, tendon sheaths present sonographically as ring-like structures: they consist of a hyperechoic outer layer, a hypoechoic rim filled with fluid, and a hyperechoic center that represents the inner layer and the tendon itself. Tendons without a synovial sheath, such as the Achilles tendon or the patellar tendon, are enveloped by loose areolar connective tissue called paratenon (FORNAGE 1986).

4.3.1.2
Artifacts

Acoustic artifacts occur with higher intensity when using high-frequency probes. In tendon imaging, two types of artifacts are important: anisotropic reflection of the sound waves and acoustic shadowing.

The principle of acoustic fiber anisotropy was first described by Dussik in 1958 (DUSSIK et al. 1958). Tendons are strongly anisotropic reflectors. They behave like mirrors so that the angle of the reflected sound wave is the same as that of the transmitted sound wave (Fig. 4.9). With smaller angles, more echos are received, yielding a better image with higher signal-to-noise ratio. However, in human tissue it is almost impossible to image a tendon in its complete course without hypoechoic areas due to anisotropic reflection. Therefore, the investigator has to be familiar with this artifact, which is often not encountered in abdominal or cardiovascular ultrasonography.

Acoustic shadowing may be the result of refraction or total reflection of the sound waves on bone or gas. Refraction occurs on the various forms of septae and other types of collagen tissue and may lead to unexpected forms of shadowing. For example, the fibrous septations on the deltoid muscle can cast acoustic shadows on the subjacent rotator cuff. The resulting hypoechoic area may simulate a lesion of the cuff.

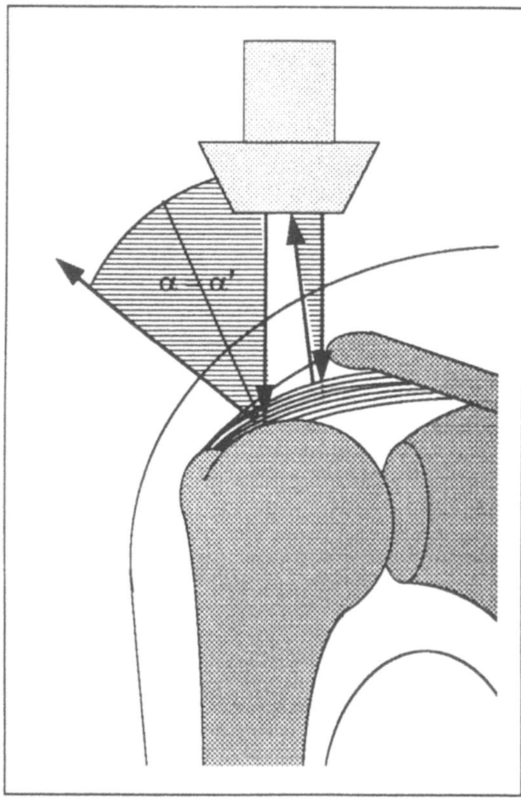

Fig. 4.9. Principle of acoustic fiber anisotropy: if the angles α and α' are small, the reflected sound waves are received by the transducer. If they increase, the ultrasound echos cannot be received by the transducer, which results in a hypoechoic appearance of the tendon

4.3.1.3
Principles of US Investigation and Equipment

Many attempts have been made to standardize US studies of tendons and muscles of the shoulder, the hand and wrist, the knee, and the ankle. Most have not been generally accepted because of differences in technical equipment and clinical access. It is, however, feasible to conduct standardized imaging in musculoskeletal ultrasound according to three principal rules: documentation of abnormalities in at least two planes, comparison of findings with the complementary structures of the contralateral side of the body, and dynamic imaging.

Because spatial resolution increases in proportion to frequency, the investigator should use probes with the highest frequencies possible (MARTINOLI et al. 1993). Therefore, US equipment should contain probes with frequencies between 5 and 13 MHz. To avoid diagnostic misconceptions due to artifacts, it is preferable to use linear probes rather than sector probes. A standoff pad should be positioned between the transducer and the skin to compensate irregularities of the body surface.

4.3.1.4
Basic US Signs

Abnormalities of tendons have to be described with regard to their structure, shape and thickness. Tendon structure may be hypoechoic, hyperechoic, inhomogeneous or calcified (with hyperechoic reflections and acoustic shadowing). The surrounding tissue with its bursae and bony insertions has to be investigated, too.

Table 4.1. Differential diagnosis of US signs in tendon diseases

US signs	Differential diagnosis
Hypoechoic lesion	Tendinitis, partial rupture, metabolic changes
Hyperechoic lesion	Rupture, metabolic changes (xanthoma)
Inhomogeneous structure	Tendinitis, rupture (chronic forms or rupture with hematoma), metabolic changes
Tendon calcification	Tendinitis, old rupture, postoperative
Tendon thickening	Tendinitis, rupture, metabolic changes, rheumatic disease
Abnormalities at tendon insertion (with or without calcification)	Fibroostitis (spur formation) due to degeneration, rheumatic disease
Disintegration of tendon fibers	Rupture

Tumors are excluded because of their rarity.
US, = ultrasound.

Degeneration of the collagen fibers plays a major role in tendon disease because all tendons of the body are prone to mechanical stress. Therefore, the US signs that reflect degenerative changes in the shape of thickening, thinning or abnormalities in structure are relatively uniform (Table 4.1). However, together with clinical symptoms and signs, ultrasonography is a valuable tool to define the type and degree of tendinous lesions (KVIST 1994).

4.3.2
Clinical Application

US has gained wide acceptance for imaging the rotator cuff of the shoulder, the patellar tendon and the Achilles tendon. Moreover, US examinations can be performed in virtually all superficial tendons and ligaments of the body including the ankle, the hand and wrist, and the cruciate ligaments. Imaging has to be done with proper technical equipment by an experienced investigator. Therefore, the application of US in these regions is limited to dedicated groups of patients such as those involved in sporting activities.

4.3.2.1
Degenerative Disease (Tendinitis)

Tendinitis is almost always attributable to chronic trauma which in many cases is the result of a high level of athletic activity (VAN HOLSBEECK and INTROCASO 1991). The sonographic findings are identical in all locations. Hypoechoic lesions with or without tendon thickening are the most common manifestations of tendinitis. With high-resolution equipment, a widening of the distance between the longitudinal fascicles may be visible (VAN HOLSBEECK and INTROCASO 1991). Due to specific types of mechanical stress, the shape and distribution of such lesions are typical of different tendons. In the rotator cuff, they mainly occur in the peripheral part of the supraspinatus tendon (Fig. 4.10; VAN HOLSBEECK et al. 1993). In the Achilles tendon, they manifest as "nodular tendinitis" typically located in the ventromedial part of the mid third. In patellar tendinitis (jumper's knee), the lesions are generally located close to the proximal insertion on the patellar apex.

Tendinitis of tendons running within a tendon sheath presents with fluid within the sheath in the form of a hypoechoic halo. Such a halo occurs only rarely in tendons without a sheath.

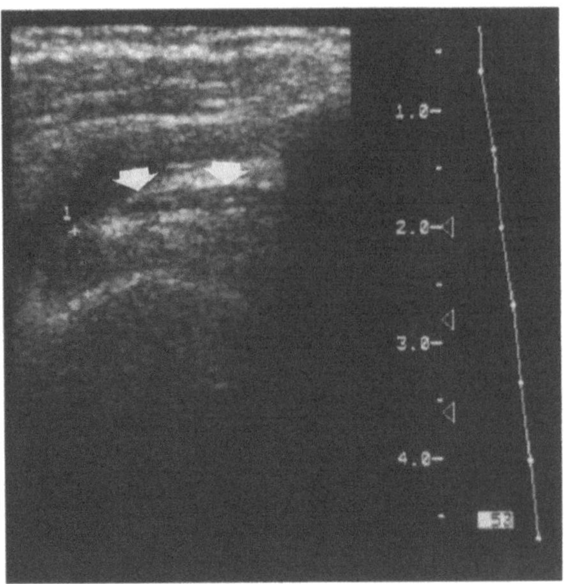

Fig. 4.10. Nodular tendinitis in the form of a hypoechoic lesion (*calipers*) with typical location in the supraspinatus tendon of a 39-year-old athlete. *Arrows* indicate a thickened hypoechoic fluid-filled subdeltoid bursa lateral of the acromion

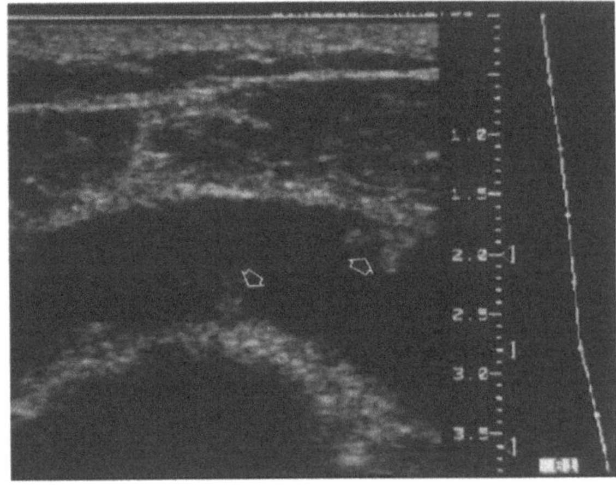

Fig. 4.11. Fresh rupture of the supraspinatus tendon with fluid-filled subdeltoid bursa and torn tendon fibers (*arrows*)

4.3.2.2
Rupture

The most specific sign of tendon rupture is disintegration of tendon fibers (Fig. 4.11). However, due to hematoma or effects of tissue reparation, this finding may be blurred and the investigator has to rely on indirect signs of rupture. These include (1) thickening of the tendon apart from the rupture site due to retracted fibers and (2) fluid accumulation

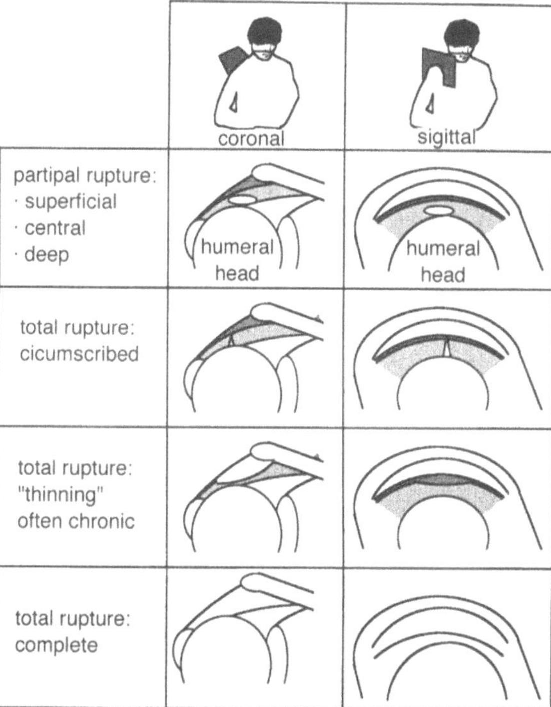

Fig. 4.12. Different forms of tendon rupture of the rotator cuff (drawing modified after WIENER and SEITZ). Sonographic appearance reflects the different macromorphologic forms of ruptures depending on their location, extent and time since the trauma

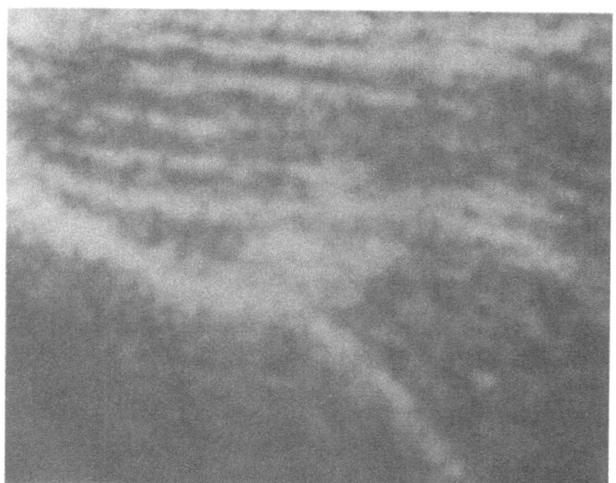

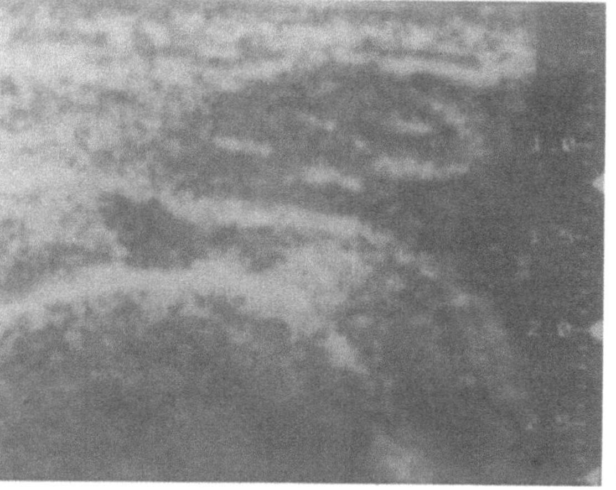

Fig. 4.13. Chronic rupture with thinning of the supraspinatus tendon in a 42-year-old patient with trauma during a game of tennis 10 years previously. **a** Coronal view, **b** sagittal view

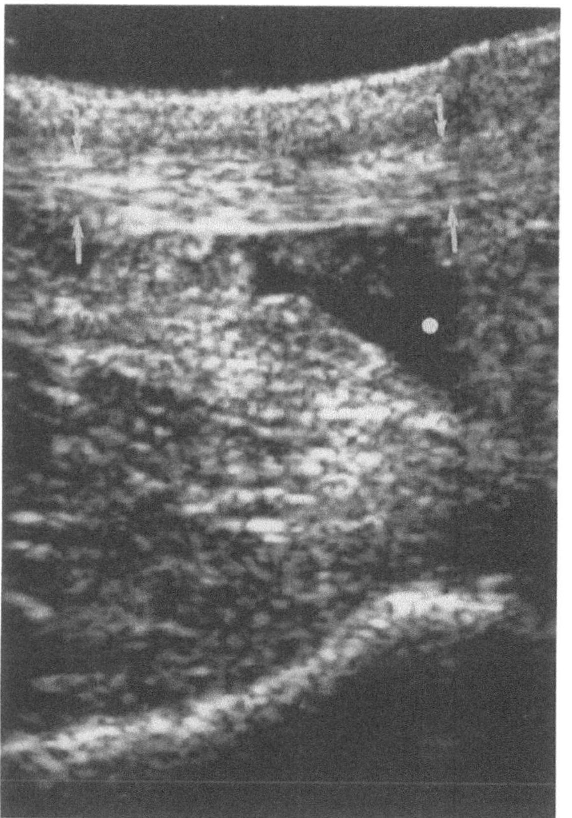

Fig. 4.14. A 28-year-old soccer player with achillodynia; relief of symptoms after local installation of corticosteroids. With US, fluid collections (*point marker*) in the pre-Achilles fat pad and surrounding the Achilles tendon (*arrows*) are visible, indicating tissue necrosis. (Reprinted with permission from KAINBERGER et al., 6-Radiologe, Jan. 1996)

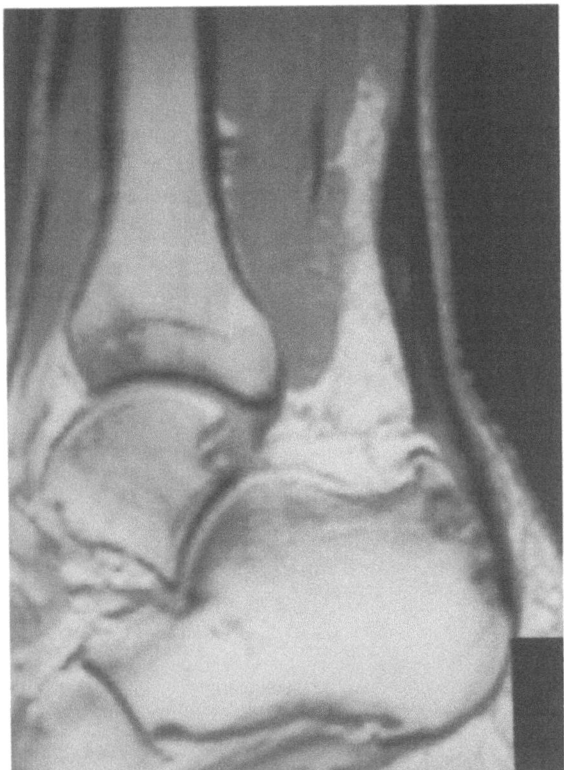

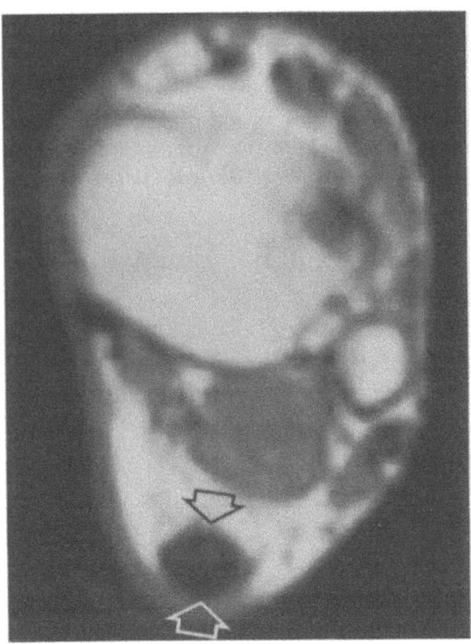

Fig. 4.15a,b. Achilles tendinitis with thickening of the Achilles tendon obtained in the sagittal plane without intratendinous lesion in **a** sagittal and **b** axial T1W SE. *SE,* spin echo

(hematoma) in the surrounding tissue or neighboring bursae. It has to be stressed that when using dynamic imaging, tendon ruptures overlooked with other imaging modalities may be demonstrated by ultrasonography.

In many tendons, ruptures are caused by tendinitis due to overuse syndromes. This may result in varying manifestations of rupture (Figs. 4.12–14; KANNUS and JOZSA 1991; WIENER and SEITZ 1993).

4.3.2.3
Inflammation

Inflammation occurs as tendovaginitis rather than in the collagen fibers. In sports medicine, it is generally the result of overuse. However, one should not overlook infectious disease as a sequela of local injury or the first manifestation of a rheumatic disease.

4.3.2.4
Metabolic and Toxic Changes

Most metabolic tendon abnormalities are the result of local or systemic application of corticosteroids. Necrosis of fibers with scar formation or rupture will occur. Sonographically, hypoechoic lesions within the tendon or its surrounding tissue and, finally, the signs of rupture can be observed (Fig. 4.15).

Of specific interest are changes due to anabolic steroids taken to enhance performance. According to animal studies, toxic changes occur in tendons after doses generally not applied to humans (KARPAKKA et al. 1991). An exception is the rotator cuff of body builders: extensive swelling of the rotator muscles may result in relative impingement and eventually lead to fiber degeneration and rupture.

4.3.2.5
Congenital Abnormalities and Tumors

Both are rare entities. In sports medicine, congenital abnormalities may lead to overuse syndromes not generally detected by clinical means alone. A typical example is the formation of an accessory soleus muscle that may cause achillodynia. Detection of the muscle is easy by documenting the characteristic muscle fibers inserting far distally in the Achilles tendon.

Tumors of the tendon and the tendon sheath include ganglions, giant cell tumors of the sheath, and some other very rare benign or malignant neoplasms. With sonography, it is sometimes difficult to

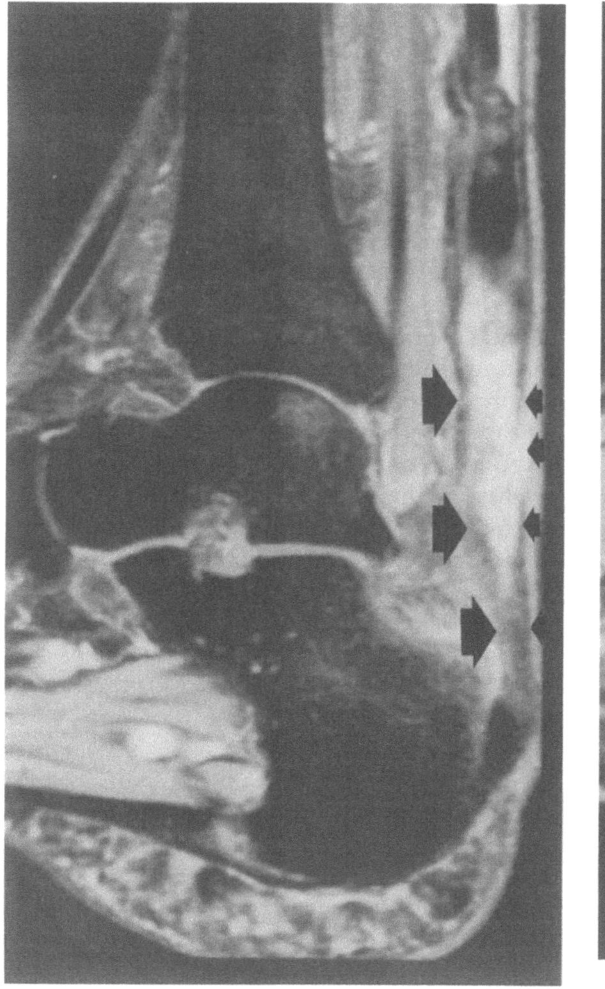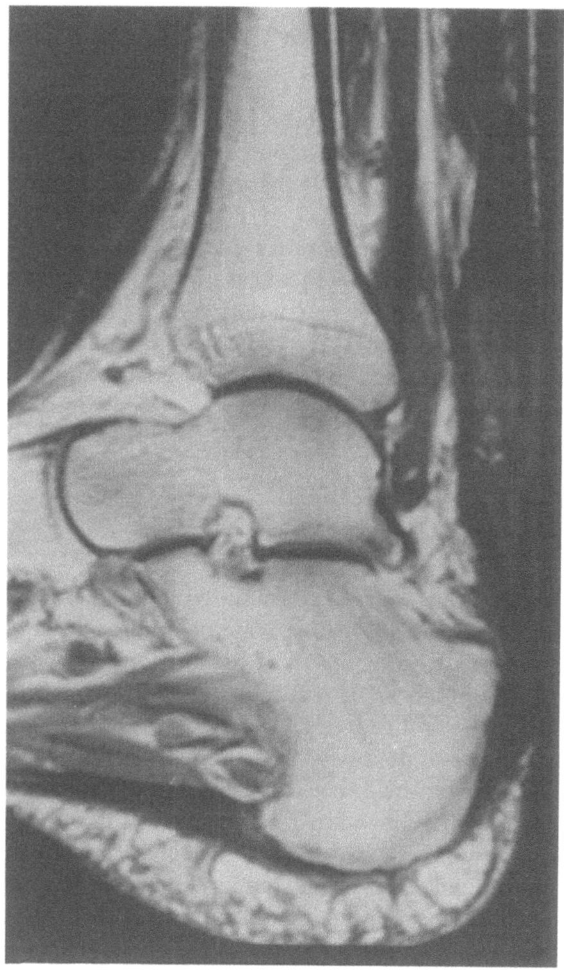

Fig. 4.16a,b. Subtotal rupture of the Achilles tendon with thickening and increased intratendinous signal, reaching the surface in **a** sagittal STIR and **b** T1W-SE

differentiate their hypoechoic appearance from focal fluid accumulations.

4.4
Magnetic Resonance Imaging

4.4.1
Principles of Imaging

Tendons are collagenous structures whose primary function is to passively transmit motion from a contracting muscle to a bone or fascia. They are relatively avascular and contain approximately 30% collagen, 2% elastin and 68% water, with collagen accounting for 70% of their dry weight. Elastin is responsible for tendon flexibility, collagen for

strength, and a basic substance for structure. Tendons consist of parallel, closely packed bundles of collagen fibers which are grouped together into fascicles surrounded by a loose connective tissue sheet containing nerves and blood vessels. They are relatively acellular. Much of the tensile strength of collagen derives from its highly organized microstructure: microfibrils of tropocollagen are arranged in fibrils which are, in turn, organized into fibers. The regularity of this structure produces an extremely short T2 relaxation time (<1 ms) to water protons constrained by collagen in tendons. Because this T2 is too rapid for even the shortest finite TE available on commercial MRI systems to detect a signal, normal tendons appear without signal on all pulse sequences (FRANKEL and NORDIN 1980; DEUTSCH and MINK 1994).

4.4.1.1
Sequences

T1-weighted images exhibit high contrast and anatomic detail, with high contrast between the dark tendon and the bright signal from the surrounding fat.

Gradient echo, inversion recovery (STIR) and T2-weighted spin echo sequences (long TR/TE) offer optimal contrast between a dark tendon and the abnormal increase in water content in the tendon and tendon sheath that characterize most pathologic processes.

4.4.1.2
Orientation

Tendon injuries are best examined in the plane perpendicular to the tendon, which allows optimal assessment of the contour of the tendon and yields images of high tissue contrast. For this purpose, the axial plane of the tendon (which may not be the true axial plane of the body) is examined.

Moreover, the degree of distension of the tendon sheath with fluid and its relationship to surrounding structures is best visualized on axial images. The full longitudinal extent of a tendon injury is best assessed in the sagittal plane (DEUTSCH and MINK 1994).

Increased signal intensity within a tendon on a T2-weighted image is always abnormal and indicative of rupture or active inflammation. Increased intratendinous signal on short-TE images, such as T1-weighted and proton-density-weighted spin echo sequences, and on all gradient echo sequences is considered to be indicative of tendinosis or myxoid degeneration. However, due to the so-called magic angle phenomenon, based on variation of tendon T2 relaxation with the orientation of the tendon relative to the B_0, the so-called angular anisotropy of T2 relaxation, the presence of intermediate signal on short-TE sequences can be a normal finding.

4.4.1.3
Magic Angle Phenomenon

This phenomenon is a manifestation of the anisotropic behavior of collagen on MR imaging. Normally, collagen, with its highly organized structure, tends to restrict the mobility of local water protons and promotes dipolar interactions among them. These dipolar interactions contribute to T2 relaxation and are responsible for the uniform loss of signal intensity exhibited by normal tendons on even short-TE sequences. The internuclear vector of this dipolar interaction is oriented along the same axis as the collagen fibers and shrinks to zero when 3 (cosinus^2 theta) $- 1 = 0$, where theta is the angle between the internuclear vector and B_0. This condition is fullfilled when theta equals 54.7°. Therefore, when tendons are oriented at approximately 55° to B_0 (B_0 = aligned along the long axis of the magnet bore in superconducting systems), T2 relaxation time increases sufficiently, i.e., more than 100-fold, to provide a signal on short-TE images. This phenomenon can be misinterpreted as tendinitis and is usually found in ankle tendons as they curve around the malleoli to enter the foot and in the critical zone of the supraspinatus tendon of the normal shoulder (ERICKSON et al. 1991, 1993; FULLERTON and CAMERON 1985).

With the exception of the magic angle phenomenon, the signal intensity of normal tendons on spin echo and gradient echo sequences with TE of more than 10 ms is very low.

In a recent report (SCHICK et al. 1995), measurements demonstrated that the transverse T2 relaxation times of water protons in tendons vary with pathologic alterations: normal collagen fibers and fibers with subtle lesions show very short T2 whereas other pathologic structures show signals that can be measured with echo times of 15 ms and more. The longest relaxation times of more than 30 ms were found with stripes inside the tendon corresponding with water protons in liquids among the collagen bundle after partial ruptures. Thus, short echo times are likely to increase sensitivity to early alterations of the tendon. The minimum echo time depends on ramp times and maximum amplitudes of the gradient system, the spatial resolution required, and the type of sequence: spin echo sequences require a longer TE than gradient echo sequences using the same gradient system and the readout time which correlates with the signal-to-noise ratio. Therefore, gradient echo sequences are superior to spin echo sequences for the identification of tendon alteration, allowing very short minimum TE for different gradient systems, and are most sensitive for all alterations of tendon tissue (KOBLIK and FREEMAN 1993; SCHICK et al. 1995). Moreover, susceptibility effects do not seem to be important for tendon imaging.

Conventional images usually allow minimum echo times of about 4 ms for gradient echo techniques with sufficient spatial resolution. Modern images just developed for echoplanar imaging and flow-rephased angiographic applications allow echo times of 2 ms and a spatial resolution beyond 1 mm in plane and 4 mm in slice thickness. These technical developments may further improve the diagnostic value of MR imaging of tendons in the near future.

4.4.2
Clinical Application

4.4.2.1
Tendon Size and Structure

Tendon thickening is the most common sign in patients with chronic tendinitis (BELTRAN et al. 1987; FORNAGE 1986; KAINBERGER et al. 1990). Tendon rupture falls into three types: (1) partial tendon rupture combined with tendon hypertrophy and thickening, (2) partial tendon rupture combined with tendon attenuation, and (3) discontinuity, i.e. complete rupture.

The tendon in the sagittal plane appears as a long thin hypointense structure due to the extremely low water content. No intratendinous signals should be available.

4.4.2.2
Acute Tendinitis

Acute tendinitis (<2 weeks) becomes symptomatic as tenosynovitis, or as peritendinitis in tendons without a synovial sheath (e.g., Achilles tendon), caused by a sudden increase in the intensity of athletic training. MR signs are fluid in the sheath or edema in the soft tissue (dark on T1- and bright on T2-weighted images) surrounding a normal tendon (CLEMENT et al. 1984).

4.4.2.3
Chronic Tendinitis

When acute tendinitis becomes chronic (>6 weeks), findings such as tendon swelling and intratendinous lesion can arise. Tendinous lesions appear as longitudinal splints in the sagittal MR images, particularly as a parallel linear signal pattern in the case of multiple lesions. The signal of those intratendinous lesions is present on T1- and proton-density-weighted images and becomes almost invisible on T2-weighted images according to foci of mucoid degeneration.

One may speculate that the pathologic signal pattern of MR imaging is due to the enlarged endotendineum septum. Endotendineum septa are the only structures to show vascularity in the inner tendon (ELLIOT 1965). Consequently, they help to activate, support and propagate inflammation within the tendon through well-known pathogenic mechanisms such as edema, angiogenesis, and remodelling of connective tissue (MARTINOLI et al. 1993). Damage of inflammatory, degenerative or traumatic origin would cause further changes in tendinous structures.

4.4.2.4
Acute Partial Tear

The differentiation of chronic tendinitis versus acute partial tear can be performed by using the signal intensity of an intratendinous lesion, since blood or edema in acute partial tear presents a higher signal intensity on T2-weighted images than on T1-weighted or proton-density images.

4.4.2.5
Old Partial Tear

Distinction between an old partial tear and chronic tendinitis is not possible unless MRI and US demonstrate surface discontinuity in the tendon (QUINN et al. 1987; BERTHOTY et al. 1989).

4.4.2.6
Complete Tendon Rupture

Large areas of signal increase on T2-weighted images fill the gap in the tendon, and the distal and proximal ends of the tendon retract, widening the contour of the remaining tendon and causing a mop-end appearance of the tendon edges. Edema and hemorrhage of the soft tissue or the tendon sheath accompany tendon rupture. Longitudinal ruptures are found in the tibialis posterior tendon and in the peroneal tendons.

Achilles tendon injuries are less obvious, with up to 25% diagnosed incorrectly (INGLIS 1976). On physical examination, swelling often obscures the presence of a palpable tendinous defect (INGLIS et al. 1976). The Thompson test may also remain negative with a partial tendinous tear (HATTRUP and

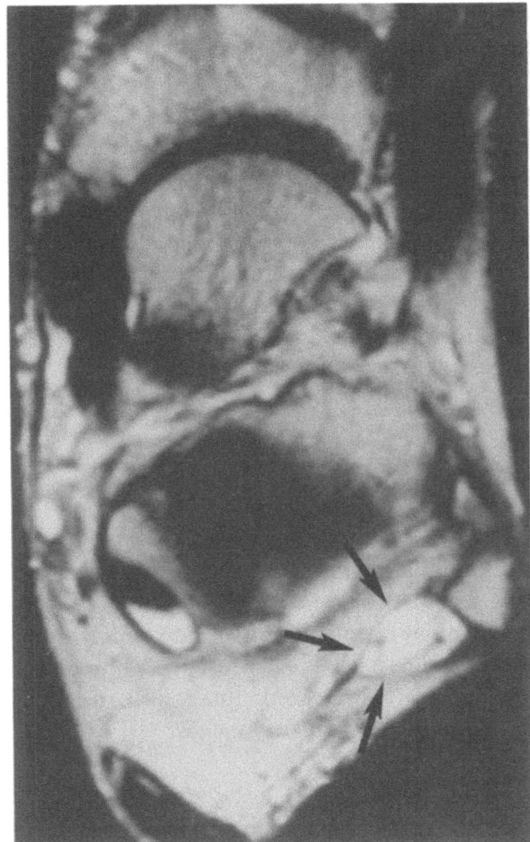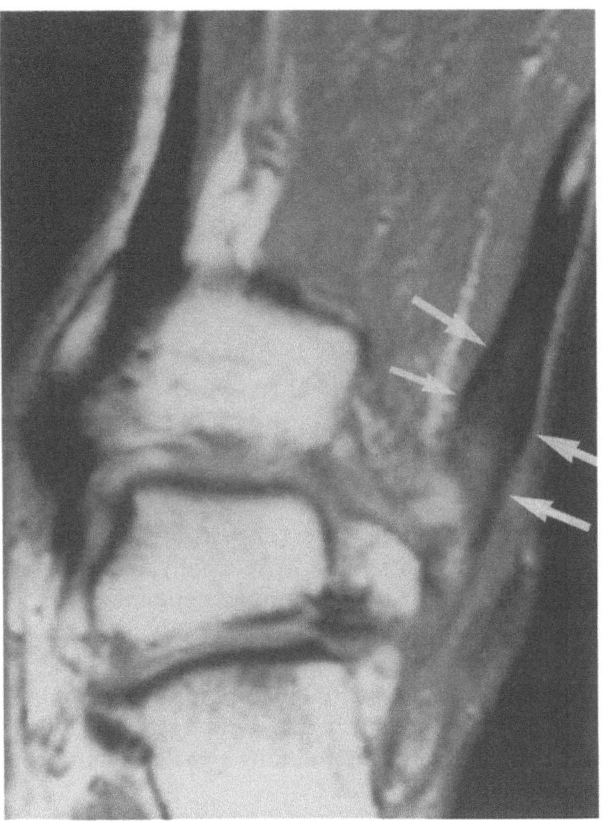

Fig. **4.17a,b. a** Rupture of the peroneal tendons with fluid in the "empty" tendon sheet in the axial T2W-SE; **b** a thickened proximal stump in the coronal T1W-SE image

JOHNSON 1985). However, prompt diagnosis is important to prevent subsequent total rupture, and a delay in treatment can result in a reduction in muscular strength and power (INGLIS and SCULCO 1981).

4.4.2.7
Postoperative Tendinitis

The structure and signal intensity of postoperative tendinitis are very similar to those of tendinitis by mechanical overstress. Furthermore, there is a significant increase in tendon diameter, and the texture of the tendon, including its surface is more irregular. In the case of acute re-ruptures, the Achilles tendon is thickened with flame-shaped intratendinous foci showing an intermediate signal on T1-weighted images, an intermediate to increased signal on proton-density images, and an increased signal on T2-weighted images (QUINN et al. 1987; LIEM et al. 1991).

4.4.2.8
Subluxation and Dislocation

Subluxation and dislocation are found at the long biceps tendon and peroneal tendons. Dislocation of the long biceps tendon is commonly combined with a rupture of the rotator cuff, based on a dysplastic intertubercular groove. On the axial plane medial of the empty bicipital groove, a thickened and even signal-increased dislocated tendon will be visible (CHAN et al. 1991). Dislocation of the peroneal tendons may be combined with tendinitis, partial tear or bone injury.

4.5
Conclusion

In the past years, new imaging modalities (MRI, sonography, CT) have changed staging and therapy strategies of tendinous sports injuries dramatically. On the one hand, it is now known that consequent conservative treatment influences the patient's outcome enormously, on the other hand numerous surgical treatments have had to be reevaluated on the basis of imaging results. This started with the cruciate ligaments and knee joint tendons and continued with Achilles tendon injuries and shoulder traumata. Without any doubt, this rapid development depends very much on collaboration between radiologists and orthopedic surgeons and has by no means levelled off.

References

Beltran J, Noto AM, Herman LJ, Lubbers LM (1987) Tendons: high-field-strength, surface coil MR imaging. Radiology 162:735–740

Berthoty D, Sartoris DJ, Resnick D (1989) Fast scan magnetic resonance of Achilles tendonitis. J Foot Surg 28:171–173

Chan TW, Dalinka MK, Kneeland JB, et al. (1991) Biceps tendon dislocation: evaluation with MR imaging. Radiology 179:649–652

Clement DB, Taunton JE, Smart GW (1984) Achilles tendinitis and peritendinitis: etiology and treatment. Am J Sports Med 12:179–184

Deutsch AL, Mink JH (1994) Tendon injuries of the lower extremity: MR assessment. Syllabus of the second meeting of the Society of Magnetic Resonance, San Francisco

Dussik KT, Fritch DJ, Kyriazidou M, Sear RS (1958) Measurements of articular tissues with ultrasound. Am J Phys Med 37:160–165

Elliot DH (1965) Structure and function of mammalian tendon. Biol Rev 40:392–421

Erickson SJ, Cox IH, Hyde SJ, Carrera GF, Strandt JA, Estkowski LD (1991) Effect of tendon orientation on MR imaging signal intensity: a manifestation of the magic angle" phenomenon. Radiology 181:389–392

Erickson SJ, Prost RW, Timins ME (1993) The "magic angle" effect: background physics and clinical relevance. Radiology 188:23–25

Fischer E (1988) Low kilovolt radiography. In: Resnick D, Niwayama G (eds) Diagnosis of bone and joint disorders. Saunders, Philadelphia, pp 108–123

Fornage BD (1986) Achilles tendon: US examination. Radiology 159:759–64

Frankel VH, Nordin M (1980) Basic biomechanics of the skeletal system. Lea and Febiger, Philadelphia

Fullerton G, Cameron I, Ord V (1985) Orientation of tendons in the magnetic field and its effect on T2 relaxation time. Radiology 155:433–435

Hattrup SJ, Johnson KA (1985) A review of ruptures of the Achilles tendon. Foot Ankle 6:34–38

Holsbeeck M van, Introcaso JH (1991) Musculoskeletal ultrasound. Mosby Year Book, St. Louis, pp 57–89

Holsbeeck M van, Kolowich PQA, Bouffard JA, Shirazi KK (1993) Partial thickness tears of the rotator cuff. Radiology 189:293–297

Inglis AE, Sculco TP (1981) Surgical repair of ruptures of the tendo Achillis. Clin Orthop 156:160–169

Inglis AE, Scott TP, Sculco TP, Patterson AH (1976) Rupture of the tendo achillis. An objective assessment of surgical and nonsurgical treatment. J Bone Joint Surg [Am] 58:990–993

Insall J, Salvati E (1976) Patella position in the normal knee joint. Radiology 101:101–104

Jelaso DV, Morris GA (1975) Rupture of the quadriceps tendon: diagnosis by arthrography. Radiology 116:621–622

Kainberger F, Engel A, Barton P, Hbsch P, Neuhold A, Salomonowitz E (1990) Injury of the Achilles tendon. Diagnosis with sonography. AJR 155:1031–1036

Kannus P, Jozsa L (1991) Histopathological changes preceding spontaneous rupture of a tendon. J Bone Joint Surg [Am] 73:1507–1525

Karpakka JA, Pesola MK, Takala TE (1992) The effects of anabolic steroids on collagen synthesis in rat skeletal muscle and tendon. A preliminary report. Am J Sports Med 20:262–266

Koblik PD, Freeman DM (1993) Short echo time magnetic resonance imaging of tendon. Invest Radiol 28:1095–1100

Kvist M (1994) Achilles tendon injuries in athletes. Sports Med 18:173–201

Liem MD, Zegel HG, Balduini FC, Turner ML, Becker JM, Caballero-Saez A (1991) Repair of Achilles tendon ruptures with a polylactic acid implant: assessment with MR imaging. AJR 156:769–773

Martinoli C, Derchi LE, Pastorino C, Bertolotto M, Silvestri E (1993) Analysis of echotexture of tendons with US. Radiology 186:839–843

Quinn SF, Murray WR, Clark RA, Cochran CF (1987) Achilles tendon: MR imaging at 1.5 T. Radiology 164:767–770

Resnick D (1988a) Arthrography, tenography and bursography. In: Resnick D, Niwayama G (eds) Diagnosis of bone and joint disorders. Saunders, Philadelphia, pp 303–440

Resnick D (1988b) Physical injury. In: Resnick D, Niwayama G (eds) Diagnosis of bone and joint disorders. Saunders, Philadelphia, pp 2757–3008

Resnick D, Goergen TG (1975) Peroneal tenography in previous calcaneal fractures. Radiology 115:211

Schick F, Dammann F, Lutz O, Claussen CD (1995) Adapted techniques for clinical MR imaging of tendons. MAGMA 3:103–107

Schneider R, Ghelman B, Kaye JJ (1975) Investigation of shoulder disability by arthrography. Radiology 114:738–745

Sommer HM (1987) The biomechanical and metabolic effects of a running regime on the Achilles tendon in the rat. Int Orthop 11:71–75

Toygar O (1947) Subkutane Ruptur der Achillessehne (Diagnostik und Behandlungsergebnisse). Helv Chir Acta 14:209–215

Wiener SN, Seitz WH Jr (1993) Sonography of the shoulder in patients with tears of the rotator cuff: accuracy and value for selecting surgical options. AJR 160:103–107

5 Acute Injuries of the Articular Surfaces

K. Bohndorf

CONTENTS

5.1
Introduction

The terms osteochondral fracture, transchondral, flake or chip fracture, osteochondritis dissecans or osteochondrosis dissecans (OCD) are often used interchangeably to describe injuries of the articular surfaces of bone. By definition, an acute osteochondral or transchondral fracture is a lesion of the articular surface of bone, produced by a force transmitted from one congruous articular surface to another through a joint space and into the underlying subchondral trabeculae (BERNDT and HARTY 1959).

This review considers the relevant anatomy, mechanisms of injury and clinical presentation of acute injuries at the articular surfaces and will not address the radiology of chronic osteochondritis

K. BOHNDORF, MD, Klinik für Diagnostische Radiologie und Neuroradiologie, Zentralklinikum Augsburg, Stenglinstrasse 2, 86156 Augsburg, Germany

dissecans. Modern imaging techniques such as MRI have increased the ability to evaluate and classify these lesions.

5.2
Anatomical Considerations: Articular Cartilage

The articular surfaces of bones are covered with hyaline cartilage, which is a nerveless, avascular, firm and yet pliable tissue. Articular cartilage is characterized on microscopic examination by its abundant shiny extracellular matrix, with sparse isolated cells located in well-defined spaces (BULLOUGH 1992). The important biomechanical properties of cartilage such as load bearing, resilience and durability depend primarily on the chemical nature and complex spatial arrangement of the cartilaginous extracellular matrix (BUCKWALTER et al. 1990). The constituent components of this matrix are water (60%–80%) and macromolecules including collagens, proteoglycans and other proteins (20%–40%). Proteoglycans bind water, while collagens form the fibrillar meshwork (BUCKWALTER et al. 1990).

Articular cartilage is a highly ordered structure. Cell shape, size and viability, collagen fibril size and orientation, and water and proteoglycan content change with increasing depth from the articular surface. Four distinct layers or zones have been described (Fig. 5.1).

The *superficial zone* is characterized by tight bundles of collagen fibers orientated parallel to the articular surface. This zone itself is separated from the joint space by a thin, cell-free layer of fine fibrils, the lamina splendens.

In the *transitional* and *deep* zones (zones 2 and 3), collagen fibers are loosely packed and homogeneously distributed. These zones differ in the size of collagen fibers and proteoglycan content, which is larger in the deep zone.

In the *calcified* zone, collagen fibers are organized perpendicular to the subchondral bone and pen-

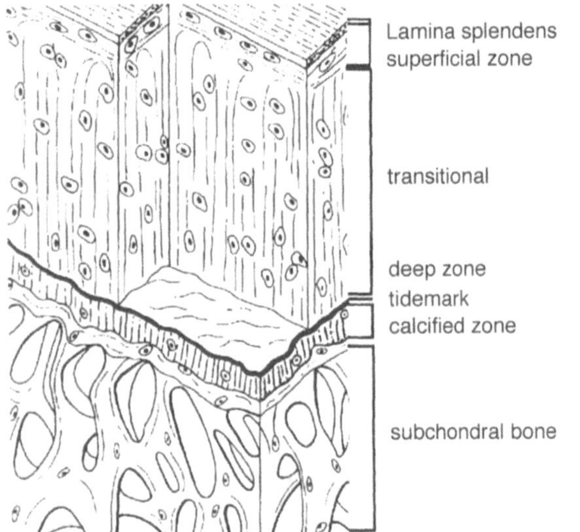

Fig. 5.1. The zones of adult articular cartilage. (Modified from Bullough 1992)

etrate directly into the calcified cartilage. The deep and calcified zones are divided by a fine line called the "tidemark", which may function as an anchor for collagen fibrils. At its base, adult articular cartilage is bordered by the subchondral bone plate. Cartilage is fitted into the irregular surface of the underlying bone somewhat like a jigsaw puzzle. This fitting is rigid, because the cartilage adjacent to the bone is calcified and has a stiffness similar to that of bone. However, there is no structural continuity between hyaline cartilage and subchondral bone. A detailed discussion of the basic composition, organisation and biomechanical properties of articular cartilage is given by Deutsch (1992).

Hyaline cartilage deforms under pressure but recovers its original shape on removal of pressure. The underlying cancellous bone also protects the cartilage by its ability to deform as a response to stress. This ability is due to the internal arrangement of mature bone tissue, in which the collagen fibers of the matrix are arranged in layers or lamellae. In each of these individual layers, the collagen bundles lie parallel to each other, but the orientation of the collagen bundles changes significantly from one layer to the next, similar to the structure of plywood (Bullough 1992). In cases of traumatic separation of cartilage and bone, this fracture takes place at the "tidemark", the junction of the calcified and non-calcified cartilage, presumably because of the considerable change in the rigidity of cartilage at this junction.

5.3
Mechanisms of Injury and Incidence

Fractures of the articular surfaces are divided into classical bony fractures, with intraarticular extension (Fig. 5.2), and fractures confined to cartilage or subchondral cancellous bone. The latter may be due to impaction caused by direct force applied vertically to the joint surface. In the case of shearing or rotational forces, pieces of articular cartilage, with or without a small segment of bone, may be knocked off the articular surface (O'Donoghue 1996; Table 5.1).

Fissuring or defects of cartilage may occur as a result of acute meniscal injury. In these cases, force is not transmitted from one joint surface to an other.

In an authoritative pathomechanical study of the ankle joint, Berndt and Harty (1959) broadened our knowledge of chondral and osteochondral fractures. In their study, *lateral* talar dome lesions were produced by a marked inversion force to a dorsiflexed foot, and *medial* dome lesions were seen with a strong inversion force to a plantar-flexed foot with external rotation of the tibia. They reasoned that the principal force causing both the medial and lateral talar dome lesions was essentially one of torsional impaction. Thus, in lateral dome lesions, the lateral talar margin impacted and compressed against the medial articular surface of the fibula. The force of impaction created a shearing and compressing component that, when strong enough, would displace the osteochondral fragment.

Concurrent osteochondral fractures of the talar dome should be suspected in all acute ankle sprains as they occur in around 2%–6% of these sprains (Shea and Manoli 1993).

Osteochondral injuries may result from a variety of transient or persistent subluxations and disloca-

Table 5.1. Fractures of articular surfaces of joints: mechanisms of injury

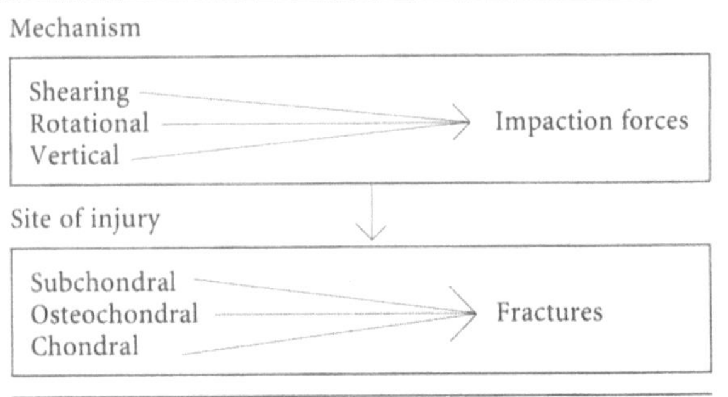

Table 5.2. Classic examples of osteochondral injuries resulting from subluxation and dislocation

- Patellar and/or lateral femoral condyle lesion due to patellar dislocation
- Glenoid surface injury of the scapula or Hill-Sachs deformity of the humeral head following anterior glenohumeral joint dislocation
- Osteochondral fracture of the femoral head due to femoral head dislocation

tions (Table 5.2) in which impaction of the opposite joint surfaces occurs. A classic example is transient lateral patellar dislocation (KIRSCH et al. 1993). Traumatic dislocation of the patella may result from a direct blow or secondary to severe rotary stress impacting on the weight-bearing knee. The site of injury is distinct from the more classical osteochonditis dissecans which arises more medially and distally on the femoral condyles. The medial facet of the patella and the lateral femoral condyle is most commonly involved. Osteochondral fractures are by no means a rare finding. In the case of acute knee injury and haemarthrosis in children, VÄHÄRSAJA and co-workers (1993) found an osteochondral fracture in 9% of their cases. In athletes with haemarthrosis of the knee joint, osteochondral fractures were the cause in 18% (MAFULLI et al. 1993).

Acute anterior cruciate ligament (ACL) tears are highly associated with concurrent bony and meniscal injury. An impaction-type osteochondral fracture directly over the anterior horn of the lateral meniscus is seen in around 20% of these patients (MINK and DEUTSCH 1990). Additionally in these cases, an osteochondral fracture or a bone bruise may be seen in the dorsal part of the tibia.

5.4
Clinical Presentation

Since the initial symptoms of injury are often obscure and immediate disability is frequently slight, an early definitive diagnosis may be difficult (O'DONOGHUE 1996; FLICK and GOULD 1985). However, the long-term consequences are significant and will be discussed below. In cases of complex joint trauma, ligamentous and capsular injuries and lesions of the fibrous cartilage (e.g. meniscal blocking) will command clinical attention. Consequently, coexistent lesions of the articular surfaces may be overlooked unless the patient is thoroughly investigated radiologically.

5.5
Imaging: Technique and Interpretation

5.5.1
Radiography

The classical sites of injury are the talus, the femoral condyles and the patella. However, almost every joint that is subject to trauma may exhibit injuries.

5.5.1.1
Talus

The minimum radiographic examination for the initial evaluation of a twisted ankle should include anteroposterior, lateral and internal oblique (mortise view) radiographs. The internal oblique view is extremely useful because the lateral talar dome is free of overlaps. The medial and lateral malleoli are parallel to the film cassette, and the talofibular joint is profiled. If a fracture is suspected, additional internal oblique views should be obtained with the ankle in different positions of flexion and extension. Because medial talar dome fractures are usually posterosuperior, plantar-flexion mortise views will show these lesions best. Lateral talar dome lesions are best seen on mortise views with the foot in dorsiflexion or in neutral position since most lateral lesions are on the anterosuperior dome.

In should be stressed that lateral fragments of the talus in the majority of cases have a thin and shallow appearance with surface fragment width greater than depth; however, there are exceptions (Figs. 5.2, 5.3).

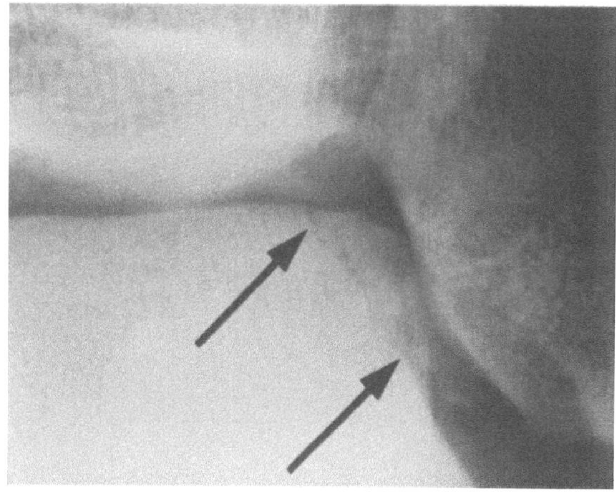

Fig. 5.2. Fracture of the lateral aspect of the superior talus with intraarticular extension. The *fracture line* involves the osteocartilaginous part of the talus dome and runs obliquely to reach the lateral aspect of the talus (*arrows*).

In contrast, medially located talar lesions generally have a deep, crater-like character. In around 70% of cases, the correct diagnosis of acute osteochondral fracture will be established by plain radiography (PETTINE and MORREY 1987). Thus, good quality plain-film radiographs remain the mainstay of diagnosis and should be employed prior to more sophisticated imaging modalities.

5.5.1.2
Patella

A "skyline view" (axial patella view) is appropriate for evaluation of the anterior aspect of the lateral femoral condyle and the articular surface of the patella, and is mandatory in cases of transient patellar dislocation (Fig. 5.4).

5.5.1.3
Femoral Condyles

In general, the fracture line parallels the joint surface, and the depth of the lesion defines the cartilaginous and osseous extent of the fragment. The main radiographic features at the femoral condyles are:

- Wafer-like area of increased density of the subchondral bone
- Irregularities of the bony contour (undulating, indented margin) or bony defect
- Gross fragmentation with total or partial separation of the fragment (Fig. 5.5)
- Free fragment (the site of origin of the fragment cannot always be located; Fig. 5.6)

Even in the case of optimal radiographic technique with recognition of subtle changes, it is a well-established fact that plain radiography may miss the lesion (O'DONOGHUE 1966; SHEA and MANOLI 1993).

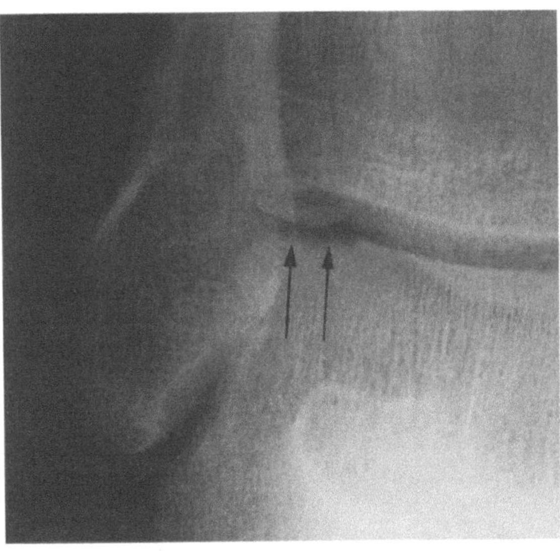

Fig. 5.3. Osteochondral fracture of the lateral talus with a thin and shallow appearance (*arrows*)

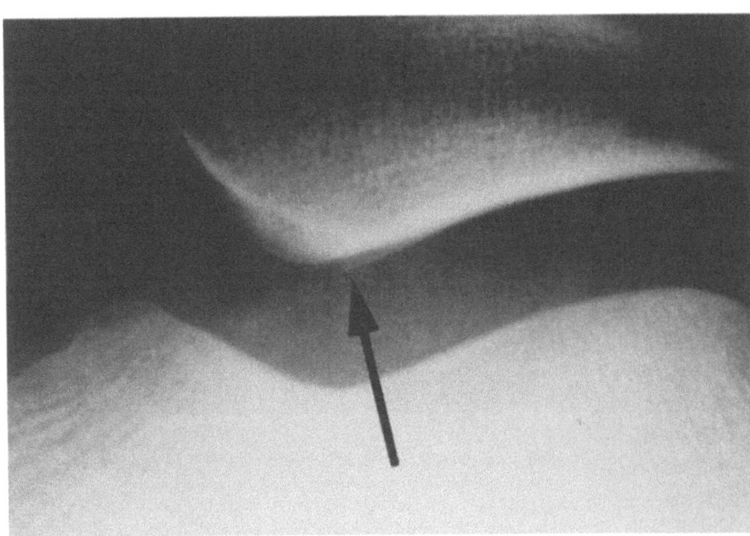

Fig. 5.4. Ostechondral fracture of the patella due to transient patellar dislocation; "skyline view". The *arrow* indicates the lateral border of the osteocartilaginous lesion. A subtle contour defect was the only radiographic sign of the fracture

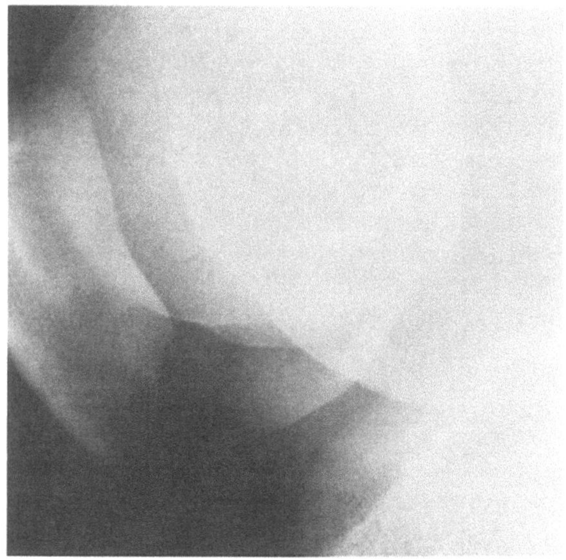

Fig. 5.5. Gross osteochondral fracture with partial separation of the fragment

5.5.2
Conventional Tomography

In all joints involved, conventional tomography still has to be considered a useful method to evaluate the osteocartilaginous junction, but with this method the solely cartilaginous or subchondral trabecular lesions will be missed. Therefore, although the definition of minor osseous abnormalities is improved by tomography, it is not the optimal tomographic modality because of poor resolution and decreased contrast.

5.5.3
Bone Scanning

Prior to the introduction of MRI, a technetium ^{99m}MDP (methylene diphosphonate) scan was the next step in the work-up of traumatic joint pathology. Bone scanning is highly sensitive as early as 12 h after injury (I. Watt, personal communication 1996) and may indicate even minor injuries to both bone and soft tissues. However, the technique cannot distinguish osteochondral fracture from subchondral microfracture and does not provide direct informa-

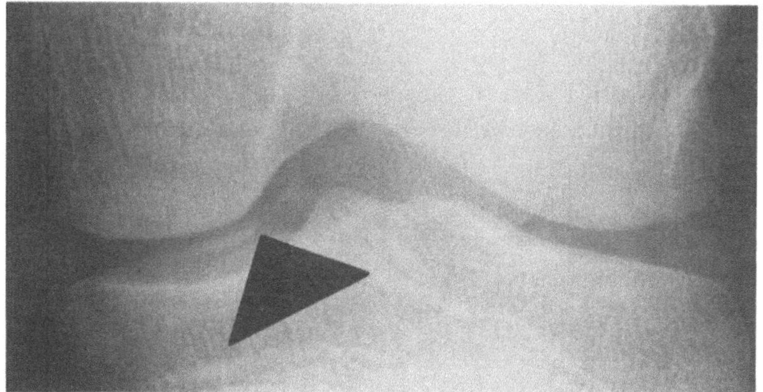

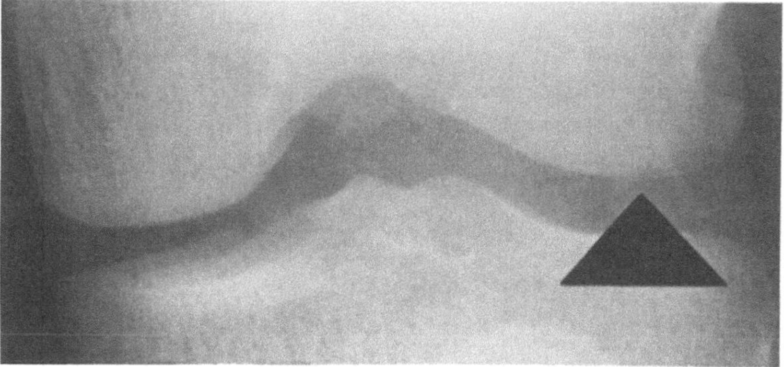

Fig. 5.6. A Osteochondral fracture of the lateral femoral condyle with a free fragment medially (*arrowhead*). The contour defect laterally was not shown in either plane. **B** After arthroscopic fixation, a thin, linear area of increased density is shown (*arrowhead*)

tion regarding articular cartilage. Nonetheless, an abnormal bone would indicate the need for further investigation, preferably MRI.

5.5.4
Computed Tomography

The identification and quantification of loose osteocartilaginous bodies or those attached to the synovial lining require a careful search of the recesses and dependent portions of the joint, which is accomplished best of all by CT (SARTORIS et al. 1985; DEUTSCH 1992). Chondral defects are not well appreciated because of the axial plane of imaging and the insufficient contrast to intraarticular fluid.

5.5.5
Magnetic Resonance Imaging

MRI is extremely sensitive in the general detection of acute traumatic lesions of most joints, including the knee and tibiotalar joint as well as other sites that escape detection with routine radiography.

5.5.5.1
Imaging Technique

MR imaging of the joint in the evaluation of acute injuries of the articular surfaces provides information on:

1. The subchondral cancellous bone
2. The junction between bone and cartilage
3. The cartilage
4. The fluid-filled joint space (if present)

Joint imaging is dependent on high resolution, which makes application of a surface coil essential in all cases.

To reach the above-mentioned goals, the use of different sequences and imaging planes is necessary. The location of the lesion and the configuration of the joint itself will determine whether coronal, sagittal or axial images are preferable.

The recommended imaging protocol consists of a short-tau-inversion-recovery (STIR) sequences, T1- and T2-weighted turbo-spin-echo (TSE) sequences and a gradient-echo (GE) technique. The STIR sequence is the primary "localizer" of the lesion and is called the "MR bone scan". This sequence employs an inversion pulse applied at an inversion time TI at the null crossing point of the longitudinal magnetization of fat to suppress the fat signal in the image, allowing sensitive depiction of all traumatic lesions in the bone and the soft tissues when edema is present. The absence of increased signal on the STIR sequence as compared to muscle has in practical experience excluded the likelihood of significant bony injury. In addition, fluid in the joint has a high signal, providing good contrast between fluid and the intermediate signal of the cartilage. We agree with DEUTSCH (1992) that the STIR sequence is reasonably effective in the assessment of the relatively thick articular cartilage of the patella, yet less successful in depicting the thinner articular cartilage overlying the talar dome.

T1-weighted spin echo (SE) images are helpful in defining the anatomy and better differentiating bone bruises from fractures, the latter running parallel or vertical to the cartilage. The interface between cartilage and bone marrow seen as a "black line" can be used to evaluate osteochondral fractures in T1-weighted images. T2-weighted TSE sequences (TR > 2500 ms, TE > 90 ms) provide excellent image quality in a reasonable time (<5 min). The articular cartilage demonstrates a decreased signal intensity. Irregularities of the contour are nicely seen when there is fluid in the joint. Free fragments are also depicted well with this sequence.

GE imaging represents a wide spectrum of 2D or 3D sequences having in common the use of a gradient reversal for signal acquisition and the application of a RF pulse of less than 90°. Image contrast is dependent not only on tissue relaxation times and the timing parameters TR and TE, but is also affected by the pulse flip angle, the presence or absence of steady-state conditions and the mode of acquisition (2D versus 3D; WEHRLI and ATLAS 1991).

GE sequences show excellent contrast between cartilage and intraarticular fluid. These sequences enable definition, in conjunction with T2-TSE and STIR, of the contour of the cartilage. Our present protocol consists of a 2D fast field echo (FFE) sequence (TR 550 ms, TE 18 ms/30°) or a 3D FFE (TR 18 ms, TE 8 ms/10°). However, these protocols have to be adapted to the equipment one is working with.

Surface detail of articular cartilage can be demonstrated by employing saline and/or gadolinium chelates intraarticularly. However, no data are reported in cases of acute injuries at the articular surfaces of bone, and the method is currently not recommended.

Table 5.3. MRI classification of acute injuries at the articular surfaces

---

I.   Injuries with disrupted articular cartilage
     - Chondral lesions
     - Osteochondral lesions
II. Injuries with intact articular cartilage
     - Subchondral impaction
     - Subchondral contusions ("bone bruises")

5.5.5.2
Imaging Results

A simple classification of osteochondral injury can be based on MRI findings, taking advantage of the ability of MRI to depict both articular cartilage and subchondral bone (Table 5.3).

5.6
Injuries of the Articular Surfaces with Disrupted Articular Cartilage

5.6.1
Chondral Lesions

Purely cartilaginous lesions may occur when chondral chips or flaps are knocked from the "tidemark". They are especially common in the knee joint, while they are rare in other joints. In most cases, displacement of the chondral lesions occurs. If large enough, they are represented by a defect in the cartilaginous lining, best seen in T2-TSE-, GE- or STIR sequences. Chondral and osteochondral lesions can be differentiated by analyzing the subchondral "black line" dividing the cartilage from the bone marrow. In part, this line represents the subchondral bone plate. However, chemical shift and edge artifacts as well as short T1 relaxation due to collagen and calcium in layer 4 are responsible for an artificial broadening of the line (ADAM et al. 1988). If there is no abnormality of this black line in shape, thickness or signal, it may be concluded that there is no fragmentation of the underlying bone. Bone marrow edema is evident in acute injury, differentiating acute chondral lesions from degeneration. However, it is well known from the extensive studies on degenerative cartilage changes that small chondral lesions may be overlooked by MRI (ADAM et al. 1994; HODLER et al. 1992). In practical terms, this seems to be of no clinical importance in the evaluation of acute joint injuries.

5.6.2
Osteochondral Lesions

Extension of injury to the underlying bone may result in a classical transchondral fracture. Comminution of the articular surface may occur with variable degrees of surface depression and production of loose osteochondral fragments. The subchondral "black line" is disrupted (Fig. 5.7). A circular, ovoid or flat osteochondral fragment with intermediate and low signal is best seen on T2-TSE-, STIR- and GE sequences. In the event that the osteochondral defect is detached, it may lie displaced elsewhere in the joint or may remain in its anatomical position. In the latter case, a high-signal-intensity cleavage plane, probably representing synovial fluid, may separate the fragment totally or partially from its bony bed.

5.7
Injuries of the Articular Surfaces with Intact Articular Cartilage

From the experimental work of BERNDT and HARTY (1959) it is well known that injuries at the articulating surfaces may result in an area of compression of subchondral bone with damage to the bony trabeculae, while the cartilage remains intact. We may speculate that impaction force applied to articular cartilage may only deform the elastic cartilage but produces hemorrhage and disruption of the "weaker" trabecular bone.

5.7.1
Subchondral Impaction

The main feature of subchondral impaction is the delineation of intact cartilage on GE-, STIR- or T2-TSE sequences. The subchondral "black line" may or may not be well depictable. Impaction parallel to the cartilage may occur with thickening of the subchondral black line (BOHNDORF 1996). Crescentic or arcuate signal losses have also been described VELLET et al. 1991; Fig. 5.8). On STIR images, a relatively large area of inhomogeneous high signal is usually seen.

5.7.2
Subchondral Contusions ("Bone Bruises")

It is believed that simple subchondral bone contusions, also referred to as "bone bruises", can be dif-

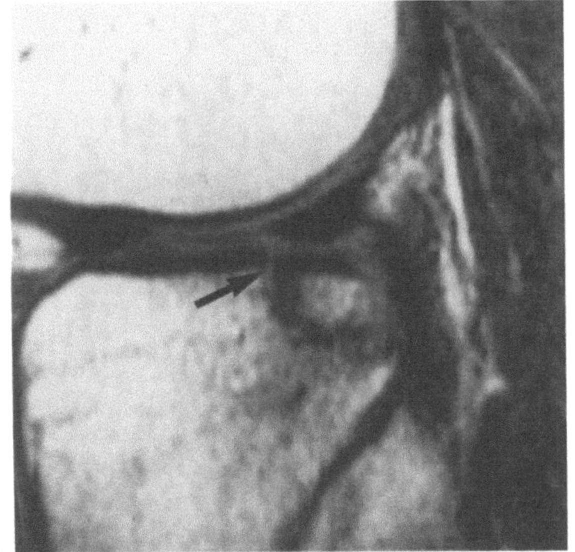

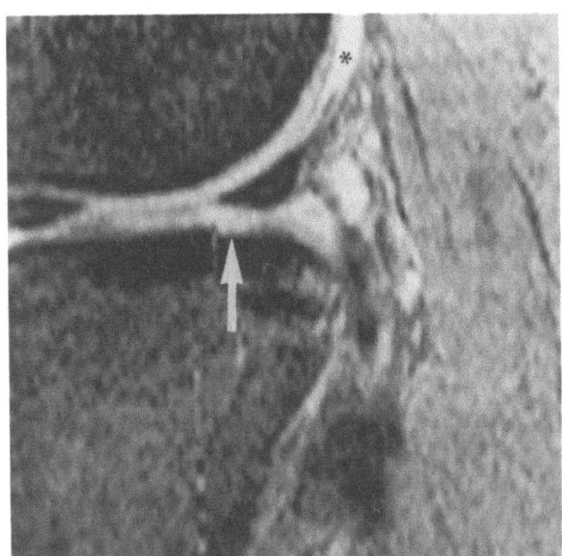

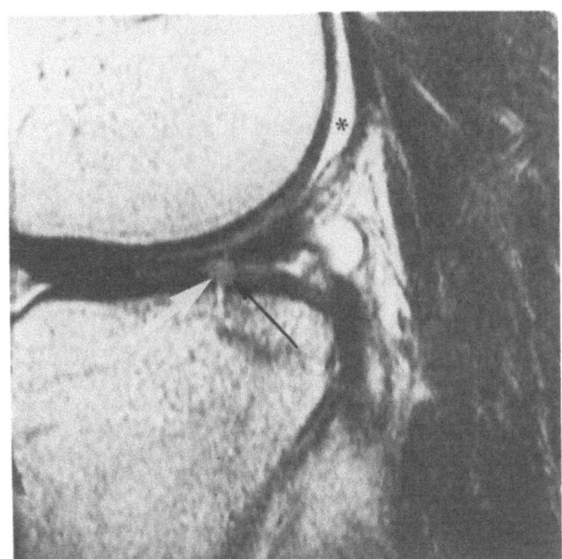

ferentiated from subchondral impaction, although the forces applied are basically the same. Bone bruises are characterized as poorly defined, reticulated inhomogeneous areas of low signal intensity in T1-weighted SE images (Fig. 5.9). STIR images demonstrate increased signal intensity, usually over a larger area than T1-weighted images.

5.8
Treatment and Prognosis

When a chondral or osteochondral fracture has been diagnosed, appropriate therapy should be instituted to deal with the mechanical effect of free fragments, to halt the progression of an acute injury to a chronic stage and to avoid early degenerative changes. The general principle of treatment of chondral and osteochondral fractures is fixation of the fragment which is usually transcartilaginous and not transosseous. Fixation is done nowadays by means of arthroscopy rather than open arthrotomy. In injuries with intact cartilage or when only a small disruption of articular cartilage is seen, conservative, nonoperative treatment may lead to good or fair clinical results (PETTINE and MORREY 1987). In cases of subchondral microfracture (bone bruise), conservative treatment by immobilization is the therapy of choice.

There is considerable evidence that improperly treated acute osteochondral fractures may progress to chronic lesions with avascular necrosis of the fragment (BERNDT and HARTY 1959; O'DONOGHUE 1966; ALEXANDER and LICHTMAN 1980; MARKS 1952). This necrotic state will persist until neovascularization occurs. Revascularization of the attached fragment is impeded by inadequate immobilization due to shearing of new capillaries growing across the fracture site (NAUMETZ and SCHWEIGEL 1980). VELLET et al. (1991) also showed convincingly that injuries of the articular surfaces with intact cartilage may progress after several months to chronic osteochondral defects although

Fig. 5.7A–C. Osteochondral-type injury of the articulating surfaces with disrupted articular cartilage. A The T1-weighted SE image reveals a crescentic signal loss in the dorsal part of the tibial plateau. The subchondral *black line* is clearly disrupted (*arrow*). B The GE technique (2D FFE 550/18/30°) does not show an obvious defect; however, the signal of the cartilage is increased (*arrow*; *asterisk* for water). C The T2-weighted TSE image helps to exclude a knocked-off cartilaginous defect. However, fissuring and swelling of the cartilage has changed the signal (*arrow*; *asterisk* for water)

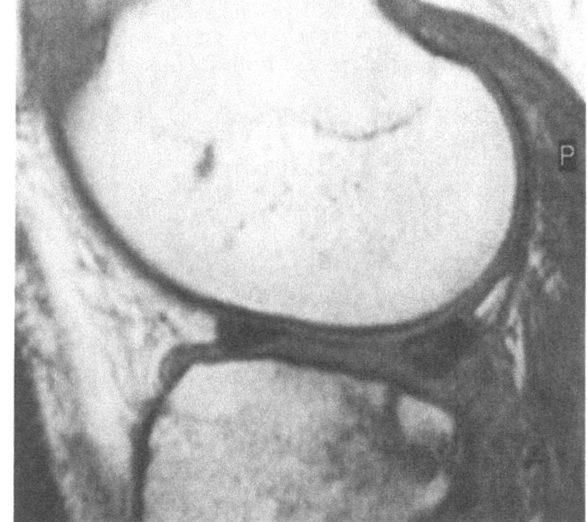

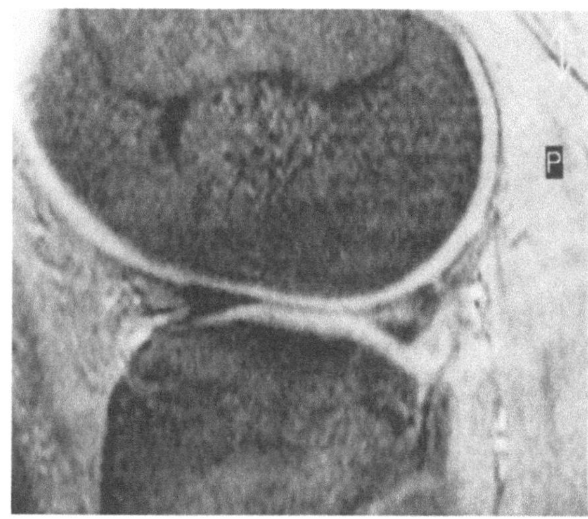

Fig. 5.8A,B. Impaction-type injury of the articular surface with intact articular cartilage. **A** The T1-weighted SE image reveals a crescentic signal loss in the dorsal part of the tibial plateau. The subchondral *black line* is not disrupted. In addition, traumatic meniscal injury is seen. **B** The GE technique (2D FFE 550/18/30°) confirms intact cartilage

no chondral abnormality was seen arthroscopically at the time of trauma.

5.9
Conclusion

Chondral and osteochondral fractures have been overlooked to a large extent in the management of injuries involving joints. This has led to recommendation of arthroscopy in all cases of radiographically negative hemarthrosis of the knee joint, because clinical experience showed that chondral or osteo-

chondral fractures were important causes of hemarthrosis not explicable on the basis of clinical or radiographic examination (VÄHÄRSAJA et al. 1993). It is likely that MRI will replace arthroscopy as a primary diagnostic tool. Although well-designed prospective studies comparing arthroscopy and MRI of *acute* injuries of the articulating surfaces need to be performed, clinical experience has shown that MRI is able to diagnose or, more importantly, to exclude osteochondral fractures. The greater potential of MRI, however, is its ability to diagnose subchondral injuries which are not seen by any other technique, including arthroscopy. The early diagnosis of these lesions may be important to avoid progression from an acute injury to a chronic condition.

O'DONOGHUE's plea of 1966 is now achievable: "My plea is that the patient is entitled to a meticulous examination at the time of his original injury; that if at all possible a definite diagnosis should be made before the ideal time for treatment has passed".

At present, there are no scientific data indicating when to recommend early MRI in the investigation of the acutely tramatized joint. However, the following may be considered reasonable indications for urgent MRI:

– Unexplained lipohemarthrosis on a radiograph
– Unexplained blood on a joint aspiration

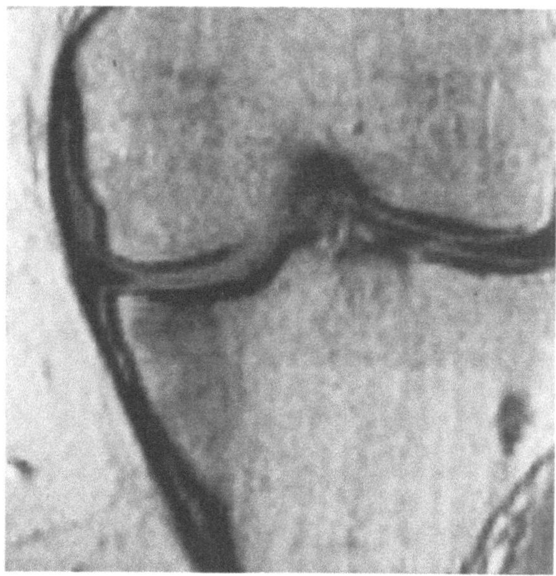

Fig. 5.9. Bone bruise. In the T1-weighted image, a faint, irregularly bordered loss of signal intensity is seen subchondrally in the lateral tibial plateau. The *black line* separating bone from cartilage is well preserved. In the STIR sequence, this area has high signal intensity (not shown)

– Suspicious sclerosis or subchondral plate irregularity on an X ray of the joints

Acknowledgement. I am grateful to Dr. Iain Watt for help in the preparation of the manuscript.

References

Adam G, Bohndorf K, Prescher A, Krasny R, Günther RW (1988) Der hyaline Gelenkknorpel in der MR-Tomographie des Kniegelenks bei 1,5T. Fortschr Röntgenstr 148:648–651

Adam G, Prescher A, Nolte-Ernsting C, Bühne M, Scherer K, Küpper W, Günther RW (1994) MRT des hyalinen Kniegelenksknorpels. Fortschr Röntgenstr 160:143–148

Alexander AH, Lichtman DM (1980) Surgical treatment of transchondral talar dome fractures. J Bone Joint Surg [Am] 62:646–652

Berndt AL, Harty M (1959) Transchondral fractures (osteochondritis dissecans) of the talus. J Bone Joint Surg [Am] 41:988–1020

Bohndorf K (1996) Injuries at the articulating surfaces of bone (chondral, osteochondral, subchondral fractures and osteochondrosis dissecans). Eur J Radiol 22:22–29

Buckwalter JA, Rosenberg LC, Hunziker EB (1990) Articular cartilage: composition, structure, response to injury and methods of faciliting repairs. In: Ewing JF (ed) Articular cartilage and knee joint function: basic science and arthroscopy. Raven, New York

Bullough PG (1992) Atlas of orthopaedic pathology, 2nd edn. Gower, New York

Deutsch AL (1992) Osteochondral injuries of the talar dome. In: Deutsch AL, Mink JH, Kerr R (eds) MRI of the foot and ankle. Raven, New York

Flick AB, Gould N (1985) Osteochondritis dissecans of the talus (transchondral fractures of the talus): review of the literature and new surgical approach for medial dome lesions. Foot Ankle 5:165–185

Hodler J, Berthiaume MJ, Schweitzer ME, Resnick D (1992) Knee joint hyaline cartilage defects: a comparative study of MR and anatomic sections. J Comput Assist Tomogr 16:597–603

Kirsch MD, Fitzgerald SW, Friedmann H, Rogers LF (1993) Transient lateral patellar dislocation: diagnosis with MR imaging. AJR Am J Roentgenol 161:109–113

Mafulli N, Binfield PM, King JBV, Good CJ (1993) Acute haemarthrosis of the knee in athletes. J Bone Joint Surg [Br] 75:945–949

Marks KL (1952) Flake fracture of the talus progressing to osteochondritis dissecans. J Bone Joint Surg [Br] 34:90–92

Mink JH, Deutsch AL (1988) Occult cartilage and bone injuries of the knee: detection, classification, and asessment with MR imaging. Radiology 170:823–829

Mink JH, Deutsch AL (1990) MRI of the musculoskeletal system. A teaching file. Raven, New York

Naumetz VA, Schweigel JF (1980) Osteocartilagineous lesions of the talar dome. J Trauma 20:924–927

O'Donoghue DH (1966) Chondral and osteochondral fractures. J Trauma 6:496–481

Pettine KA, Morrey BF (1987) Osteochondral fractures of the talus. J Bone Joint Surg [Br] 69:89–92

Sartoris DJ, Kursunoglu S, Pineda C (1985) Detection of intra-articular osteochondral bodies in the knee using computed arthrotomography. Radiology 155:447–453

Shea MP, Manoli A (1993) Osteochondral lesions of the talar dome. Foot Ankle 14:48–55

Vähärsaja V, Kinnunen P, Serlo W (1993) Arthroscopy of the acute traumatic knee in children. Acta Orthop Scand 64:580–582

Vellet AD, Marks PH, Fowler PJ, Munro TG (1991) Occult posttraumatic osteochondral lesions of the knee: prevalence, classification, and short-term sequelae evaluated with MR imaging. Radiology 178:271–276

Wehrli FW, Atlas SW (1991) Fast imaging: principles, techniques and clinical application. In: Atlas SW (ed) Magnetic resonance imaging of the brain and spine. Raven, New York

6 The Radiological Imaging of Shoulder Instability

A.M. Davies[1] and P.N.M. Tyrrell[2]

CONTENTS

6.1
Introduction

The shoulder joint has the greatest range of movement of all the joints in the body. Because of this it is also the joint most susceptible to instability. Stability problems, notably recurrent subluxation and/or dislocation, are most common in athletes participating in sports utilising a wide range of shoulder movements such as discus throwing, shot putting and contact sports. The diagnosis of shoulder instability is essentially clinical. The value of imaging is to determine the nature of the underlying injury in order to facilitate treatment which frequently includes surgical repair.

Various imaging techniques are available for assessment of the joint capsular mechanism and labral ligamentous complex. The choice of techniques has increased in recent years with the advent of magnetic resonance (MR) imaging. MR imaging, after initial enthusiasm, lost some favour with considerable debate regarding the relative merits of computed tomographic arthrography (CTA) and MR imaging. Recently, MR arthrography has been gaining in popularity. This has resulted in an alteration in prac-

tice in some imaging departments from the non-invasive technique of MR imaging without contrast medium to an invasive technique, similar in many respects to CTA. The various techniques and their relative merits and limitations in the assessment of shoulder instability are reviewed.

6.2
Pathophysiology and Anatomy

Shoulder instability is a condition manifest by recurrent subluxation or dislocation which most often develops following trauma to the shoulder such as a fall on the outstretched hand or a direct blow to the shoulder, frequently resulting in an acute anterior dislocation. Congenital and developmental anomalies about the shoulder may contribute to the occurrence of instability, but it is rare for the condition to develop in the absence of a primary traumatic event. In the athletic population, subtle instabilities may develop as a result of repetitive micro-injury.

Shoulder instability, which refers to instability of the glenohumeral articulation, can be traumatic or atraumatic, acute, recurrent or fixed and may be classified according to its direction. This may be anterior, posterior, inferior or multidirectional. Anterior glenohumeral instability is the most common, followed by multidirectional instability. Posterior and inferior instability are uncommon. The majority of anterior dislocations occur during abduction and external rotation, and in the acute situation the diagnosis is usually obvious. Subtle subluxations, however, particularly when recurrent, can be difficult to diagnose. The critical determining factor in whether a patient with an acute dislocation will develop a recurrent problem is the patient's age. The highest risk group is between the ages of 15–25 years, where the chance of recurrence following initial dislocation is 50–70%. Other factors involved in prognosis include the presence of an associated fracture and severe trauma causing the initial dislocation; these

[1] A.M. Davies, MD, MRI Centre, The Royal Orthopaedic Hospital, Birmingham B31 2AP, UK
[2] P.N.M. Tyrrell, MD, The Robert Jones & Agnes Hunt Orthopaedic Hospital, Oswestry, Shropshire SY10 7AG UK

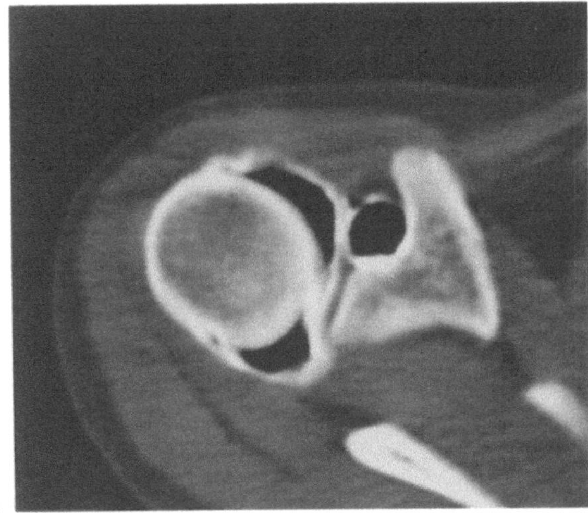

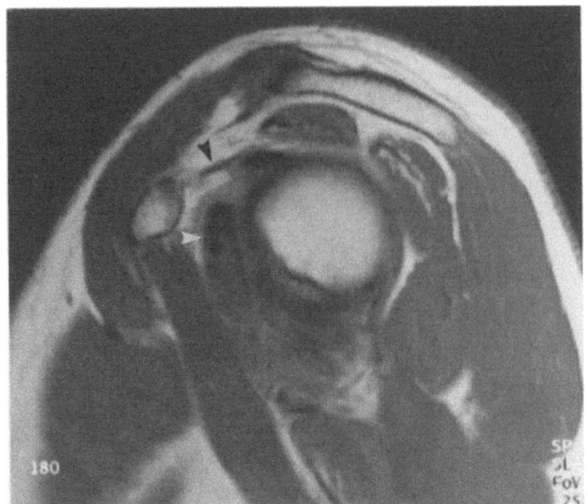

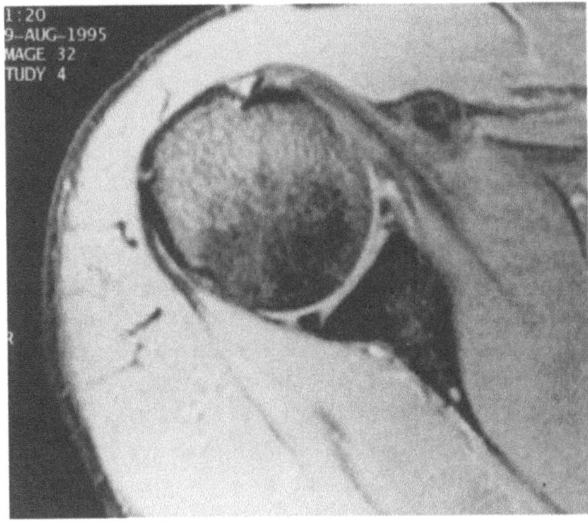

Fig. 6.1. a CTA at the level of the coracoid showing an intact superior labrum and SGHL lying anteriorly. b Axial gradient-echo MR image through the mid-glenoid showing undercutting of the glenoid labrum. The MGHL is seen lying between the anterior labrum and the subscapularis tendon. c Sagittal oblique T1W MR image (TR 690, TE 12) through the medial humeral head showing the coracohumeral ligament (*black arrowhead*) with the subscapularis tendon inferiorly (*white arrowhead*). *CTA*, computed tomographic arthrography; *SGHL*, superior glenohumeral ligament; *MR*, magnetic resonance; *MGHL*, middle glenohumeral Ligament

features are surprisingly associated with a lower rate of recurrence (HAWKINS and MOHTADI 1991).

The shoulder joint is shallow and inherently unstable, with much of the stability depending on the surrounding soft tissue structures. Glenohumeral stability is primarily dependent on the glenoid labrum, the joint capsule and its anteriorly located thickened condensations, the superior, middle and inferior glenohumeral ligaments, the coracohumeral ligament and the subscapular tendon of the rotator cuff (Fig. 6.1). These structures together form a capsular unit called the anterior capsular mechanism (MOSELEY and OVERGAARD 1962). The specific structures responsible for stability at any given time depend on the position and action of the shoulder.

Injuries associated with glenohumeral instability include tears (including avulsions) of the bony and cartilaginous glenoid, commonly referred to as a Bankart lesion (BANKART 1938), tears of the glenohumeral ligaments, stripping of the anterior capsule from the glenoid and tears of the subscapularis

tendon. These injuries may all give rise to recurrent instability, particularly if there has been an avulsion of the glenohumeral ligament complex at its insertion into the glenoid labrum. Abnormal glenoid and humeral version, glenoid hypoplasia (MANNS and DAVIES 1991; WIRTH et al. 1993; TROUT and RESNICK 1996), loss of glenoid concavity (LAZARUS et al. 1996) and subscapularis laxity (SYMEONIDES 1972) may be contributory factors on occasion. Associated bone injuries of the humeral head, notably a Hill-Sachs fracture and trough-line fractures, may also occur.

Numerous reports have attempted to identify the "essential" lesion responsible for recurrent dislocation. This may be an oversimplification of the problem. Most consider this to be a torn or detached glenoid labrum, with or without a fracture of the glenoid rim. A number of investigators have disputed the concept of the glenoid labrum as an important stabilising factor, attributing the success of Bankart's surgical procedure to reattachment of the fibrous capsule to the glenoid rim (ROWE and PATAL 1978; TOWNLEY 1950). In this view, stability is mainly dependent on the ability of the capsule to act as an effective barrier against projection of the humeral head in external rotation. The labral lesion is then considered a result rather than the cause of recurrent instability. In these patients, especially early in the course of the disorder, labral damage may be minimal and the detection of capsular anomalies may be the only clue to its accurate diagnosis.

The shallow surface of the glenoid is deepened by the glenoid labrum, a fibrocartilaginous rim which is attached around the margin of the glenoid cavity. Its attachment to the margin of the glenoid is sometimes deficient in parts. Cadaver studies have shown that the labrum is loosely attached to the glenoid particularly in its anterosuperior quadrant (COOPER et al. 1992). Apparent detachments in this area may be a normal phenomenon (see below). The fibrous capsule is attached medially to the circumference of the glenoid cavity beyond the glenoid labrum; above, it encroaches onto the root of the coracoid process so as to include the long head of the biceps tendon within the joint; laterally it is attached to the anatomical neck of the humerus except on the medial side where it descends for rather more than 1 cm onto the shaft of the bone. Three types of insertion of the capsule medially are recognised (Fig. 6.2; MOSELEY and OVERGAARD 1962; ZLATKIN et al. 1988). In Type 1, the capsule inserts directly onto the labrum. In Type 2, the insertion is at the middle third of the scapular neck. In Type 3, the insertion is at the medial third of the scapular neck. The capsule is more capacious the more medially located its medial insertion. Types 1 and 2 occur as normal variants. It is not clear whether Type 3 occurs as a developmental anomaly or if it is secondary to capsular stripping, but it is associated with an increased predisposition to anterior dislocation.

The superior, middle and inferior glenohumeral ligaments represent localised thickenings of the capsule anteriorly. At their scapular ends they all attach to the upper part of the medial margin of the glenoid cavity and are intimately connected with the glenoid labrum. The superior glenohumeral ligament (SGHL) originates from the superior glenoid labrum, anterior to the biceps tendon, courses along the medial edge of the tendon and is attached to a small depression above the lesser tubercle of the humerus (Fig. 6.1). Its primary function is to limit inferior motion of the humerus. The middle glenohumeral ligament (MGHL) originates from the upper margin of the glenoid, courses obliquely anterior to the glenoid labrum and inserts into the lower part of the

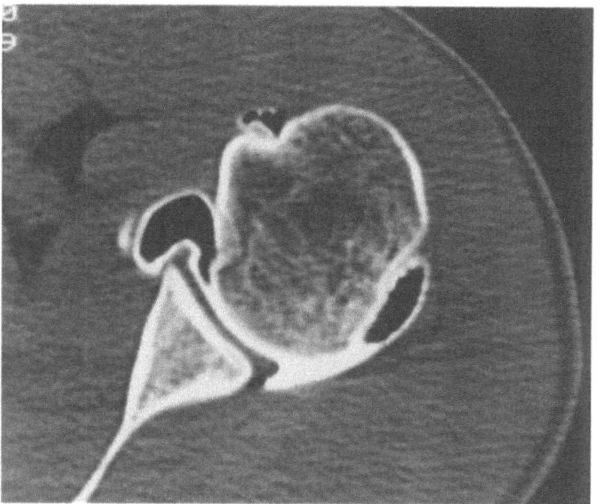
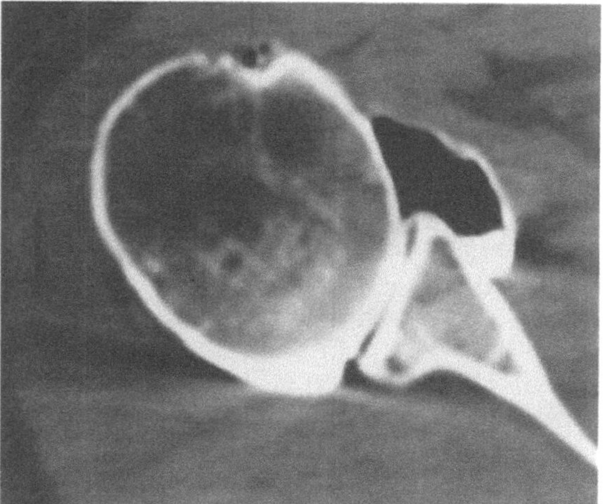
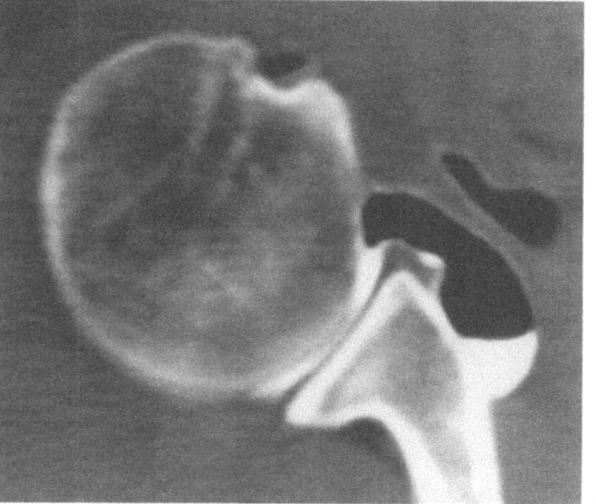

Fig. 6.2. a CTA through the mid-glenoid demonstrating a Type 1 capsule insertion. **b** A Type 2 with a deficient anterior labrum and **c** a Type 3 capsule insertion

lesser tubercle of the humerus. It aids in limiting inferior translation of the glenohumeral joint. The inferior glenohumeral ligament (IGHL), considered by many to be the most important component of the anterior capsular mechanism contributing to stability, has two major components – the axillary pouch and the superior band. In the axillary pouch the ligament is ill-defined and the fibres blend with the axillary recess of the capsule. More superiorly the fibres of the IGHL become a distinct cord-like structure known as the superior band which arises from the upper half of the anterior glenoid labrum; it is closely related to and may blend with labral tissue. Through most of the course of the ligament, it runs adjacent to and parallel with the anterior glenoid labrum.

There are a number of anatomical variants and anomalies which can give rise to confusion in image interpretation. Such anomalies include congenital absence of either the MGHL or the IGHL, which can occur in up to 25% of cases. Difficulties that may be experienced in image interpretation as a result of complex anatomy will be referred to, as appropriate, in the text.

6.3
Radiography

Despite the introduction of the newer, more sophisticated imaging techniques, the radiograph remains the initial investigation of choice for the shoulder. As with all trauma, adequate evaluation of the shoulder requires two views: a film parallel to the glenohumeral joint and one at 90° tangential to the shoulder joint.

A true anteroposterior (AP) radiograph of the shoulder is not optimal as the scapula is seen at an angle and the glenohumeral joint is partially obscured by the overlapping bony structures. The AP radiograph is best obtained with the patient in a 40° posterior oblique position. Acute anterior dislocation, classified as subcoracoid, subglenoid, subclavicular and rarely intrathoracic, is easily detected on the AP radiograph (Fig. 6.3). The uncommon posterior dislocation, constituting less than 5% of all shoulder dislocations, is overlooked on the initial radiographic examination in over 50% of cases (Fig. 6.4; McLaughlin 1952). It is for this reason, with the consequent spectre of litigation, that some form of lateral projection is mandatory. The literature describes numerous different methods of obtaining a lateral projection of the shoulder. The axillary projection (Lawrence 1915) is arguably the easiest to interpret but is frequently difficult to obtain in trauma due to the degree of abduction required. The transthoracic projection (Vastamaki and Solonen 1980) is probably best avoided as it can be difficult to interpret and necessitates a significant radiation dose to the trunk. It is not the purpose of this chapter to advocate a particular alternative projection. It seems prudent to advise consistency within an imaging department irrespective of the type of lateral employed. This will ensure that the radiographer is fully conversant with the technique necessary to obtain a satisfactory result and that the requesting clinician is familiar with his interpretation. These views include the posterior oblique scapular (Neer 1970), apical oblique projection (Garth et al. 1984; Richardson et al. 1988) and lateral scapular Y-view (Rubin et al. 1974).

The purpose of radiography in the patient with instability, presumed due to recurrent dislocation, is to delineate the typical Hill-Sachs compression fracture of the posterolateral aspect of the humeral head and fracture of the anterior glenoid rim. The Hill-Sachs lesion, otherwise known as the hatchet deformity, appears as a flattened or indented area of the posterolateral aspect of the head of the humerus at the level of the greater tuberosity with dense medial and inferior borders due to compressed bone. The defect may be identified in over three-quarters of patients with a history of recurrent dislocation (Hill-Sachs 1940; Adams 1950) but has also been reported following a single dislocation (Adams 1950; Rowe and Sakellarides 1961). In recurrent posterior dislocation the hatchet deformity may be seen on the anterolateral aspect of the humeral head (Arndt and Sears 1965) and is termed a reverse Hill-Sachs lesion. The bony Bankart lesion indicative of recurrent dislocation comprises fractures of the antero-inferior rim of the glenoid, periosteal new bone formation due to capsular stripping from the neck of the scapula and rounding or eburnation of the glenoid margin (Eyre-Brook 1948).

Projections described in the literature to demonstrate the bony sequelae of recurrent dislocation include the Didiee position (Didiee 1930), the exaggerated external-rotation axillary shoulder position (Rafert et al. 1990), the Stripp axial projection (Horsfield and Jones 1987), the Stryker notch position (Hall et al. 1959), the modified Stryker position (Horsfield 1991) and the Westpoint view (Rokous et al. 1972). In the uncommon inferior subluxation of the glenohumeral joint, the hammock projection is helpful (Horsfield 1991).

Fig. 6.3. a Anteroposterior (*AP*) radiograph showing a subcoracoid anterior dislocation. b AP radiograph showing a sub-glenoid anterior dislocation

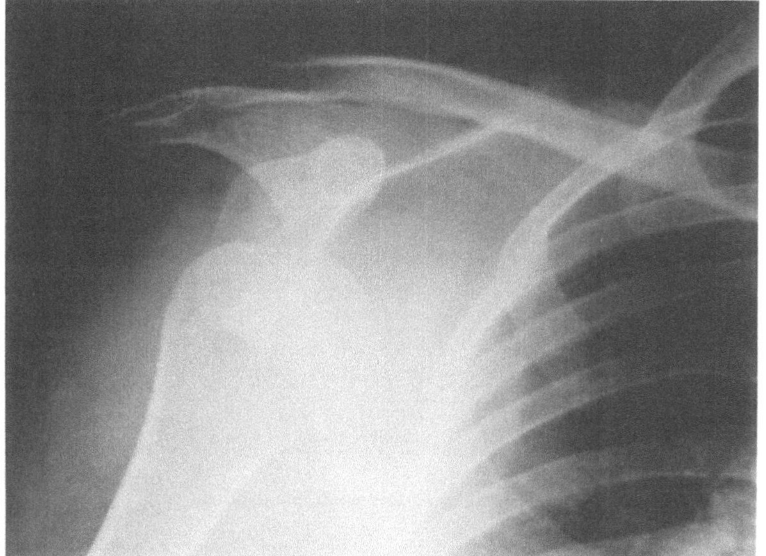

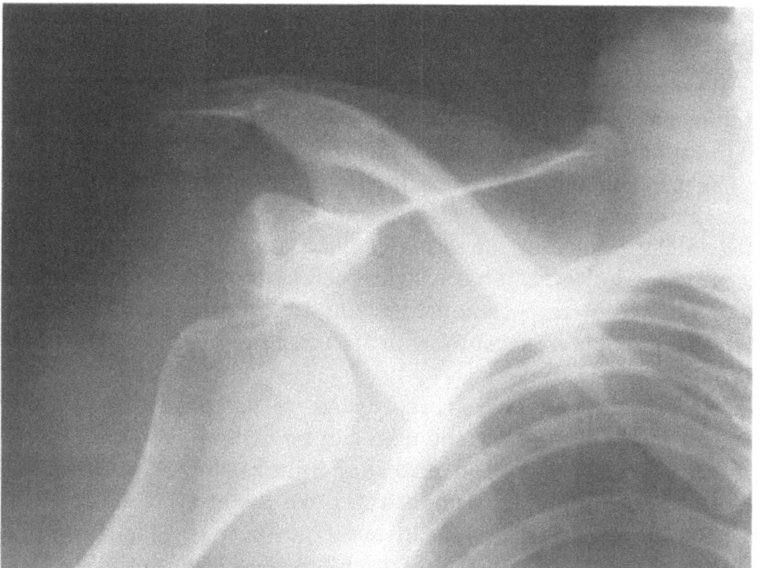

6.4
Arthrography

Arthrography is usually performed via an anterior approach. With the arm by the side and externally rotated to increase the space between the glenoid labrum and the humeral head, a 22-gauge (22G) needle is introduced vertically into the joint under fluoroscopic control. Satisfactory location of the needle within the joint is indicated by the rapid flow of positive contrast medium away from the needle tip. Approximately 12 ml of iodinated contrast medium is injected in the single contrast technique, 4 ml of contrast medium followed by 10–15 ml of air in the double contrast technique. In the presence of capsular stripping, the joint may require a rather larger volume of contrast medium to achieve satisfactory distension. In the normal examination, the articular cartilage is identified and contrast medium outlines the glenoid labrum and fills the posterior pouch and the subscapularis recess. The proximal 2 cm of the biceps tendon is usually visualised and the extent of the joint capsule is defined, typically terminating at the anatomical neck of the humerus where it forms a smooth well-defined line. The subdeltoid/subacromial bursa is separated from the

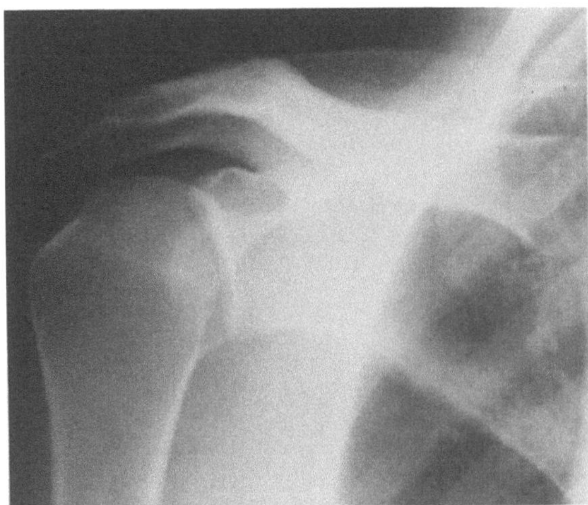

Fig. 6.4. AP radiograph showing a chronic posterior dislocation which was missed

shoulder joint by the rotator cuff, and under normal circumstances, contrast medium or air does not enter the subdeltoid/subacromial structures.

The principal indication for arthrography is in the assessment of rotator cuff disease, but it has been used in the evaluation of shoulder dislocation. In recent years, however, it has usually been employed as an adjunct to cross-sectional imaging techniques such as CT and, more recently, with MR imaging (see below).

The differences between acute and recurrent anterior dislocation of the shoulder can be demonstrated by arthrography and associated injuries also identified. Arthrography demonstrates two distinct sequelae of acute dislocation. In one type there is rupture of the capsule anteriorly or anteroinferiorly with free leakage of fluid into the axillary tissues. In the second type the glenoid labrum or the adjacent capsule becomes detached from the glenoid margin, which allows fluid to flow beneath the subscapularis in the region of the subscapularis bursa. In recurrent dislocation, the subscapular bursa may be enlarged and loss of definition of the translucent area of the glenoid labrum corresponding to a Bankart lesion may be found at operation (REEVES 1966). In one study, all patients with recurrent anterior dislocation had an enlarged subscapular bursa and in 62% the axial view showed a lack of definition of the anterior translucent labrum (REEVES 1966). The remaining 38% showed an attenuated labrum at operation which was separated from the anterior capsule. There were similar findings in recurrent non-

traumatic posterior dislocation with a large posterior pouch and an ill-defined or absent translucent triangle of the labrum. Tijnes and co-authors demonstrated an enlarged but intact capsule in 58% of acute dislocations, and this finding was more common in patients with recurrent dislocation, occurring in 77% (TIJNES et al. 1979). The high frequency of enlarged but intact shoulder capsules after an initial dislocation suggested that the humeral head does not routinely rupture the capsule during dislocation but rather tears the glenoid labrum at its bony attachment and dislocates subperiosteally, dissecting a false pouch below the periosteum and under the subscapularis. In this study Hill-Sachs lesions occurred in 28% of patients, fractures of the greater tuberosity in 22% and of the coracoid process in 2%. Rupture of the rotator cuff is more frequent in initial dislocation than in recurrent dislocation (REEVES 1966). Arthrography can detect abnormalities not visible on radiographic examination, particularly the cartilaginous Bankart lesion (GOLDMAN and GHELMAN 1978). There can be technical difficulties involved in accurately delineating the labrum. Axial hypocycloidal tomography may be employed in an attempt to improve visualisation but this can be a difficult position for the patient to maintain and technically difficult to achieve optimal exposures. Arthrotomography of the shoulder in this day and age has been largely superseded by CT arthrography and MR imaging.

6.5
Computed Tomography

Plain computed tomography (CT), that is, without intraarticular contrast medium, is of value in the acute traumatic setting by identifying the position and extent of fracture fagments and their precise location to the joint surfaces (Fig. 6.5). In recurrent dislocation, it can show a Hill-Sachs lesion and/or a bony Bankart lesion (Fig. 6.6). There is insufficient soft tissue contrast to identify intraarticular soft tissue structures with any degree of accuracy, and thus concomitant arthrography is often employed to improve visualisation and interpretation.

Three-dimensional computed tomography (3DCT) does produce aesthetically pleasing images, but is of little value in radiological diagnostic interpretation. Those involved in management, notably orthopaedic surgeons, may however find these images helpful by improving visualisation of the deformity following complex fractures.

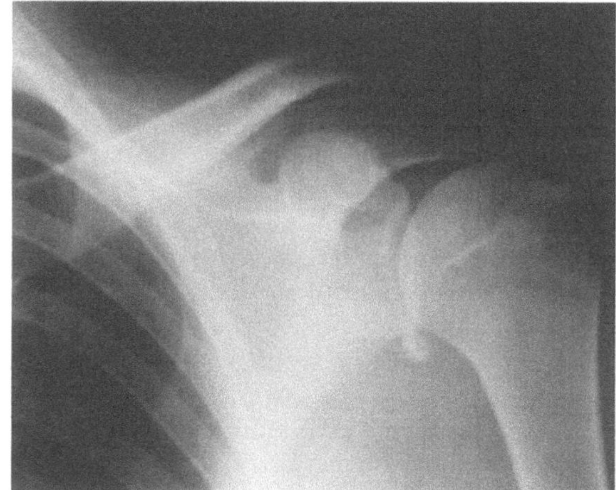

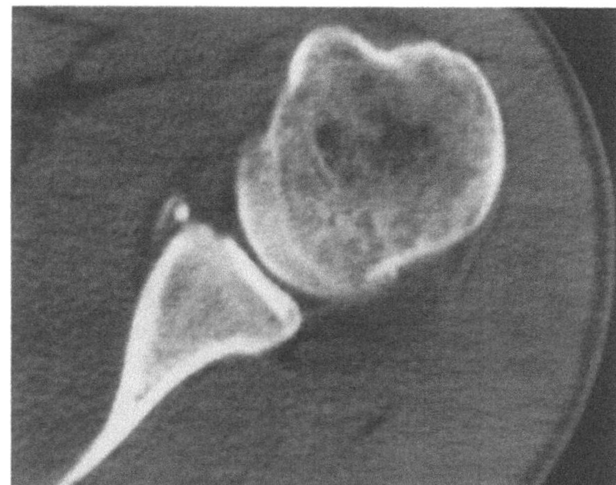

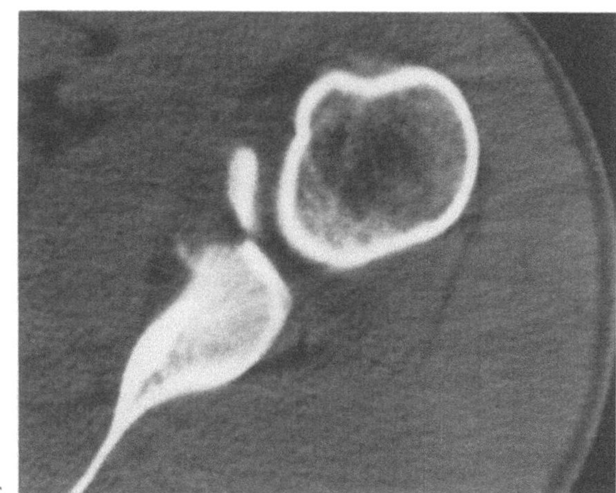

Fig. 6.5. a AP radiograph following reduction of a dislocation showing a loose body in the axillary recess and loss of the anteroinferior cortex of the glenoid. **b** Axial CT of the same patient showing a fracture of the anterior glenoid rim. **c** Axial CT of same patient showing a fragment of bone in the axillary recess. *CT*, computed tomography

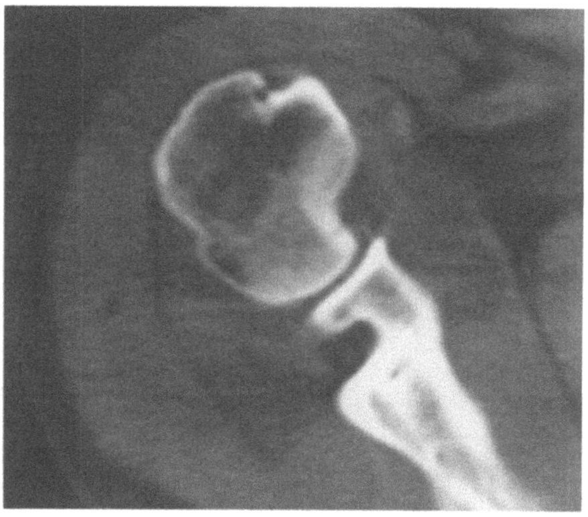

Fig. 6.6. Axial CT showing a reverse Hill-Sachs lesion due to recurrent posterior dislocation

6.6
Computed Tomographic Arthrography

A standard arthrographic technique can be combined with CT, the cross-sectional display greatly enhancing the demonstration of the intraarticular structures. The technique is similar to that of standard arthrography but with the use of less iodinated contrast medium (approximately 1.5 ml) together with approximately 10 ml of air it is the preferred double contrast technique. In addition, 0.1 ml of a 1:1000 solution of adrenaline can also be added to delay absorption of the contrast medium that may occur if the patient cannot proceed immediately to the CT suite.

Computed tomographic arthrography (CTA) is more sensitive than arthrography in the detection of labral tears (DEUTSCH et al. 1984). This is largely because of the improved visualisation and definition of the capsulo-labral complex afforded by the axial sections. The advantages of CTA are that it is a reproducible and accurate procedure and there is a relatively low radiation dose. Positioning of the patient is simple, a major advantage if the patient is in pain. Supine examination usually produces adequate images of the anterior and posterior labrum. However, the prone oblique position on the scan table has been found to enhance evaluation of the labrum (Fig. 6.7; TURNER et al. 1994). There is also the potential for sagittal and coronal reconstruction of the images if so desired, but image quality is usually suboptimal. Spiral CTA may overcome this problem. Direct sagittal CTA has been described (BELTRAN et al. 1986).

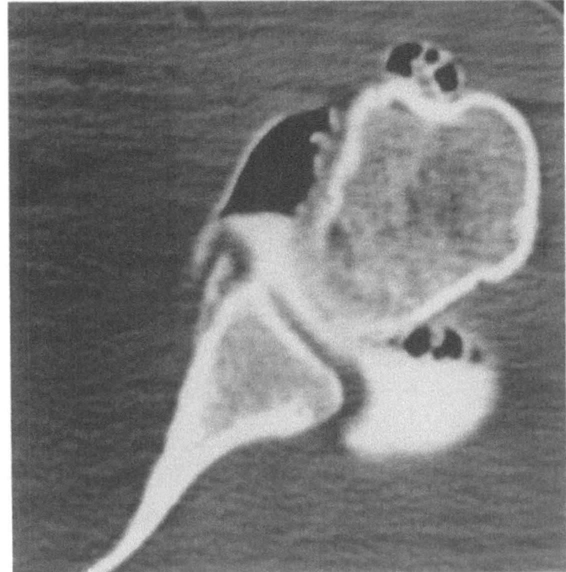

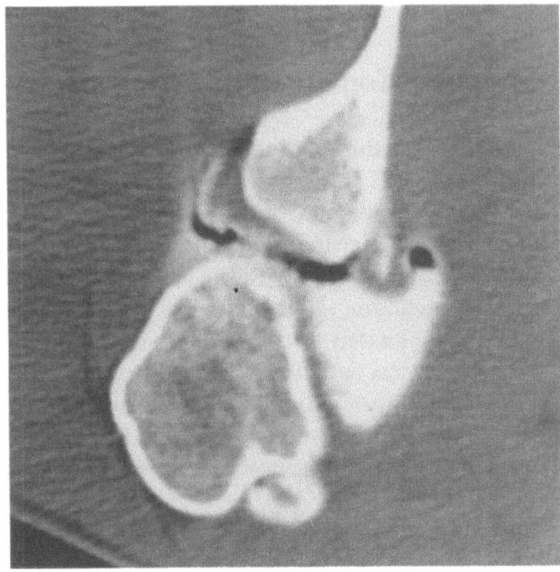

Fig. 6.7. a CTA in the supine position showing elevation of the anterior labrum with periosteal new bone due to stripping. **b** Prone oblique CTA at the same level showing a bare area on the anterior glenoid outlined by air

This proved less accurate than axial CTA, detecting only six of eight Bankart lesions as compared to 100% with the axial technique. The two false-negative results occurred from the exclusion of the glenoid labrum in one case and volume averaging in the other. The patient position required for direct sagittal CTA is both difficult to achieve and maintain.

Potential problems associated with CTA of the shoulder which may result in poor image quality include the presence of a joint effusion, which can dilute the contrast medium, and a delay of more than 20 min between injection of contrast medium and the CT scan (a problem which can be minimised by the addition of adrenaline, see above); an extra-articular injection of contrast medium may impair image quality.

The normal glenoid labrum typically has a triangular configuration but may also appear slightly rounded and smooth. The anterior and posterior labra are approximately equal in size (Fig. 6.2a,c). Normal variants of the anterior labrum, as seen on CTA, include a deficient labrum, a small yet well-defined labrum and a sulcus between the labrum and the glenoid articular cartilage which may frequently be misdiagnosed as a tear (McNIESH and CALLAGHAN 1987). Abnormalities that can be readily visualised on CTA include irregular blunting or attenuation of the labral lip (Fig. 6.2b), discontinuities of the labral lip, and separation or displacement of a part of the labrum (Fig. 6.7). Stripping of the joint capsule may also be observed. The site of insertion of the capsule is usually optimally visualised independent of the degree of joint distension or the amount of contrast medium injected. The capsular insertion onto the anterior glenoid is seen on CTA as a smooth reflection of the contrast-coated synovium that blends with the lateral surface of the labrum. It is distinguished from the cortical bone by a thin band of soft tissue that includes the periosteum of the glenoid. The posterior insertion of the capsule along the glenoid rim is more constant and formation of a synovial recess in this region is rare. The three different types of capsular insertion on the glenoid and scapula can be readily identified by CTA (Fig. 6.2). In Types 2 and 3, there may be an associated underdevelopment of the MGHL and IGHL, and this may also be associated with a large subscapularis recess with no passive restraint to anterior dislocation. Rafii and co-authors noted capsular abnormalities in all patients in their study with instability (RAFII et al. 1986). The most common abnormalities involved the region of the capsular insertion onto the glenoid. This determination was based on the distorted appearance of the capsular reflection with either loss or thickening of the intervening soft tissue layer over the scapular margin. An association with periosteal new bone arising from the glenoid (Figs. 6.7, 6.8) and an enlarged subscapularis bursa were also noted.

Various patterns of injury on CTA in recurrent instability have been reported (SINGSON et al. 1987). A full 96% of patients in Singson and co-workers'

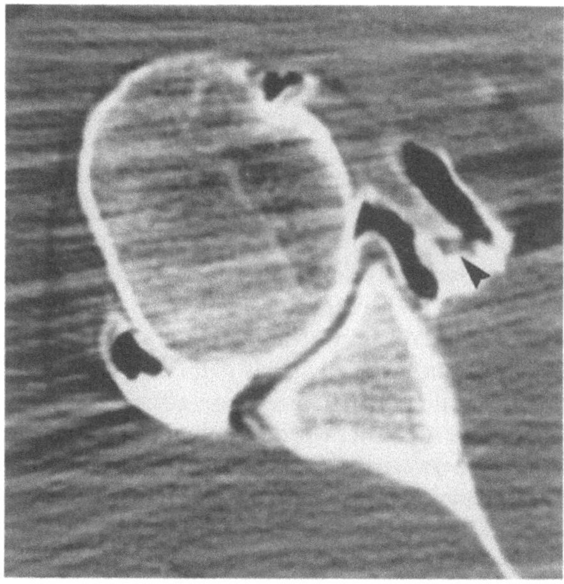

Fig. 6.8. Adult male with anterior instability showing evidence of periosteal new bone posteriorly and partial rupture of the subscapularis tendon (*black arrowhead*)

study demonstrated anterior glenoid tears, a figure similar to that noted by Resch and colleagues of 89% (SINGSON et al. 1987; RESCH et al. 1989). Other labral abnormalities include labral detachments, an attenuated or absent labrum (Figs. 6.2b, 6.7), and a partial labral detachment or tear at a site opposite to that expected for the direction of instability (Fig. 6.8; RAFII et al. 1987). Anterior capsular lesions defined by CTA have included marked medial scapular insertion, glenoid marginal stripping or detachment, and tears or loss of intervening scapular marginal soft tissues (SINGSON et al. 1987). A widened or rounded capsular reflection or enlarged redundant synovial recess is common. An actual tear of the capsule is uncommon in recurrent dislocators (RAFII et al. 1987). Capsular abnormalities tend to be more common and severe in those with recurrent dislocation than subluxation (SINGSON et al. 1987).

The GHLs can be difficult to visualise on CTA. Rafii and co-authors visualised the SGHL in all cases of instability (Fig. 6.9; RAFII et al. 1989). The MGHL and IGHL were seen in 60% and 50% of cases of instability, respectively. The GHLs often had an irregular outline. A Hill-Sachs deformity was an infrequent finding in this study. However, in 34% of patients, the findings on CTA were critical in making the diagnosis as the condition could not be confirmed clinically.

Subscapularis muscle and/or tendon abnormalities include tears and irregularities with widening of the subscapularis bursa (Fig. 6.8). Posterior instability is frequently associated with posterior labral or capsular tears and/or a wide recess well visualised at CTA. Distinct tears of the upper half of the posterior labrum may also be seen. Singson and co-authors noted anterior labral tears in 100% of those with posterior instability, and posterior labral abnormalities or posterior capsular tears were seen in a proportion of those with major anterior or anteroinferior instability (SINGSON et al. 1987).

Although labral tears are frequently associated with instability, they may be found in clinically stable shoulders, often associated with other pathology but also on occasion in isolation. The range of abnormalities is similar to that seen in unstable shoulders. The extent of injury to the labrum depends on the effect of pressure and grinding forces as the head slides out of the socket. The relationship of the radius of curvature of the humeral head to the glenoid and the angle of glenoid inclination relative to the bony socket can be assessed on CT. The angle of glenoid inclination changes greatly in the presence of damaged rim cartilage and may thus contribute to instability (RESCH et al. 1988).

In the athlete without shoulder instability, a superior labral tear due to the biceps pulling upon the labrum has been suggested. These lesions have been associated with the violent act of throwing as a result

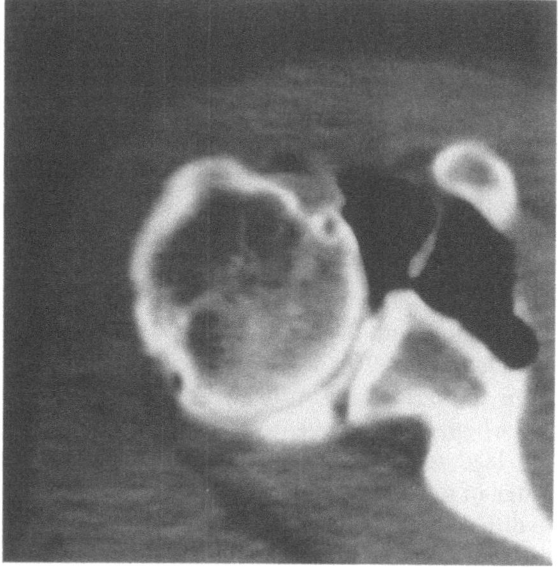

Fig. 6.9. Absent anterosuperior labrum and deficient origin of the SGHL. Compare with the normal appearances in Fig. 1a

of the contraction of the bicipital tendon on the labrum with which it shares a common insertion onto the supraglenoid tubercle. The inner margin of the labrum is not strongly attached to the glenoid, predisposing it to detachment. Labral separations are associated with degeneration and aging, and "athletic" use may accelerate the degenerative process. Anterior labral tears may also derive from an impingement between the humeral head and the subscapularis tendon during the act of throwing. Tears of the superior labrum, anterior and posterior (SLAP lesions), have assumed a greater importance in recent years. These are not easy to demonstrate on CTA despite what the literature claims (Fig. 6.9). Criteria for four different grades of lesion with arthroscopic correlation have been described (HUNTER et al. 1992). The changes, as seen on CTA, begin just below the insertion of biceps onto the supraglenoid area. Careful attention to the capsular reflection onto the anterior aspect of the base of the coracoid process is essential in identifying the SLAP lesion. Air abutting the bone without intervening soft tissue should suggest the diagnosis of a SLAP lesion.

6.7
Magnetic Resonance Imaging

Magnetic resonance (MR) imaging was initially heralded as a major advance in shoulder imaging because of its capabilities of multiplanar imaging and superb soft tissue contrast. Its acceptance as a diagnostic technique has, however, lagged behind MR imaging of other areas such as the knee for a variety of reasons. The shoulder is a technically difficult area to image. It is displaced from the isocentre of the magnet in the periphery of the field. There is no ideal surface coil as the shoulder is not suited to a circular design. The early magnets could only scan in the orthogonal planes which differ from the planes of the important structures in the shoulder. The area is prone to artefacts from the thorax including the cardiac rhythm and the respiratory cycle. Coil burnout can also occur. This is due to excessive high signal from the tissues immediately adjacent to the coil. Since high signal frequently indicates pathology, this can lead to diagnostic confusion. There is a wide range of normal variants, and there can be difficulty in differentiating the normal from the abnormal and the symptomatic from the asymptomatic.

The technique protocol can vary and will largely depend on the magnet and the individual preference of the supervising radiologist. The patient is positioned supine with the arm along the side of the body, ensuring that it does not actually rest on the abdomen as this will incur respiratory motion artefact. The arm is positioned in slight external rotation. A series of sequences is then obtained in three planes. Axial images are used in the specific evaluation of the glenoid labrum, the capsule, the GHLs and the humerus for a Hill-Sachs deformity. T1-weighted (T1W) images to define anatomy and T2-weighted (T2W) spin-echo images are obtained. The T2W sequence is particularly helpful in demonstrating intraarticular structures if an effusion is present (Fig. 6.10). A gradient-echo sequence provides good contrast between the labrum and other structures. The coronal oblique sequence is oriented along the plane of the supraspinatus tendon and is helpful in evaluation of the superior labrum and bicipital tendon and more specifically in the evaluation of the rotator cuff for tears, impingement or tendinopathy. Gradient-echo sequences are particularly susceptible to the magic angle phenomenon in the rotator cuff area and thus may give rise to some diagnostic confusion. The sagittal image lies perpendicular to the supraspinatus tendon and parallel to the glenoid and is specifically useful in the evaluation of the coracoacromial arch and subacromial structures (Fig. 6.1c). It may also provide valuable information on the state of the superior labrum. A short-tau inversion-recovery sequence (STIR) is valuable in acute injuries in the assessment particularly of a bone "bruise" in the humeral head. Further external rotation of the shoulder, especially during the acquisition of the axial images, may lead to a slight increase in the diagnostic sensitivity regarding the detection of tears of the anteroinferior labrum (TUITE et al. 1994).

MR imaging appearances of the normal shoulder, normal variants and potential pitfalls in interpretation are well described (KAPLAN et al. 1992; LIOU et al. 1993; NEUMANN et al. 1991). "Undercutting" the base of the glenoid labrum by the articular cartilage is a known pitfall simulating a tear on MR (KAPLAN et al. 1992; Fig. 6.1b). Although it was originally stated that undercutting does not normally extend through the full thickess of the labral base, in contrast to a labral tear which does, LIOU and co-authors (1993) showed a full-thickness undercutting in the majority of cases, thus questioning the reliability of this sign. This study also showed that the SGHL is infrequently identified probably due to its small size and its course paralleling the plane of imaging. Its proximity to the biceps tendon also makes differen-

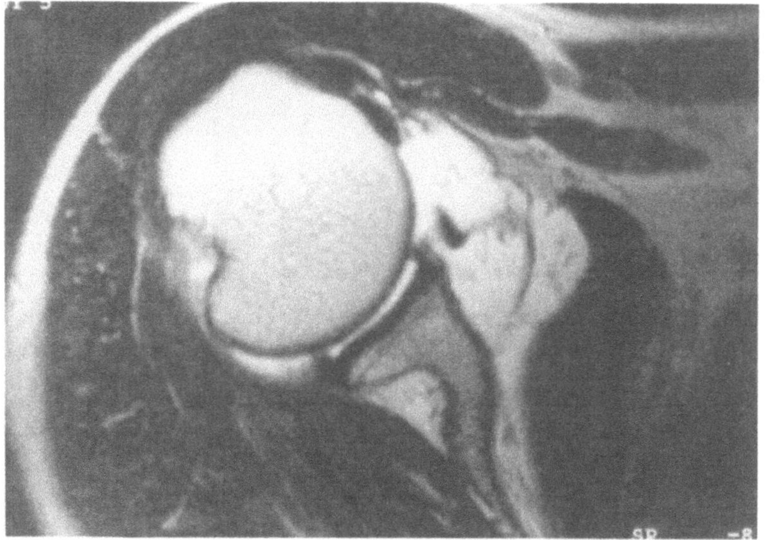

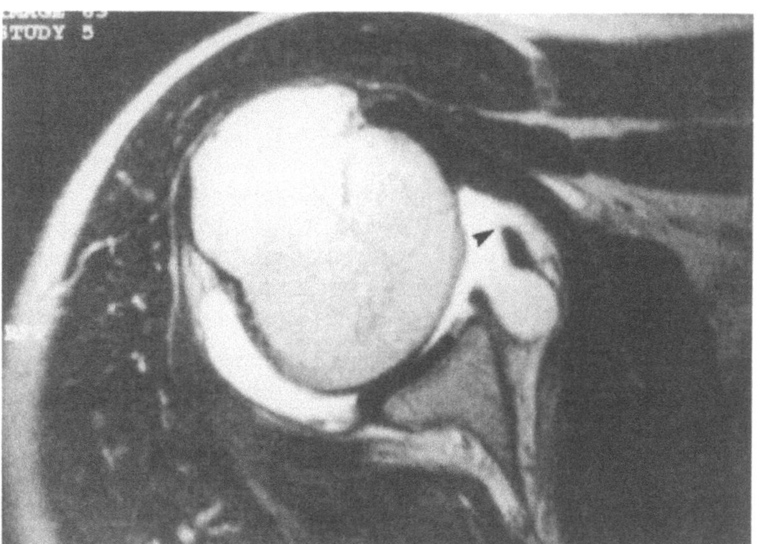

Fig. 6.10. a Axial T2W MR image in the presence of a joint effusion showing a Hill-Sachs deformity and anterior capsular stripping. **b** Axial T2W MR image (same patient as in **a**) showing elevation of the anterior labrum with a torn MGHL (*black arrowhead*)

tiation of these two structures at MR imaging difficult. The MGHL and the IGHL may be congenitally absent in 25% of patients. LIOU and colleagues (1993) also suggested that normal GHLs could be confused as representing labral tears to those unfamiliar with the location and appearance of the GHLs (Fig. 6.1b). This difficulty in interpretation has been in large part overcome by the more recent introduction of MR arthrography (see below). Proton density images demonstrate the GHLs more frequently than other imaging sequences. These ligaments are seldom seen on T2W images because of the low signal-to-noise ratio. The IGHL labral complex is easily confused with a labrum that has a signal extending to its surface. This complex anatomy may be one rea-

son for discrepancies reported by different authors for the accuracy of MR imaging in the diagnosis of labral tears. Other factors contributing to difficulties in assessment have included the close apposition of the GHLs to the anterior labrum and also the variability in the size and shape of the normal labrum.

NEUMANN and co-authors (1991) reported various anterior labral appearances in asymptomatic shoulders at MR imaging, with absence of the labrum in 6% of cases. Intrinsic labral signal was noted on proton density images but never on T2W images.

The range of labral abnormalities associated with glenohumeral instability can be depicted on MR imaging. These include labral tears, detachments and labral attenuation (Fig. 6.11). Labral degeneration is

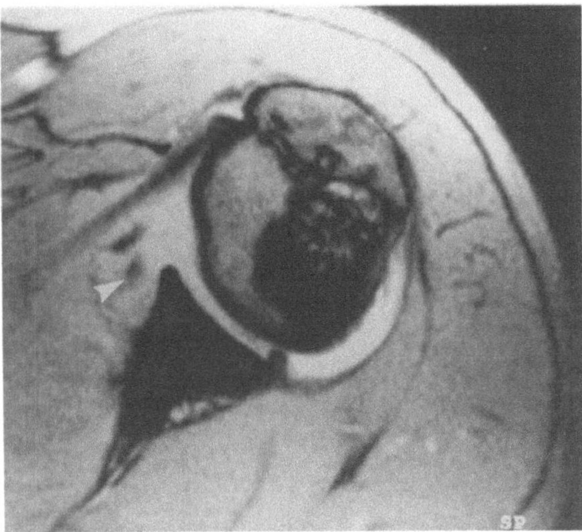

Fig. 6.11. Axial gradient-echo MR image showing a detached anterior labrum (*white arrowhead*) lying immediately posterior to the MGHL. A compression fracture of the greater tuberosity is also present

also apparent. Disruptions in the shape, location or signal intensity of the labrum help to identify the abnormality. Glenoid labral tears are characterised by areas of linear or complex increased signal intensity extending through the labrum on T1W or gradient-echo (GRE) T2*-weighted (T2W*) images (GROSS et al. 1990). Labral fraying without a discrete tear may be indicative of degenerative change.

The ability to accurately define labral lesions is important because treatment of shoulder problems varies according to specific aetiology. Labral tears have been shown to cause mechanical symptoms, while a detachment of the glenoid-labrum-inferior glenohumeral ligament complex results in instability. Complete labral degeneration may cause instability but, unlike a detached labrum, is not repairable by arthroscopic techniques. MRI has been used for evaluation of the labrum and capsuloligamentous complex with varying success. The gold standard is usually taken as arthroscopy. GREEN and CHRISTENSEN (1994) reported a sensitivity of 75%, a specificity of 100%, positive and negative predictive values of 100% and 41%, respectively, and an accuracy rate of 79% in the diagnosis of labral tears on MR imaging. However, correlation of the findings at MR imaging with a surgical classification defined by arthroscopy enabled accurate classification with MRI in only 21% of labra with the precision necessary to affect surgical planning, leading to the conclusion that MRI was not useful in surgical planning

for most patients with obvious anterior instability. GROSS and colleagues (1990), however, noted an excellent correlation between surgical findings and MRI although they did not specificaly seek to compare a surgical classification with that of the MR findings.

Capsular stripping may not be well appreciated on MR imaging owing to the lack of distension of the subscapularis recess. However, separation of the capsule from the bony glenoid can be readily detected if a joint effusion is present (Fig. 6.10; KIEFT et al. 1988; COUMAS et al. 1992). Alternatively, performing an arthrogram, by distending the joint, may enhance and facilitate diagnostic interpretation and this has remained an important advantage of CTA over MR imaging (KIEFT et al. 1988). However, in the presence of a rotator cuff tear, which may be present with instability, there can be difficulty with CTA in evaluating the labrum and capsular structures due to extravasation of contrast medium and air. This problem does not occur with MR imaging (HABIBIAN et al. 1989).

The bone changes seen in instability can be readily depicted on MRI, including the bony Bankart's lesion and the Hill-Sachs lesion (Figs. 6.12–6.14). MR imaging also allows assessment of bone changes in both the acute and chronic situation. In an acute dislocation, fluid within the joint may distend the capsule and optimally demonstrate capsular stripping, readily identify labral tears and detachments, and show increased signal within a

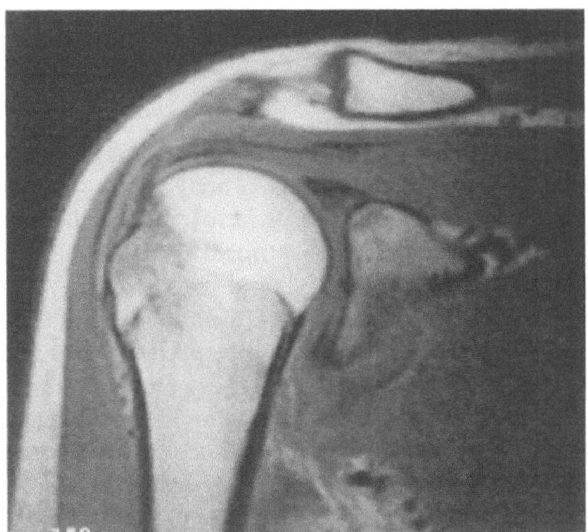

Fig. 6.12. Coronal oblique T1W MR image following acute anterior dislocation showing the compression fracture of the greater tuberosity

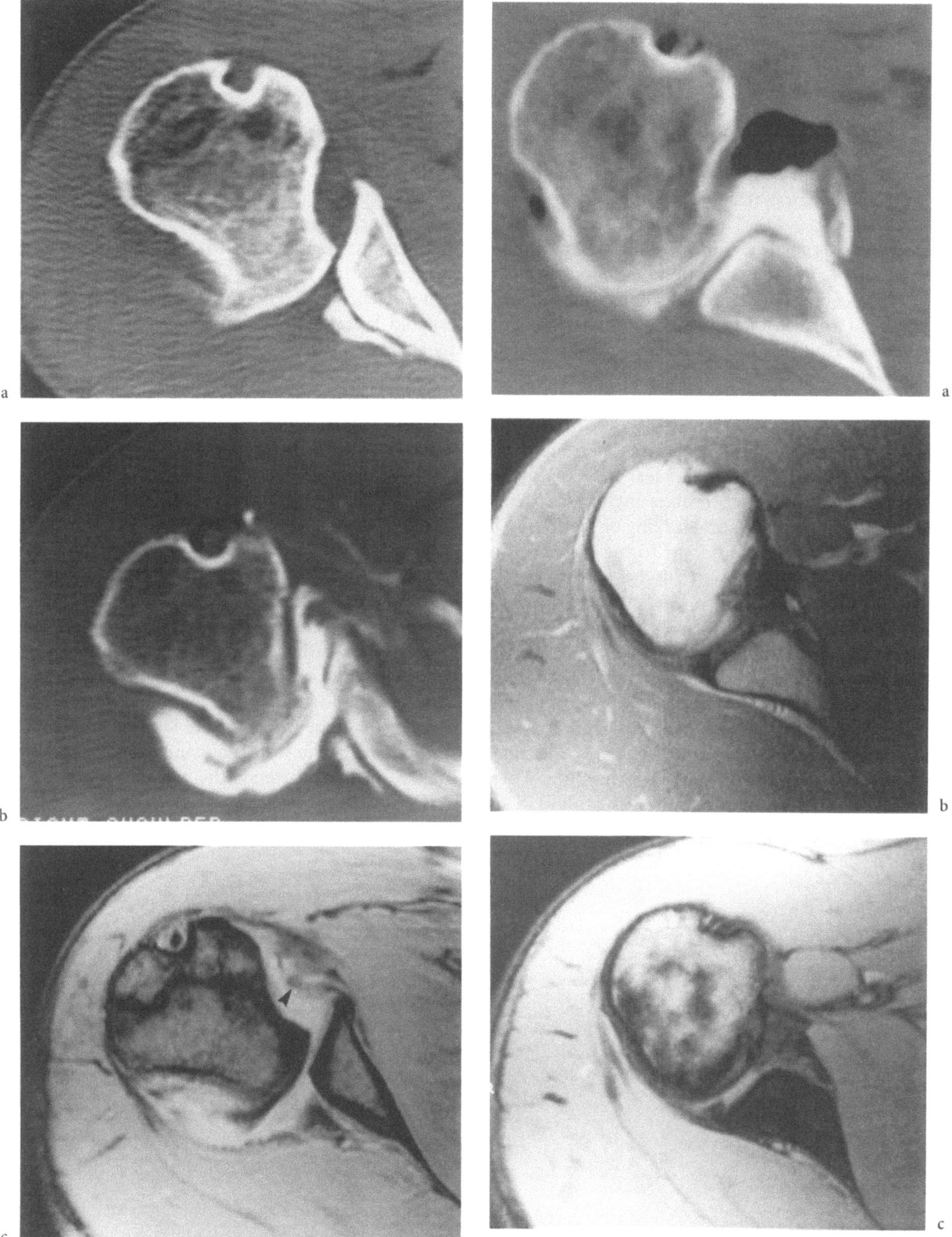

Fig. 6.13. a,b CTA pre- and post-arthrographic contrast medium showing chronic multidirectional instability with normal and reversed Hill-Sachs defects and a fracture of the posterior glenoid. The posterior labrum is absent. c Axial gradient MR image showing comparable bony anatomy to a and b. A lax MGHL is also shown (*black arrowhead*)

Fig. 6.14. a CTA showing a fracture of the anterior glenoid with displacement of the bone and labrum. b Axial proton density MR image of the same patient as in a showing bony changes, but the labrum cannot be clearly identified. c Axial gradient-echo MR image of the same patient as in a demonstrating the bony changes, but again the anterior labrum cannot be clearly identified

Hill-Sachs defect. High signal intensity (SI) on T1W may also be identified with a haemarthrosis. Trough-line compression fractures and other bone injuries including bone bruises may also be seen.

Glenoid labral cysts, often located in the spino-glenoid or suprascapular notch, are associated with glenoid labral tears and shoulder instability (TIRMAN et al. 1994). The presence of a Hill-Sachs lesion has prognostic significance regarding the like-lihood of recurrent dislocation and may indicate prior dislocation. The Hill-Sachs defect must be dif-ferentiated from an anatomic indentation in the pos-terolateral aspect of the humerus, and this can be readily achieved on MR imaging (WORKMAN et al. 1992; RICHARDS et al. 1994).

Labral pathology as an isolated source of shoulder pain is being increasingly recognised, particularly in throwers, swimmers and athletes participating in overhead activities. Such lesions include flap tears and those tears seen as labral fraying or separation in the anatomical region adjacent to the long head of the biceps. The attachment of the labrum to the glenoid anteriorly and also particularly superiorly may be loose, and central detachments in the region of the biceps interval are well described. In the ab-sence of instability and labral deficiency, their clini-cal significance has been questioned (SCHWEITZER 1994). These superior labral anterior and posterior (SLAP) lesions are being more frequently identified as a result of improved imaging techniques. These lesions are relatively uncommon, being found in ap-proximately 3.9% of all arthroscopies (SNYDER et al.

1990). The coronal oblique plane can be the most useful in their identification, with intermediate to high signal of "Y" or "T" shape traversing the glenoid labrum (MONU et al. 1994). The MR findings re-ported as being characteristic of these lesions in-clude increased signal intensity in the glenoid labrum with or without extension into the biceps tendon anchor and cleavage in the superior part of the glenoid labrum which is best seen on coronal images as high signal intensity extending into the glenoid labrum (Fig. 6.15; CARTLAND et al. 1992). Isolated labral lesions can be treated with surgical debridement via the arthroscope. It is important, however, to ensure that the labral tear is not associ-ated with other evidence of instability since, if the destabilising lesion is not treated in addition, there is likely to be a recurrence of symptoms (PAYNE 1994).

In the absence of intraarticular contrast medium anterior labral lesions are reported with sensitivities varying from 44% to 95% and specificities of 67%–86% (Fig. 6.14; GARNEAU et al. 1991; IANOTTI et al. 1991; LEGAN et al. 1991). Superior labral tears are detected with less reliability (LEGAN et al. 1991). There is also a reduced sensitivity for the detection of posterior labral tears. The potential reasons for this have been alluded to above, including normal varia-tions in the appearance of the labrum and also the variability in the capsuloligamentous attachment sites. Joint fluid distends the capsule, separates the GHLs, fills labral tears and displaces detached labra, and thus greatly facilitates visualisation and conse-

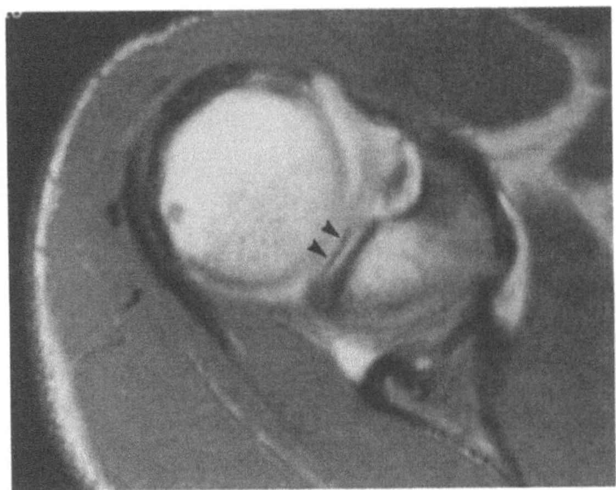

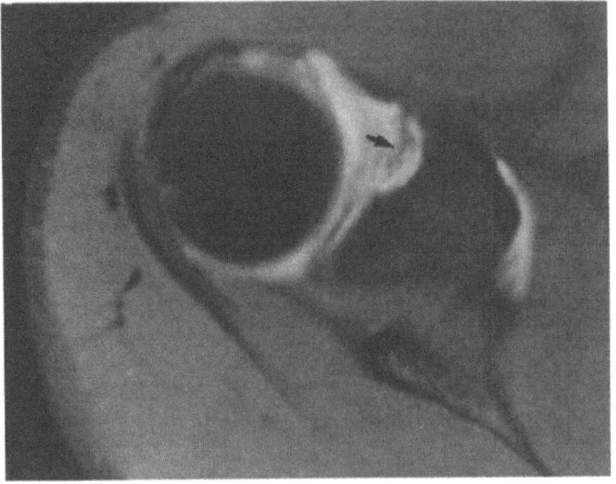

Fig. 6.15. a T1W and **b** T1W fat saturation MR images show-ing separation of the superior labrum from the rim of the glenoid (SLAP) lesion (*arrowheads*). This can be more clearly identified on the axial fat saturation T1W image (**b**) than on the conventional T1W sequence (**a**). The adjacent SGHL is clearly damaged (*black arrow*). *SLAP*, superior labrum, ante-rior and posterior

quently interpretation and diagnosis. In the absence of an effusion the reintroduction of arthrography has improved the opportunity for accurate diagnosis (Fig. 6.10).

6.8
Magnetic Resonance Arthrography

In the early 1990s there was much debate about the usefulness or otherwise of MR imaging in evaluation of glenohumeral instability and indeed rotator cuff tears of the shoulder. The results of MR imaging were disappointing, and confidence in image interpretation was variable. More recently an increasing number of studies have appeared in the literature looking at results with MR arthrography. This technique, although invasive, combines the advantages of standard MR imaging, that is multiplanar imaging and high contrast resolution, with joint distension and the benefits which that incurs, notably excellent visualisation of many of the intraarticular structures (Fig. 6.16; FLANNIGAN et al. 1990; PALMER et al. 1995).

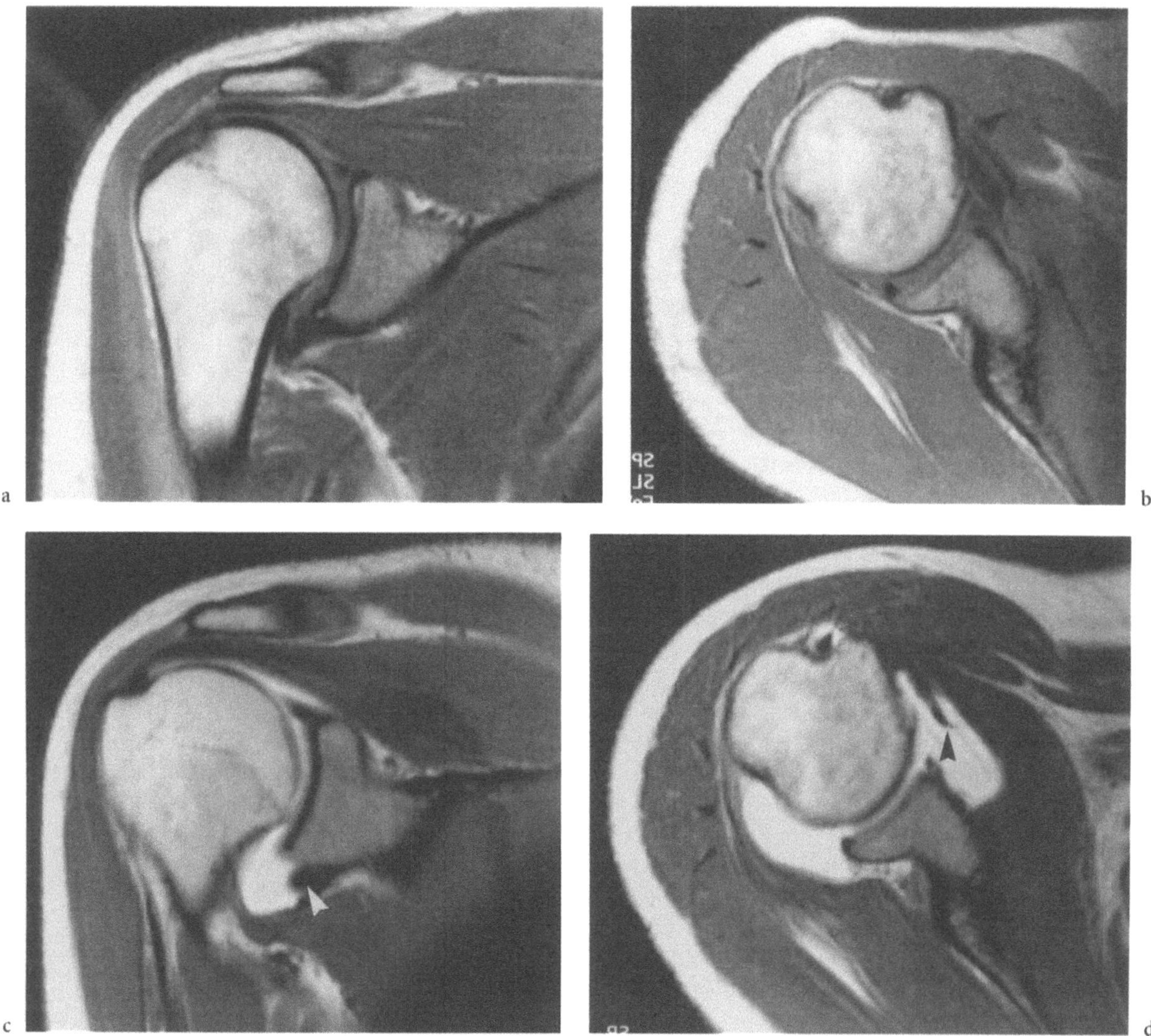

Fig. 6.16a–d. Coronal oblique and axial T1W MR images pre- (a, b) and post-arthrogram (c, d). The anteroinferior Bankart lesion is better demonstrated on the post-arthrogram scans (c, d). In particular, the displacement of the inferior labrum can be seen on the coronal oblique image (c; *white arrowhead*), and the deficient MGHL is seen on the axial image (d; *black arrowhead*)

The actual technique of arthrography is similar to that described above, but the nature of the contrast medium, its concentration and volume differ. Many radiologists will initially inject a small amount of iodinated contrast medium to ensure a satisfactory intraarticular location of the needle tip, and then follow this with a variable amount of gadopentetate dimeglumine. The volume used may vary, but a total volume of 12–15 ml of saline should ideally be employed in a single contrast technique to distend the joint satisfactorily. Larger volumes may sometimes be used, particularly when there has been capsular stripping and the joint is capacious. The patient will invariably indicate if the joint distension is proving uncomfortable, but adhesive capsulitis is not usually a problem in these patients. Air is not used in MR arthrography since it tends to cause artefact and interfere with image interpretation. Different concentrations of gadopentetate dimeglumine in saline have been tried, ranging from 2.5 to 45 mmol/l (KOPKA et al. 1994). The interaction between both the iodinated contrast agent and the gadopentetate will determine the contrast-to-noise ratio and the ultimate signal intensity achieved. The imaging sequence protocol will be determined by the preference of the individual radiologist. We have used T1W and a T1W with fat-saturation spin-echo sequence in all three planes with satisfactory results (Figs. 6.15, 6.16). A small amount of adrenaline (0.1 ml of a 1:1000 solution) can be injected intraarticularly during the procedure, as in CTA, to delay absorption of the contrast medium if MR imaging is not to be immediate. It should be noted that in certain countries there is as yet no licence for the intraarticular injection of gadopentetate, and a check with the oppropriate regulatory authority may be required before using this contrast agent in this way for the first time.

MR arthrography can overcome many of the potential sources of error found with conventional standard MR imaging of the shoulder. Hyaline cartilage has a lower signal intensity than the contrast solution and a potential pitfall on conventional MR imaging of hyaline cartilage undercutting the labrum simulating a pseudo-ear does not occur. This is because contrast material fills tears and outlines the contours of deficient labra (Fig. 6.16). The GHLs are separated from the glenoid margin and labrum by the distended joint capsule and thus can be readily differentiated from labral fragments, and the GHLs can be followed to their capsular insertions. Abnormalities and tears of the GHLs themselves can be more readily appreciated (Figs. 6.15, 6.16). Normal sublabral sulci, however, remain a source of diagnostic confusion (PALMER et al. 1995). Normal sulci may occur at the base of either the superior labrum at its junction with the bicipital tendon, or in the anterosuperior labrum between the origins of the MGHL and the IGHL. A sublabral region of contrast medium confined to these locations is not diagnostic of a tear unless the labrum is displaced from the hyaline cartilage (PALMER et al. 1994).

The GHLs are more frequently identified at MR arthrography than on conventional MR imaging (Figs. 6.15, 6.16). CHANDNANI et al. (1995) identified the SGHL, the MGHL and the IGHL in 85%, 85% and 91% of patients, respectively. In the diagnosis of tears of the GHLs, MR arthrography had a sensitivity of 100%, 89% and 88%, respectively, with a specificity of 94%, 88% and 100%, respectively. Labral tears in the superior, inferior, anterior and posterior regions had sensitivities of 89%, 97%, 92% and 100%, respectively, with specificitieis of 88%, 86%, 100% and 100%, respectively. Similar sensitivities and specificities for labral tears of 91% and 93% were found by Palmer and co-authors (PALMER et al. 1994), with these figures being reproduced in a further study (PALMER and CASLOWITZ 1995). Inferior labral-ligamentous lesions enabled prediction of anterior instability with 76% sensitivity and 98% specificity. It was also found in this important study that capsular insertion sites had no role in the prediction of capsular instability.

A comparative study of MR imaging, MR arthrography and CTA showed MRI and MR arthrography to be more sensitive in the detection of labral tears than CTA. MR arthrography was the most sensitive for detached labral fragments and labral degeneration and also best visualised the inferior part of the labrum and the IGHL (CHANDNANI et al. 1993).

The capability of MR arthrography to accurately demonstrate the precise sites of abnormalities of the labrum and/or the GHLs is clinically important. Preoperative knowledge of these lesions may be useful in guiding the surgical approach.

6.9
Management of Shoulder Instability

Treatment of a primary dislocation usually involves a period of immobilisation with restriction of athletic activities involving the joint and physiotherapy of the muscles about the joint. These conservative measures are unlikely to prevent recurrence. The development of recurrent instability appears to be a multifactorial scenario. There has been much discussion about the "essential" lesion in recurrent instability. As we have seen from the earlier discussion, there are many factors that may be responsible for or at least contribute to recurrent instability. Management is directed towards trying to correct or repair the traumatic lesion. In the past this was felt to be most frequently due to a bony Bankart lesion. However, with advances in imaging particularly of the soft tissues, increasing attention is being focussed on the inferior glenohumeral ligament-labral complex as the area most prone to damage. Arthroscopic repair of torn labra and damaged or disrupted ligaments is attractive because it decreases trauma to the joint and reduces the risk of losing motion, specifically external rotation after the repair. However, despite various studies comparing techniques, arthroscopic repair does not compare favourably with open repair for preventing post-operative recurrence of stability problems. This is usually because the entire defect has not been repaired or indeed visualised satisfactorily at the first procedure.

As experience in arthroscopy increases, many surgeons are employing the technique as a diagnostic procedure with therapeutic options either through the arthroscope or proceeding to an open procedure, depending on the findings. As a result of this, the amount of pre-operative imaging of the unstable shoulder has decreased considerably in some centres.

6.10
Conclusion

The principal pathology in shoulder instability is frequently a combination of labral and capsular damage with, more specifically, implication of damage to the IGHL. Improvement in imaging techniques has resulted in better visualisation and delineation of intraarticular structures with consequent increase in accuracy and confidence of diagnostic interpretation. Arthroscopy is likely to remain the gold standard, purely because of direct visualisation, but as with all techniques, its accuracy will be operator-dependent.

Arthrography, whether combined with CT or MRI, is probably the imaging modality of choice. MRI without intraarticular contrast, but with careful attention to technique including thin sections and appropriate selection of sequences is satisfactory in experienced hands. Distension of the joint with fluid, however, enhances anatomical and pathological delineation. The final choice of technique will depend on local availability of equipment and ultimately on individual preference.

Acknowledgement. The authors would like to thank the Medical Photography Department of the Robert Jones & Agnes Hunt Orthopaedic Hospital for preparing the illustrations.

References

Adams JC (1950) The humeral head defect in recurrent anterior dislocation of the shoulder. Br J Radiol 23:151–156

Arndt JG, Sears AD (1965) Posterior dislocation of the shoulder. AJR Am J Roentgenol 94:639–645

Bankart ASB (1938) The pathology and treatment of recurrent dislocation of the shoulder joint. Br J Sung 26:23–29

Beltran J, Gray LA, Bools JC, Zuelzer W, Weis LD, Unverferth LJ (1986) Rotator cuff lesions of the shoulder: evaluation by direct sagittal CT arthrography. Radiology 160:161–165

Cartland JP, Crues JV III, Stauffer A, Nottage W, Ryu RKN (1992) MR imaging in the evaluation of SLAP injuries of the shoulder. AJR Am J Roentgenol 159:787–792

Chandnani VP, Yeager TD, DeBerardino T (1993) Glenoid labral tears: prospective evaluation with MR imaging, MR arthrography and CT arthrography. AJR Am J Roentgenol 161:1229–1235

Chandnani VP, Gagliardi JA, Murnane TG, Bradley YC, DeBerardino TA, Spaeth J, Hansen MF (1995) Glenohumeral ligaments and shoulder capsular mechanism: evaluation with MR arthrography. Radiology 196:27–32

Cooper DE, Arnoczky SP, O'Brien SJ, et al. (1992) Anatomy, histology and vascularity of the glenoid labrum: an anatomical study. J Bone Joint Surg [Am] 74:46–52

Coumas JM, Waite RJ, Goss TP, Ferrari DA, Kanzaria PK, Pappas AM (1992) CT and MR evaluation of the labral capsular ligamentous complex of the shoulder. AJR Am J Roentgenol 158:591–597

Deutsch AL, Resnick D, Mink JH, et al. (1984) Computed and conventional arthrotomography of the glenohumeral joint: normal anatomy and clinical experience. Radiology 153:603–609

Didiee J (1930) Le radiodiagnostic dans le luxation récidivante de l'épaule. J Radiol Electrol 14:209–218

Eyre-Brook AL (1948) Recurrent dislocation of the shoulder: lesions discovered in 17 cases, surgery employed and intermediate report on results. J Bone Joint Surg [Br] 30:39–46

Flannigan B, Kursunoglu-Brahme S, Snyder J, Karzel R, Del Pizzo W, Resnick D (1990) MR arthrography of the shoulder: comparison with conventional MR imaging. AJR Am J Roentgenol 155:829–832

Garneau RA, Renfrew DL, Moore TE, El-Khoury GY, Nepola JV, Lemke JH (1991) Glenoid labrum: evaluation with MR imaging. Radiology 179:519–522

Garth WP, Slappey CE, Ochs CW (1984) Roentgenographic demonstration of instability of the shoulder: the apical oblique projection – a technical note. J Bone Joint Surg [Am]66:1450–1453

Goldman AB, Ghelman B (1978) The double contrast shoulder arthrogram. Radiology 127:655–663

Green MR, Christensen KP (1994) Magnetic resonance imaging of the glenoid labrum in anterior shoulder instability. Am J Sports Med 22:493–498

Gross ML, Seeger LL, Smith JB, Mandelbaum BR, Finerman GAM (1990) Magnetic resonance imaging of the glenoid labrum. Am J Sports Med 18:229–234

Habibian A, Stauffer A, Resnick D, et al. (1989) Comparison of conventional and computed arthrotomography with MR imaging in the evaluation of the shoulder. J Comput Assist Tomogr 13:968–975

Hall RH, Isaac F, Booth CR (1959) Dislocation of the shoulder with special reference to accompanying small fractures. J Bone Joint Surg [Am] 41:489–494

Hawkins RJ, Mohtadi NGH (1991) Clinical evaluation of shoulder instability. Clin J Sports Med 1:59–64

Hill HA, Sachs M (1940) The grooved defect of the humeral head: a frequently unrecognised complication of dislocation of the shoulder joint. Radiology 35:690–700

Horsfield D (1991) Radiography of the shoulder. In: Watson MS (ed) Surgical disorders of the shoulder. Churchill Livingstone, Edinburgh, p 83

Horsfield D, Jones SN (1987) A useful projection in the radiography of the shoulder. J Bone Joint Surg [Br] 69:338

Hunter JC, Blatz DJ, Escobedo EM (1992) SLAP lesions of the glenoid labrum: CT arthrography and arthroscopic correlation. Radiology 184:513–518

Ianotti JP, Zlatkin MB, Esterhai JL, Kressel HY, Dalinka MK, Spindler KP (1991) Magnetic resonance of the shoulder. J Bone Joint Surg [Am] 73:17–29

Kaplan PA, Bryans KC, Davick JP, Otte M, Stinson WW, Dussault RG (1992) MR imaging of the normal shoulder: variants and pitfalls. Radiology 184:519–524

Kieft GJ, Bloem JL, Rozing PM, Obermann WR (1988) MR imaging of recurrent anterior dislocation of the shoulder: comparison with CT arthrography. AJR Am J Roentgenol 150:1083–1087

Kopka L, Funke M, Fischer U, Keating D, Oestmann J, Grabbe E (1994) MR arthrography of the shoulder with gadopentetate dimeglumine. AJR Am J Roentgenol 163:621–623

Lawrence WS (1915) New position in radiography of the shoulder. AJR Am J Roentgenol 2:728–730

Lazarus MD, Sidler JA, Harryman DT II Matsen FA (1996) Effect of a chondral labral defect on glenoid concavity and glenohumeral stability. J Bone Joint Surg [Am] 78:94–102

Legan JM, Burkhard TK, Goff WB II (1991) Tears of the glenoid labrum: MR imaging of 88 arthroscopically confirmed cases. Radiology 179:241–246

Liou JTS, Wilson AJ, Totty WG, Brown JJ (1993) The normal shoulder: common variations that simulate pathologic conditions at MR imaging. Radiology 186:435–411

Manns RA, Davies AM (1991) Glenoid hypoplasia: assessment by computed tomographic arthrography. Clin Radiol 43:316–320

McLaughlin HL (1952) Posterior dislocation of the shoulder. J Bone Joint Surg [Am] 34:584–590

McNiesh LM, Callaghan JJ (1987) CT arthrography of the shoulder: variations of the glenoid labrum. AJR Am J Roentgenol 149:963–966

Monu JUV, Pope TL Jr, Chabon SJ, Vanarthos WJ (1994) MR diagnosis of superior labral anterior posterior (SLAP) injuries of the glenoid labrum. AJR Am J Roentgenol 163:1425–1429

Moseley HF, Overgaard B (1962) The anterior capsular mechanism in recurrent anterior dislocation of the shoulder. J Bone Joint Surg [Br] 44:913–927

Neer CS (1970) Displaced proximal humeral fractures. Classification and evaluation. J Bone Joint Surg [Am] 52:1077–1089

Neumann CH, Petersen SA, Jahnke AH (1991) MR imaging of the labral capsular complex; normal variations. AJR Am J Roentgenol 157:1015–1021

Palmer WE, Caslowitz PL (1995) Anterior shoulder instability: diagnostic criteria determined from prospective analysis of 121 MR arthrograms. Radiology 197:819–825

Palmer WE, Brown JH, Rosenthal DI (1994) Labral-ligamentous complex of the shoulder: evaluation with MR arthorgraphy. Radiology 190:645–651

Palmer WE, Caslowitz PL, Chew FS (1995) MR arthrography of the shoulder: normal intraarticular structures and common abnormalities. AJR Am J Roentgenol 164:141–146

Payne LZ (1994) Tears of the glenoid labrum. Orthop Rev 23:577–583

Rafert J, Long BW, Hernandez EM, Kreipke DL (1990) Axillary shoulder with exaggerated rotation; the Hill-Sachs defect. Radiol Technol 62:18–25

Rafii M, Firooznia H, Golimba C, Minkoff J, Bonamo J (1986) CT arthrography of capsular structures of the shoulder. AJR Am J Roentgenol 146:361–367

Rafii M, Firooznia H, Bonamo JJ, Minkoff J, Golimba C (1987) Athlete shoulder injuries: CT arthrographic findings. Radiology 162:559–564

Rafii M, Minkoff J, Bonamo JJ, Firooznia H, Jaffe L, Golimba C, Sherman O (1988) Computed tomography (CT) arthrography of shoulder instabilities in athletes. Am J Sports Med 16:352–361

Reeves B (1966) Arthrography of the shoulder. J Bone Joint Surg [Br] 48:424–435

Resch H, Helweg G, Zur Nedden D, Beck E (1988) Double contrast computed tomographic examination techniques in habitual and recurrent shoulder dislocation. Eur J Radiol 8:6–12

Richards RD, Sartoris DJ, Pathria MN, Resnick D (1994) Hill-Sachs lesion and normal humeral groove: MR imaging features allowing their differentiation. Radiology 190:665–668

Richardson JB, Ramsay A, Davidson JK, Kelly IG (1988) Radiographs in shoulder trauma. J Bone Joint Surg [Br] 70:457–460

Rokous JR, Feagin JA, Abott HG (1972) Modified axillary roentgenogram. Clin Orthop 82:84–86

Rowe CR, Patal D (1978) The Bankart procedure; a long-term end result study. J Bone Joint Surg [Am] 60:1–16

Rowe CR, Sakellarides HT (1961) Factors relating to recurrence of anterior dislocation of the shoulder. Clin Orthop 20:40–47

Rubin SA, Gray RL, Green WR (1974) The scapular "Y": a diagnostic aid in shoulder trauma. Radiology 110:725–726

Schweitzer ME (1994) MR arthrography of the labral ligamentous complex of the shoulder. Radiology 190:641–647

Singson RD, Feldman F, Bigliani L (1987) CT arthographic patterns in recurrent glenohumeral instability. AJR Am J Roentgenol 149:749–753

Snyder SJ, Karzel RP, Del Pizzo W, Ferkel RD (1990) SLAP lesions of the shoulder. Arthroscopy 6:274–279

Symeonides PP (1972) The significance of the subscapularis muscle in the pathogenesis of recurrent anterior dislocation of the shoulder. J Bone Joint Surg [Br] 54:476–483

Tirman PFJ, Feller JF, Lanzen DL, Peterfy CG, Bergman AG (1994) Association of glenoid labral cysts with labral tears and glenohumeral instability: radiologic findings and clinical significance. Radiology 190:653–658

Tijnes J, Loyd HM, Tullos HS (1979) Arthrography in acute shoulder dislocations. South Med J 72:564–567

Townley CO (1950) The capsular mechanism in recurrent dislocation of the shoulder. J Bone Joint Surg [Am] 32:370–380

Trout TE, Resnick D (1996) Glenoid hypoplasia and its relationship to instability. Skeletal Radiol 25:37–40

Tuite MJ, De Smet AA, Norris MA, Orwin JF (1994) MR diagnosis of labral tears of the shoulder: value of T2*-weighted gradient-recalled echo images made in external rotaion. AJR Am J Roentgenol 164:941–944

Turner PJ, O'Connor PJ, Saifuddin A, Williams J, Coral A, Butt WP (1994) Prone oblique positioning for computed tomographic arthrography of the shoulder. Br J Radiol 67:835–839

Wirth MA, Lyons MB, Rockwood CA (1993) Hypoplasia of the glenoid. J Bone Joint Surg [Am] 75:1175–1183

Workman TL, Burkhard TK, Resnick D, Goff WB II, Balsara ZN, Davis DJ, Lapoint JM (1992) Hill-Sachs lesion – comparison of detection with MR imaging, radiography and arthroscopy. Radiology 185:847–852

Vastamaki M, Solonen K (1980) Posterior dislocation and fracture dislocation of the shoulder. Acta Orthop Scand 51:479–484

Zlatkin MB, Bjorkengren AG, Gylys-Morin V, et al. (1988) Cross-sectional imaging of the capsular mechanism of the glenohumeral joint. AJR Am J Roentgenol 150:151–158

7 Instability of the Elbow and Wrist

E.R. Tjin A Ton[1], R.C. Fritz[2], and W.R. Obermann[3]

CONTENTS

7.1
Introduction

Interpreting radiographs and other diagnostic modalities of patients with carpal instability can be difficult. The anatomy and kinematics of the wrist are complex. The highly mobile wrist is composed of multiple interlocking bones bridged by intrinsic and extrinsic ligaments that allow complex motion and give stability to the joint. There is a spectrum of carpal injuries that ranges from sprains, carpal instability, fractures and (sub)luxations to fracture dislocation. Misdiagnoses can be minimized by understanding of the anatomy, kinematics and injury patterns of this joint. It is also useful to know the statistical frequency of injury at various sites and the orthopedic classifications of such injuries.

The diagnosis and treatment of elbow instability has caused considerable confusion in the past but has recently become better understood. There have been significant advances in both clinical and basic research regarding the stability of the elbow joint. There is currently a greater understanding of the pathoanatomy, kinematics, injury mechanisms, signs and symptoms, imaging diagnosis, and management of elbow instability. Sections. 7.5 and 7.6 will focus on MR imaging in the diagnosis of elbow instability.

7.2
Wrist Anatomy

The osseous structures of the wrist consist of the distal radius and ulna, carpal bones, and the bases of the metacarpal bones. The carpus is composed of eight bones arranged in proximal and distal rows. The proximal carpal row consists of the scaphoid, the lunate, the triquetrum and the pisiform. Although the pisiform bone traditionally is considered part of the proximal carpal row, actually it is a sesamoid bone of the flexor carpi ulnaris tendon and does not participate in carpal motion. The distal carpal row consists of the trapezium, the trapezoid, the capitate and the hamate.

According to arthrographic studies, the wrist contains three major separate joint compartments: the distal radioulnar, the radiocarpal and the midcarpal joints. The midcarpal compartment communicates with the carpometacarpal joints 2–5. Usually the first carpometacarpal joint is a separate compartment. OBERMANN (1994) found in 68% of cases that the pisotriquetral joint communicates with the radiocarpal compartment.

The ligamentous anatomy of the wrist is complex, allowing dorsovolar flexion, radioulnar deviation and circumduction, and also stabilizes the wrist. Contributions of TALEISNIK (1976), MAYFIELD et al. (1976), KAUER (1979), PALMER and WERNER (1981), BERGER and LANDSMEER (1990) and ROMINGER et al. (1993) were the most notable. The ligaments are named for the bones from which they originate and

[1] E.R. Tjin A Ton, MD, Department of Radiology, Leiden University Hospital, P.O. Box 9600, 2300 RC Leiden, The Netherlands
[2] R.C. Fritz, MD, National Orthopedic Imaging Associates, University of California at San francisca, San Francisco, California, USA
[3] W.R. Obermann, MD, Department of Radiology, Leiden University Hospital, P.O. Box 9600, 2300 RC Leiden, The Netherlands

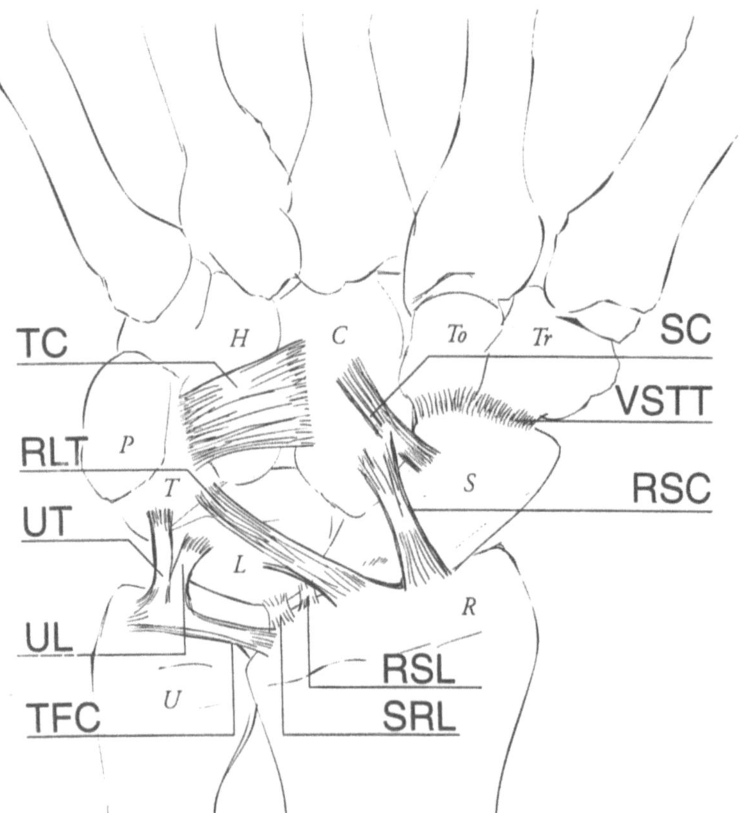

Fig. 7.1. Schematic drawing of the two inverted volar V-shaped ligamentous groups. The proximal inverted V-shaped group is formed by ulno-triquetral (*UT*), ulnolunate (*UL*) and radiolunotriquetral (*RLT*) ligaments. The distal-inverted V-shaped group is formed by triquetrocapitate (*TC*), radioscaphocapitate (*RSC*) and scaphocapitate (*SC*) ligaments. Radioscapholunate (*RSL*), short radiolunate (*SRL*) and volar scaphotrapeziotrapezoid (*VSTT*) ligaments. *TFC*, triangular fibrocartilage; *P*, pisiform; *H*, hamate; *C*, capitate; *To*, trapezoid; *Tr*, trapezium; *S*, scaphoid; *L*, lunate; *T*, triquetrum; *U*, ulna; *R*, radius

into which they insert. There are extrinsic and intrinsic ligaments of the wrist. Extrinsic ligaments are focal thickenings of the joint capsule; they are intracapsular and course between the carpal bones and the radius, the ulna, triangular fibrocartilage (TFC, also known as the articular disc) or the metacarpals. The articular surface of the distal radius slopes in volar and ulnar direction. Therefore, under normal axial loading the carpus tends to slide in volar and ulnar direction. This is counteracted by the extrinsic volar and dorsal radiocarpal ligaments. Intrinsic ligaments connect carpal bones to each other.

Although there is a difference in the nomenclature and configuration schemes of the ligaments, basically on the volar side there are two inverted V-shaped ligamentous groups, and on the dorsal side there is one transversely orientated V-shaped ligamentous group. The volar ligaments are thicker and stronger than the dorsal ligaments.

The triquetrum bone is at the apex of the proximal volar inverted V-shaped ligamentous group (Fig. 7.1). It is composed medially of the extrinsic ulnotriquetral (UT) and ulnolunate (UL) ligaments and laterally of the extrinsic radiolunotriquetral (RLT) ligament; it stabilizes the lunate and thereby also the proximal carpal row. The capitate bone is at

the apex of the distal volar V-shaped ligamentous group. It is composed medially of the intrinsic triquetrocapitate (TC) ligament and laterally of the extrinsic radioscaphocapitate (RSC) and intrinsic scaphocapitate (SC) ligaments; it stabilizes the capitate and thereby also the distal carpal row. The capsule between the two volar inverted V-shaped arches is thin and is called the "space of Poirier". In addition to these two inverted volar V-shaped ligamentous groups, there are the radioscapholunate (RSL) ligament, which actually is a neurovascular structure, and the short radiolunate (SRL) ligament (Fig. 7.1), which stabilizes the lunate.

The dorsal ligaments are less thick and biomechanically less important than the volar ligaments; the dorsal radiolunotriquetral (DRLT) ligament is the major structure that extends from the distal radius to the lunate and triquetrum. The triquetral bone is the apex of the transversely orientated dorsal V-shaped ligamentous group (Fig. 7.2). It is composed proximally of the extrinsic DRLT ligament and distally of the intrinsic dorsal intercarpal (DIC) ligament, which extend from triquetrum to scaphoid and trapezium. They prevent ulnar translation of the wrist and also stabilize the proximal carpal row.

The intrinsic carpal ligaments are primarily joint stabilizers. There are volar, dorsal and interosseous

Fig. 7.2. Schematic drawing of the transversely orientated dorsal V-shaped ligamentous group. *DRLT*, dorsal radiolunotriquetral ligament; *DIC*, dorsal intercarpal ligament; *H*, hamate; *C*, capitate; *To*, trapezoid; *Tr*, trapezium; *S*, scaphoid; *L*, lunate; *T*, triquetrum; *U*, ulna; *R*, radius

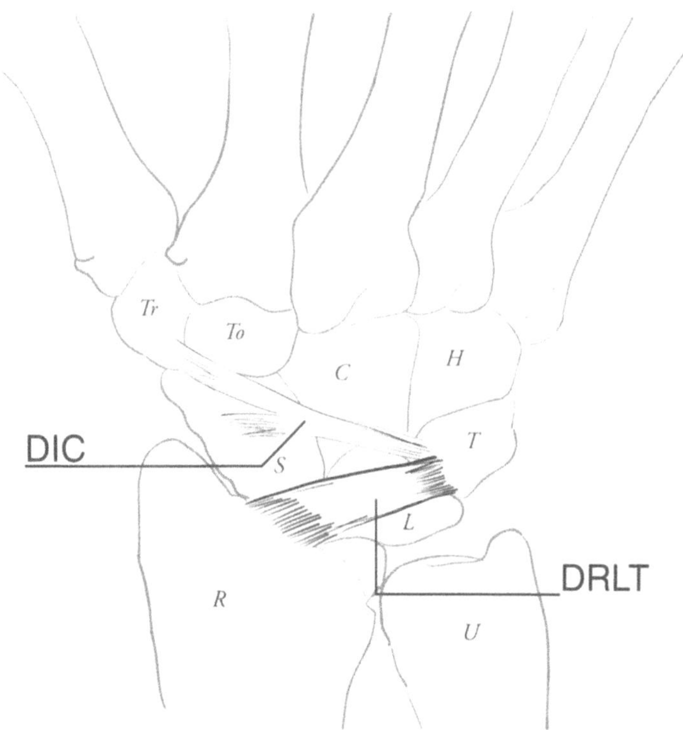

intrinsic carpal ligaments. The scapholunate (SL) interosseous and lunotriquetral (LT) interosseous ligaments connect the proximal carpal row extending from the volar to dorsal capsules at the proximal articular surface (Fig. 7.3). They separate the radiocarpal from the midcarpal compartment and are the most important intrinsic carpal ligaments. They stabilize the proximal carpal row and allow some motion, which is greater between the scaphoid and lunate than between lunate and triquetrum. The SL interosseous ligament can be divided into three biomechanically and anatomically different segments: the dorsal and volar segments are strong with attachments to the capsular ligaments and insert via Sharpey's fibers into the scaphoid and lunate bones. More Sharpey's fibers insert into the lunate; therefore, the SL interosseous ligament tears mostly from the weaker insertion of the scaphoid. The central third is a thin membrane with a weaker insertion into the hyaline cartilage of the scaphoid and lunate. The LT interosseous ligament, similar to the SL interosseous ligament, has stronger fibrous volar and dorsal segments which are biomechanically more important than the central membranous segment. The intrinsic scapho-trapezio-trapezoid (STT) ligaments are volarly thicker and stabilize the STT joint.

KAUER (1979) pointed out that ulnar and radial deviation precludes the presence of static radial and ulnar collateral ligaments. Collateral stability is "dynamically" warranted by muscles. During dorsovolar flexion on the ulnar side the extensor carpi ulnaris muscle, and on the radial side the abductor pollicis longus and extensor pollicis brevis muscles, contract isometrically; the muscles act as an "adjustable collateral system."

The triangular fibrocartilage complex (TFCC) stabilizes the distal radioulnar joint and ulnocarpal articulation. The components of the TFCC are the TFC (Fig. 7.1), the ulnocarpal meniscus, the ulnotriquetral and ulnolunate ligaments, the extensor carpi ulnaris tendon sheath, and the volar and dorsal distal radioulnar ligaments. The TFC separates the distal radioulnar joint from the radiocarpal compartment. Both the ulnocarpal meniscus and the TFC originate from the dorsoulnar aspect of the radius. The ulnocarpal meniscus runs ulnar-volarly around the wrist to insert into the triquetrum. The TFC extends horizontally to insert into the base of the ulnar styloid process. Between the ulnocarpal meniscus and the TFC is the prestyloid recess. The distal radioulnar joint is also stabilized by the sigmoid notch of the distal radius, the pronator quadratus

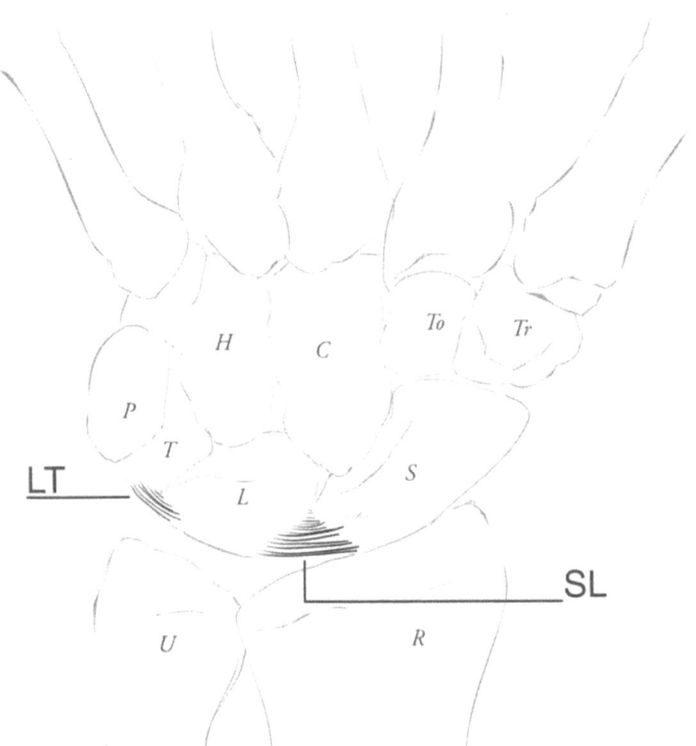

Fig. 7.3. Schematic drawing (volar aspect of the wrist) of the scapholunate (*SL*) interosseous and lunotriquetral (*LT*) interosseous ligaments. *P*, pisiform; *H*, hamate; *C*, capitate; *To*, trapezoid; *Tr*, trapezium; *S*, scaphoid; *L*, lunate; *T*, triquetrum; *U*, ulna; *R*, radius

muscle and the interosseous membrane between the radius and ulna.

7.3
Wrist Kinematics

The wrist joint is very mobile and nevertheless stable. Wrist stability depends on the bony elements, articular cartilage, and musculotendinous and ligamentous structures. Carpal motion is due to muscles and tendons that cross the carpus, thereby also generating axial loading upon the carpal bones.

There are several different mechanical models to describe the movements of the wrist. No single model can totally explain the carpal motion or the pathokinematic and force transmission of the hand to forearm.

Initially it was assumed that the carpus consists of two rigid horizontal rows, the proximal row (scaphoid, lunate, triquetrum and pisiform) and distal row (trapezium, trapezoid, capitate and hamate), that could move in relation to each other and in relation to the distal radius and ulna. The proximal carpal row moves as a unit and was considered an intercalated segment to which no tendons attach; it is situated between the radius and distal carpal row.

There is no direct motor control of the proximal carpal row which moves by indirect forces transmitted by the wrist ligaments and radiocarpal and intercarpal joints. In this mechanical model, only the movement of the carpus relative to the forearm was described; there was no assessment of intercarpal motion.

KAUER (1986, 1996) described the specific geometries and the interdependent motion of the carpal bones. The triquetrum and the lunate and proximal part (which lies between the capitate and radius) of the scaphoid are wedge-shaped in the sagittal plane, being thinner dorsally. Because of this specific geometry and the volar sloping of the distal-radius articular surface, under axial loading they tend to rotate dorsally (distal articular surface faces dorsally). The distal part of the scaphoid is interposed between the radius and the trapezium and trapezoid, volar to the flexion-extension axis, so under axial loading the distal part of the scaphoid tends to rotate volarly. Furthermore, in radial deviation and volarflexion the radial styloid and trapezium approach each other, the sagittal space for the scaphoid decreases and the scaphoid has to rotate volarly. The lunate and triquetrum follow the scaphoid and also rotate volarly, via the intact SL and LT interosseous ligaments. The triquetrum can move only slightly distally to the lunate, resulting in a slight step-off of the triquetrolunate articular surface in maximum radial deviation. From flexion to extension there is more intracarpal motion between the proximal carpal bones. The proximal articular surface of the scaphoid curves sharper in the dorsovolar direction than the lunate; therefore, the scaphoid rotates more with flexion and extension. The scaphoid also displaces proximally to the lunate with volar flexion. In volarflexion the lunate translates dorsally to the radius and volarly to the capitate. In a normal wrist, when the lunate is more or less in a neutral position, the triquetrum is slightly dorsiflexed and the scaphoid circa 45° volarflexed. The tendency of the distal scaphoid to volarflex and the dorsiflexion tendencies of the proximal scaphoid, lunate and triquetrum are balanced by the primary wrist stabilizers (the SL and LT interosseous ligaments).

RUBY et al. (1988) found that the wrist functions as two carpal rows, with the distal row tightly bound and moved as a unit with little intracarpal motion. The proximal row also moves as a unit, but there is significant motion between scaphoid, lunate and triquetrum; therefore, it functions as a variable-geometry intercalated segment. Because of the variable geometry, the proximal carpal row fits between the distal carpal row and the distal radius and TFC to keep the joints congruent. There is a great range in flexion and extension motion in normals, but the range is about the same radiocarpally and midcarpally. The midcarpal joint contributes more to radioulnar deviation than does the radiocarpal joint.

From radial to ulnar deviation in neutral flexion, the proximal carpal row primarily rotates from volarflexion to dorsiflexion. The proximal carpal row also pronates relative to the capitate, and translates volarly to the radius and distal carpal row. In ulnar deviation, the ulnar head and hamate approach, and the triquetrum translates ulnarly and distally to the hamate. The capitate remains collinear with the radius and third metacarpal for optimal force transmission from the hand to forearm.

TALEISNIK (1976, 1985) advocated a concept of three longitudinal columns with a central flexion-extension column which consists of the distal carpal row and the lunate. The axis of the central column is the radius, lunate and capitate. The scaphoid bone forms the "mobile" lateral column and stabilizes the lunatocapitate joint because the scaphoid bridges the proximal and distal carpal row. The triquetrum bone forms the "rotation" medial column to which ligaments converge and around which hand rotation takes place.

LICHTMAN (LICHTMAN et al. 1981; LICHTMAN and MARTIN 1988) proposed a "ring" model because the longitudinal columnar concept failed to explain the transverse (perilunate), transverse midcarpal and proximal carpal instabilities. The carpus is an oval transverse ring, formed by the proximal and distal carpal row which are connected by mobile ulnar and radial links. The "radial link" is the mobile scapho-trapezio-trapezoid joint, and the "ulnar link" is the rotatory triquetrohamate joint. Radial deviation compresses the STT joint, forcing the scaphoid into volarflexion and thereby also the proximal carpal row. Ulnar deviation forces the triquetrum to slide into dorsiflexion and thereby also the proximal carpal row.

WEBER (1988) stressed the transmission of forces from the hand to forearm in a longitudinal direction. The carpal intercalated system is controlled by ligaments (only at the extremes of joint motion do ligamentous constraints provide stability) and contact surface of the carpal joints. He proposed a force-bearing column (the distal radius, the lunate, the proximal two thirds of the scaphoid, the capitate, the trapezoid, and the second and third carpometacarpal joints) that transmits forces from the hand to forearm. A second ulnar control column (the distal ulna, the ulnocarpal complex, the triquetrum, the hamate, and the fourth and fifth carpometacarpal joints) provides rotational control. The third thumb-axis mobile column (the distal third of the scaphoid, the trapeziotrapezoid joint and first carpometacarpal joint) allows independent motion of the first digit. The proximal articular surface of the hamate is helicoid; this combined with the saddle-shaped articular surface of the triquetrum forms the rotatory hamatotriquetral articulation which controls the proximal carpal row. The triquetrum tends to extend and translates ulnar-volarly and distally to the hamate under axial loading due to the rotatory hamatotriquetral joint. Axial forces on the ulnar column and thumb-axis column are transmitted to the central force-bearing column.

7.4
Carpal Instability

7.4.1
Classification

Traumatic instability of the wrist is defined as "a carpal injury in which loss of normal alignment of the carpal bones develops early or late"either at rest (static instability) or under the influence of axial loading or certain wrist motions (dynamic instability). LINSCHEID et al. (1972, 1983) recognized four major groups: dorsiflexion, volarflexion, ulnar translocation and dorsal subluxation.

Most wrist injuries occur during a fall on an outstretched hand with the wrist dorsiflexed. The type and severity of wrist injury are determined by the exact position of the wrist during impact, the age of the patient, and the magnitude and direction of the force. The wrist injury can therefore range from minor sprains to major fracture dislocations.

Carpal bone pathomechanics can cause carpal instability. Ligamentous injury or laxity is often to blame; other causes are fractures and various articular disorders (e.g., rheumatoid arthritis) leading to disturbance of the normal osseous-cartilaginous-ligamentous relations. Most instability patterns are caused by various combinations and severity of ligamentous injury and/or laxity. It is possible to develop an instability between the proximal and distal carpal row, and between any articulation of the carpal bones.

There is at present no consensus on a single classification of carpal instability patterns, mainly because there is no single operation technique clearly superior either theoretically or practically for carpal instabilities. There are different concepts of wrist kinematics for classifying and different indications for operating carpal instabilities, leading to different techniques for ligament repair, reconstruction or arthrodesis. The ideal treatment would be to restore the normal wrist kinematics and anatomy.

Because of the central location of the lunate, instabilities are generally described relative to the position of the lunate. Volar, dorsal, ulnar and radial translation of the lunate are therefore termed volar, dorsal, ulnar and radial translation instabilities, respectively. The lunate is considered an intercalated segment between the radius and capitate. The lunate can be flexed (volarflexed intercalated segment instability, VISI) or extended (dorsiflexed intercalated segment instability, DISI).

AMADIO (1991) was the first to determine the direction (volar, dorsal, ulnar and radial translation; VISI and DISI) and severity (static, dynamic; subluxation and dislocation) of the instability pattern and then the location of ligament abnormality. Carpal instability-dissociative (CID) instability is caused by disruption of the SL or LT, or both interosseous ligaments. Instability due to disruption of the radiocarpal and/or midcarpal ligaments is called carpal instability-nondissociative (CIND). Both CID and CIND may not change lunate position

and may cause VISI or DISI, and the two may coexist. Instabilities can be primarily radiocarpal, midcarpal, or combined radiocarpal-midcarpal. In CIND the routine radiographs are often normal.

The spectrum of SL interosseous ligament injury can vary from biomechanically insignificant partial tears (which may cause pain) to SL dissociation, scaphoid rotatory subluxation, DISI, and eventually degenerative changes [scapholunate advanced collapse (SLAC) or SLAC wrist]. MAYFIELD et al. (1976) observed that disruption of the volar radiocarpal ligaments was also needed, with an SL interosseous ligament tear, to produce a scapholunate separation. RUBY et al. (1987) stressed the importance of the dorsal portion of the SL interosseous ligament for normal scapolunate kinematics.

Similar to SL interosseous ligament, injuries to the lunotriquetral interosseous ligament can vary from (a)symptomatic partial tears to complete disruption with triquetral instability, lunotriquetral dissociation, VISI, and finally degenerative changes on the ulnar side of the wrist. VIEGAS et al. (1990) found that partial or complete LT interosseous ligament tears produce no clinical or radiographic VISI; disruption of the volar lunotriquetral ligament and also of the dorsal radiocarpal (of the scaphoid and lunate portion) ligaments was necessary for clinical and radiographic evidence of dynamic and static VISI, respectively. HORII et al. (1991) demonstrated with stereoradiographic methods that the disruption essential for producing a static VISI was sectioning of the dorsal radiotriquetral and dorsal scaphotriquetral ligaments in association with LT interosseous ligament sectioning; volar ligamentous disruption was not necessary to produce a VISI instability. LT interosseous ligament sectioning alone increased the mobility of the lunotriquetral joint which is difficult to detect on radiographs. Although the increased lunotriquetral motion is small, the abnormal kinematics may produce synovitis and wrist pain.

7.4.2
Diagnosis

The patients who are clinically suspected of having a carpal instability usually have pain and instability symptoms of the wrist. Patients with a dynamic instability often can elicit a snap or pop. The first diagnostic step is to obtain posteroanterior (PA) and lateral radiographs in neutral position with metal markers at the site of the pain; generally, static instability patterns are diagnosed. In static instability there are abnormal angles between bones, abnormal translations and abnormal projected shapes of carpal bones.

On the PA view the shapes of the carpal bones, symmetry of the joint spaces and the three normally smooth carpal arcs are evaluated. The first two carpal arcs are the proximal convex and distal concave curvatures of the proximal carpal row. The third carpal arc is the proximal convex curvature of the capitate and hamate. On the true (i.e., without deviation or flexion) lateral radiograph of the wrist, the radio-luno-capitate third metacarpal alignment and the angles between the carpal bones are evaluated. Dorsiflexion of the distal bone on the proximal bone is considered a positive angulation, and volarflexion of the distal bone a negative angulation. The angle between the lunate (axis of the lunate is perpendicular from a line drawn between the volar and dorsal distal end of the lunate) and the radius (longitudinal axis of the radius), the LR angle, varies between +15° and −20° (Fig. 7.4A). The angle between the capitate (the long axis of the capitate) and the lunate, the CL angle, is similar to the LR angle, varying between +15° and −20°. The angle between scaphoid (axis of the scaphoid is a line connecting its distal and proximal volar margins) and radius, the SR angle, ranges from −38° to −67°, with a mean of −53°. The angle between triquetrum (line bisecting the proximal articular surface of the triquetrum passing through the distal angulation of the triquetrum) and lunate, the TL angle, ranges from −31° to +3°, with a mean of −14°. The angle between the scaphoid and lunate, the SL angle, ranges from 30° to 60°, with an average of 50°. On a lateral view DISI is defined by a dorsal angulation of the lunate, and the LR angle is greater than +15° (Fig. 7.4C). The scapholunate angle is often greater than 70°. VISI is defined by a volar angulation of the lunate, and the LR angle is greater than −20° and the SL angle often less than 30° (Fig. 7.4B). On a PA view the lunate has an elongated trapezoidal shape (representing the distal volar margin) and elongated triangular shape (representing the distal dorsal margin) in a DISI and VISI instability pattern, respectively. Ulnar translocation is defined by ulnar displacement of the carpus; more than half of the lunate lies ulnar to the radius, and the space between the radial styloid and scaphoid is increased. Dorsal carpal (sub)luxation is defined by a (sub)luxation of the carpus dorsal to its normal alignment in relation to the radius, mostly as a result of a malunited fracture of the distal radius involving the dorsal rim and styloid process. Rarely, the carpus (sub)luxates volarly and is mostly a sequela of a malunited fracture of the distal volar rim of the ra-

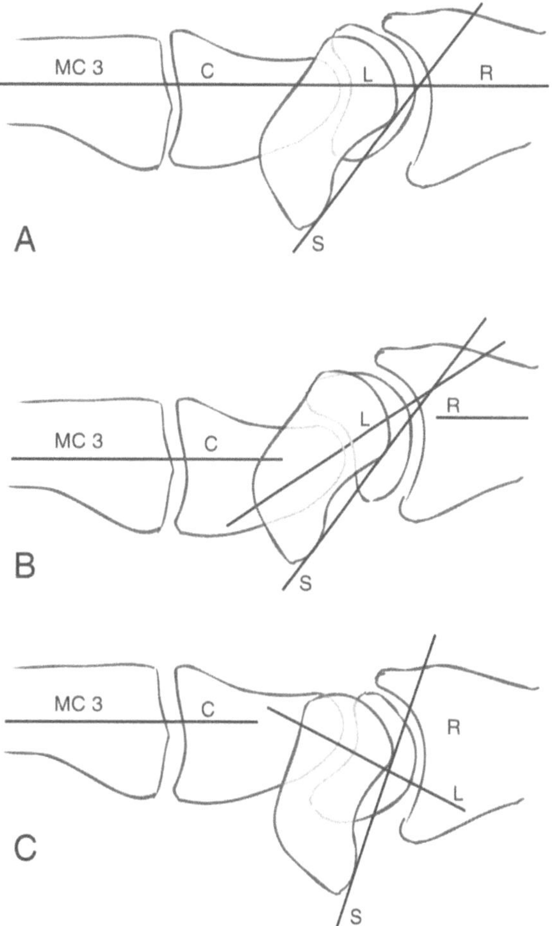

Fig. 7.4A–C. Schematic lateral projections of the wrist. In the normal wrist (**A**), a *straight line* can be drawn through the axes of third metacarpal, the capitate, the lunate and the radius. In VISI (**B**), the SL angle is often less than 30°, the CL- and LR angle are greater than 15°. In DISI (**C**), the SL angle is often greater than 70°, the CL- and LR angle are greater than 20°. *VISI*, volar-flexed intercalated segment instability; *DISI*, dorsiflexed intercalated segment instability; *MC 3*, longitudinal axis of third metacarpal; *C*, axis of capitate; *L*, axis of lunate; *R*, axis of radius; *S*, axis of scaphoid

dius. If the PA and lateral radiographs are normal or there is a dynamic instability, fluoroscopy of carpal motion is indicated. Fluoroscopic monitoring can detect transient subluxations (if necessary with the application of stress) of the carpal bones.

Wrist arthrography is used to diagnose TFC tears and SL and LT interosseous ligament tears. Accurate monitoring of the injected contrast medium with digital subtraction technique, fluoroscopy or video is necessary. LEVINSOHN et al. (1991) found tricompartment injections necessary because of some defects that only allow unidirectional flow. MANASTER (1991) did not detect additional communicating de-

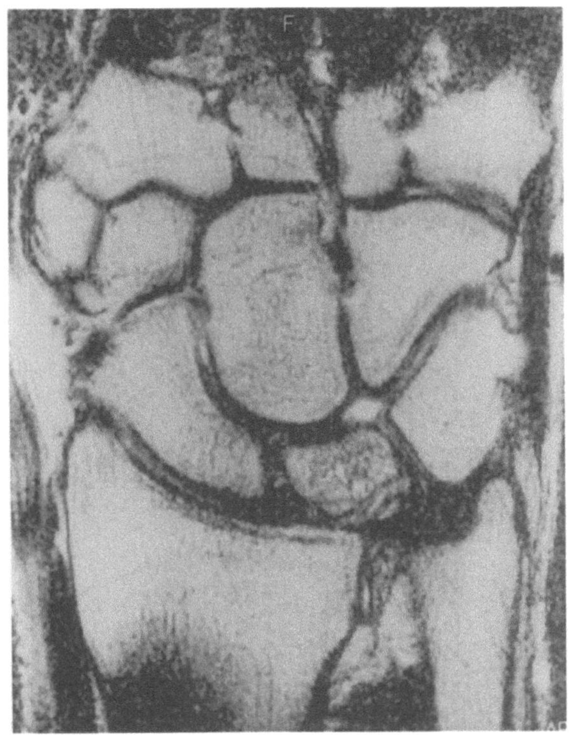

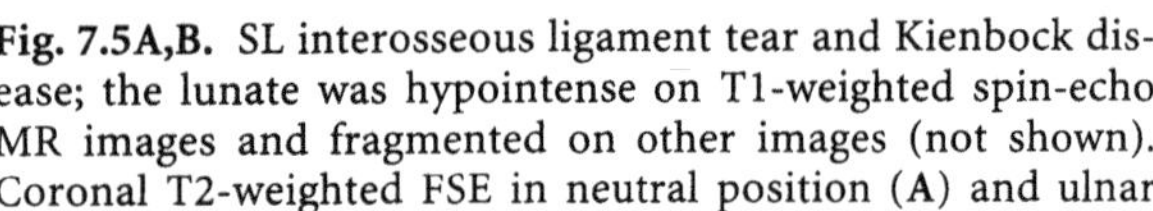

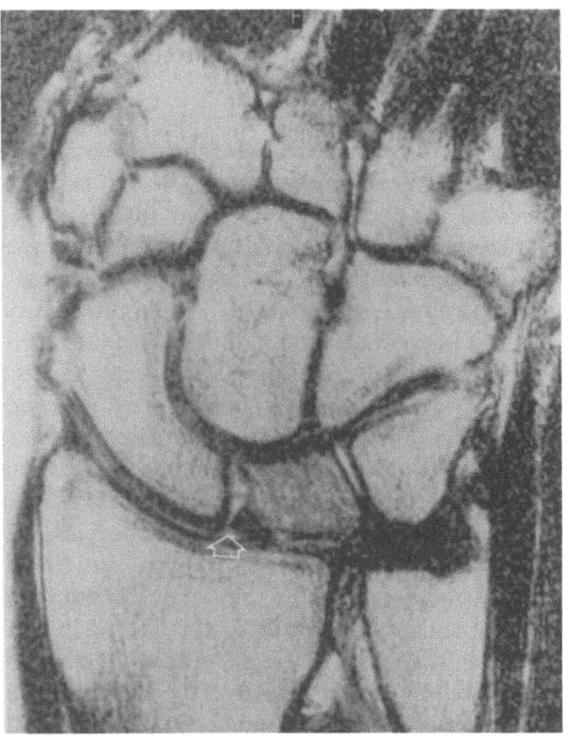

Fig. 7.5A,B. SL interosseous ligament tear and Kienbock disease; the lunate was hypointense on T1-weighted spin-echo MR images and fragmented on other images (not shown). Coronal T2-weighted FSE in neutral position (**A**) and ulnar stress deviation (**B**). Only ulnar stress deviation shows the SL interosseous ligament tear (*arrow*). *MR*, magnetic resonance; *FSE*, fast spin echo. (From TJIN A TON et al. 1995)

fects with tricompartment arthrography that would alter patient treatment and management compared to radiocarpal injections alone. Many communicating defects on wrist arthrography are depicted only after wrist motion. However, such communicating defects may be neither related to the injury nor symptomatic, and there is a high prevalence of symmetric lesions in the opposite asymptomatic wrist. The incidence of communicating defects increases with age. METZ et al. (1993) proposed bilateral arthrograms to identify asymmetric and therefore probably symptomatic lesions.

MR imaging is the only modality to noninvasively directly visualize the intrinsic and extrinsic wrist ligaments. In addition, MR imaging may reveal other diseases that may contribute to a patient's symptoms. A dedicated wrist coil and a high-field-strength magnet are necessary to obtain good signal-to-noise ratios and spatial resolution. On MR images interosseous ligament tears of the proximal carpal row are depicted as absence, discontinuity or morphologic disruption of the SL and LT interosseous ligaments. TJIN A TON et al. (1995) suggested that

stress deviation increases the accuracy of MR (Figs. 7.5, 7.6A,B), especially radial stress deviation for LT interosseous ligament tears which so far are the most difficult to detect with MRI. Because of the small wrist ligaments and their oblique orientation, three-dimensional gradient-echo (3D GRE) sequences were used to obtain high-resolution and multiplanar reconstructions by TOTTERMAN et al. (1993) and SMITH (1993). However, there is limited contrast between normal and abnormal ligaments using 3D GRE imaging. The coronal plane is best suited for evaluating the interosseous ligaments of the proximal carpal row, using a T2-weighted fast spin echo (FSE) or GRE. The sagittal plane is useful for evaluating the TFC and radiocarpal wrist ligaments, and for detecting a DISI or VISI pattern.

Although any combination of ligamentous-cartilaginous-osseous injury can theoretically occur, certain instability patterns are particularly frequent. The more common scapholunate dissociation, pseudoarthrosis of the scaphoid, triquetrolunate dissociation, ulnar translocation and dynamic instability will be described.

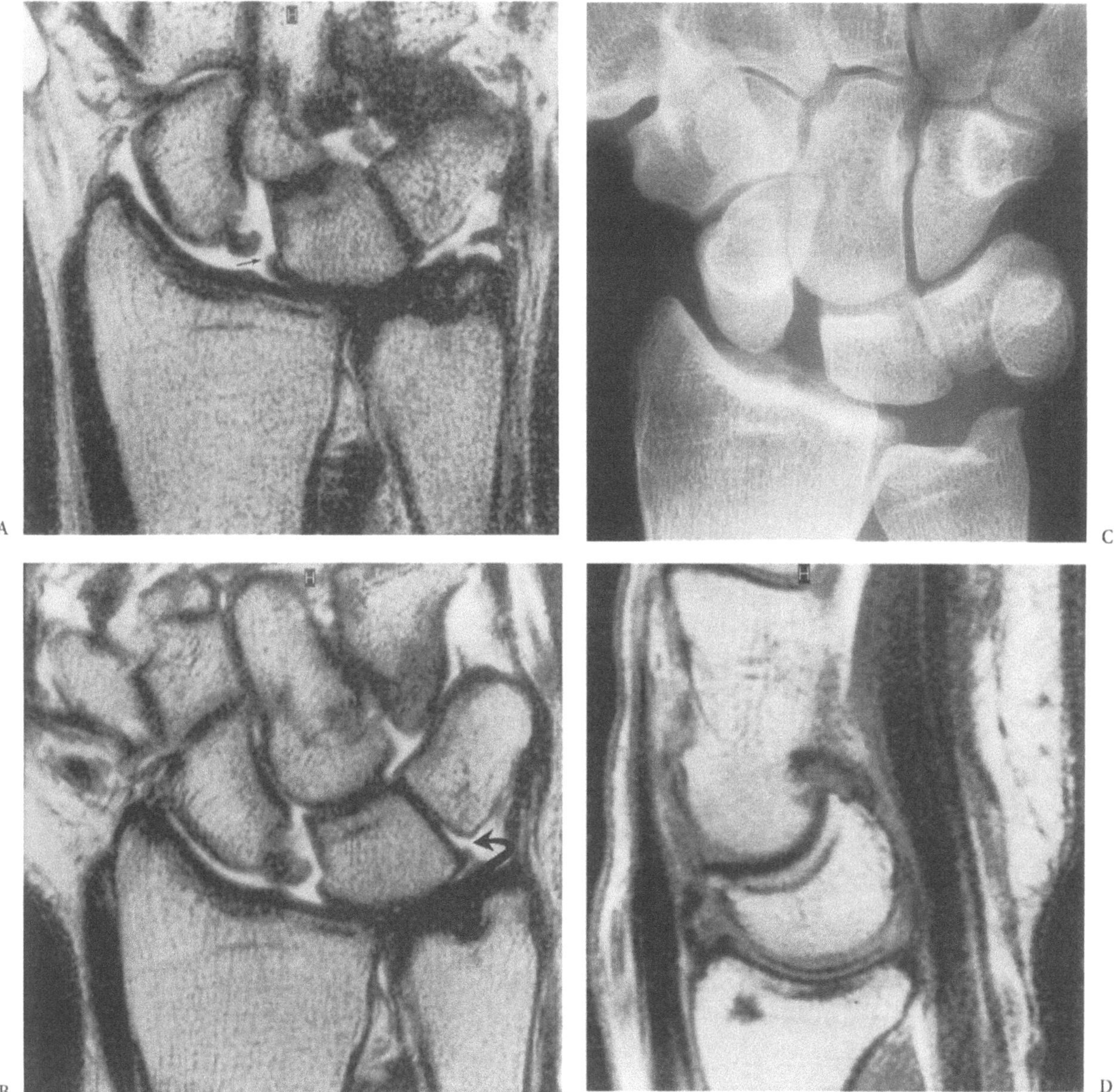

Fig. 7.6A–D. SL and LT interosseous ligament tears with DISI instability pattern. Coronal T2-weighted FSE in neutral (**A**) and in radial stress deviation (**B**). (From TJIN A TON et al. 1995). SL interosseous ligament tear (*straight arrow*) is seen in both positions, but only radial stress deviation shows the LT interosseous ligament tear (*curved arrow*). PA view in neutral position (**C**) demonstrates cortical ring sign of the scaphoid, a wide SL gap, and elongated trapezoidal shape of the lunate. Sagittal T1-weighted spin echo (**D**) depicts an extended and volar-translated lunate bone with an LR angle greater than 15°. *PA*, posteroanterior

7.4.2.1
Scapholunate Dissociation

Wrist injury at the radial side usually occurs during hyperextension and supination of the wrist. The scapholunate interosseous ligament is disrupted. BERGER et al. (1982) found that a disruption of the volar radiocarpal ligaments is also necessary to produce the instability. On the posteroanterior radiograph the scaphoid is foreshortened and volarflexed (because of the natural tendency of the scaphoid to volarflex), and the cortex of the distal pole is seen end-on producing a cortical "ring sign" (Fig. 7.6C). The capitate tends to displace dorsally and slide between the scaphoid and lunate, and displace the two bones. Scapholunate dissociation is suggested when the scapholunate distance is greater than 2mm (Terry Thomas sign); however, in some cases there is a wide scapholunate joint space without a scapholunate interosseous ligament tear. CAUTILLI and WEHBE (1991) found a scapholunate distance up to 5mm in normal individuals; however, none of them had a "ring sign." With axial loading (clenched fist) and ulnar and radial deviation, the scapholunate gap may continue to widen in scapholunate dissociation. The scaphoid translates dorsally (rotatory subluxation of the scaphoid); BURGESS (1987) showed that the radioscaphoid contact area shifts dorsally and is reduced, which leads to degenerative arthritis of the wrist. The lunate tends to extend and often there is a DISI pattern (Fig. 7.6D). SL interosseous ligament tears can progress from

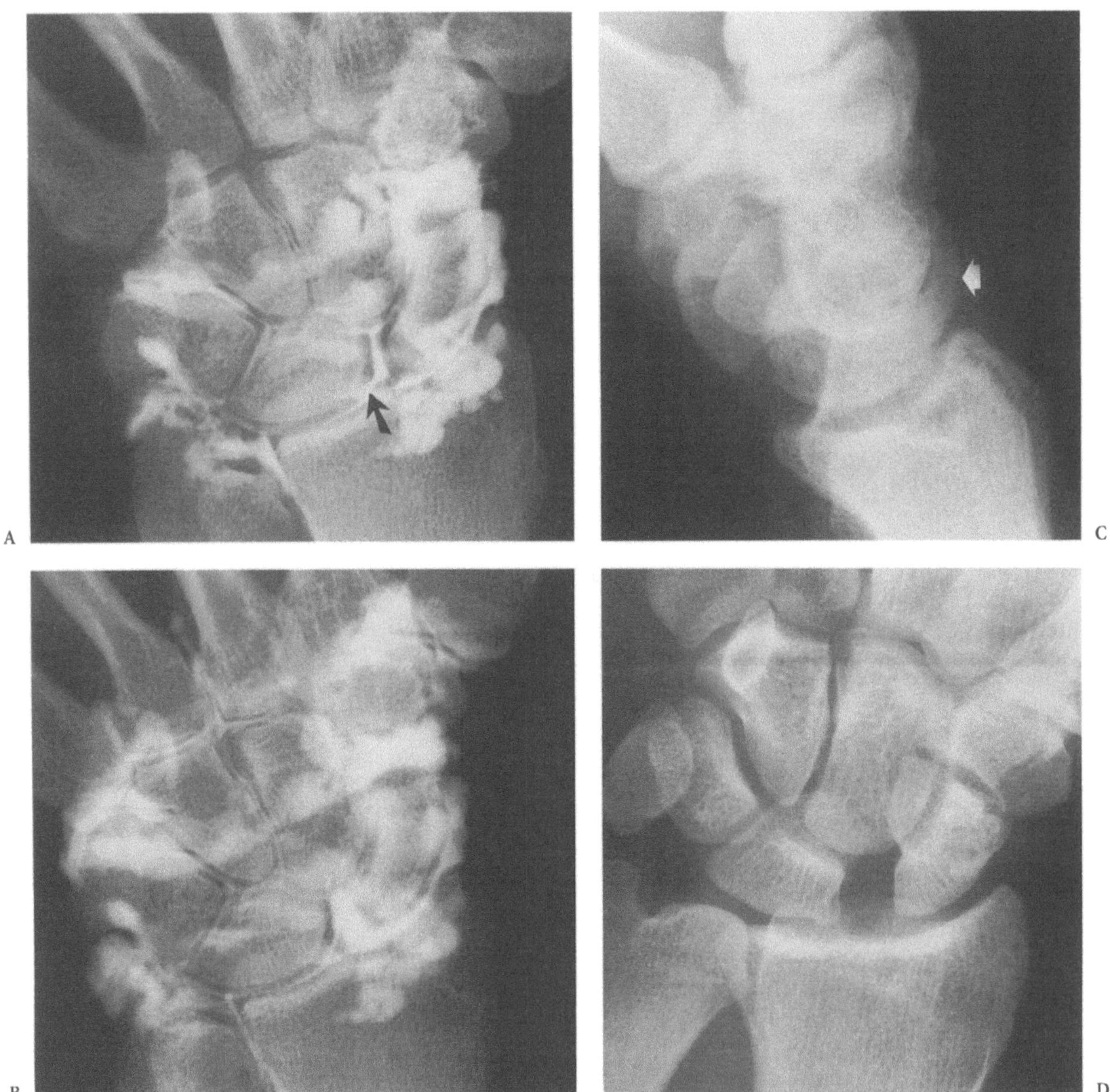

Fig. 7.7A–D. Patient with progressive tearing of the SL interosseous ligament. Wrist arthrogram (A) demonstrates a small biomechanically insignificant SL interosseous ligament tear (*arrow*). One year later the wrist arthrogram showed SL dissociation (B). The lateral view (C) demonstrates an extended lunate and dorsally translated proximal pole of the scaphoid (*arrow*). PA view (D) depicts SL diastases, foreshortening of the scaphoid and trapezoidal shape of the lunate

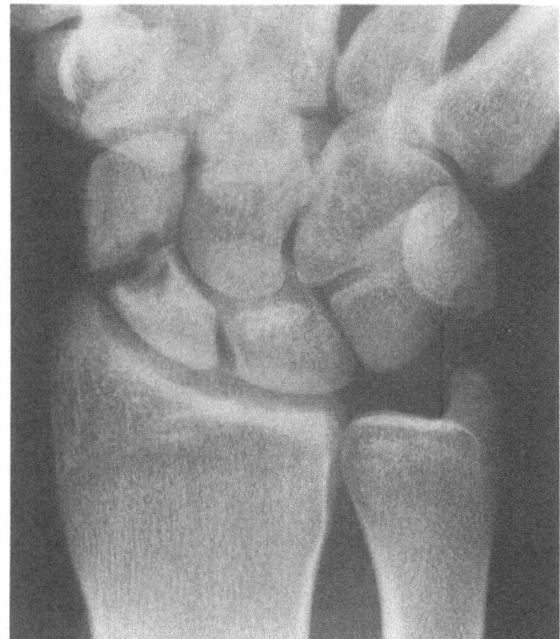

A

biomechanically insignificant tears to SL dissociation and rotatory subluxation of the scaphoid (Fig. 7.7).

7.4.2.2
Pseudoarthrosis of the Scaphoid

Rotatory subluxation of the scaphoid can be secondary to scaphoid nonunion (Fig. 7.8) and other causes, i.e., Kienbock's disease. An unstable fracture (a malunion or nonunion) of the scaphoid may result in a DISI. After a waist fracture of the scaphoid, the distal pole (because of the axial loading of the trapezium) tends to volarflex, and the proximal pole (following the dorsiflexion tendency of both the lunate and triquetrum via intact SL and LT interosseous ligaments) tends to dorsiflex.

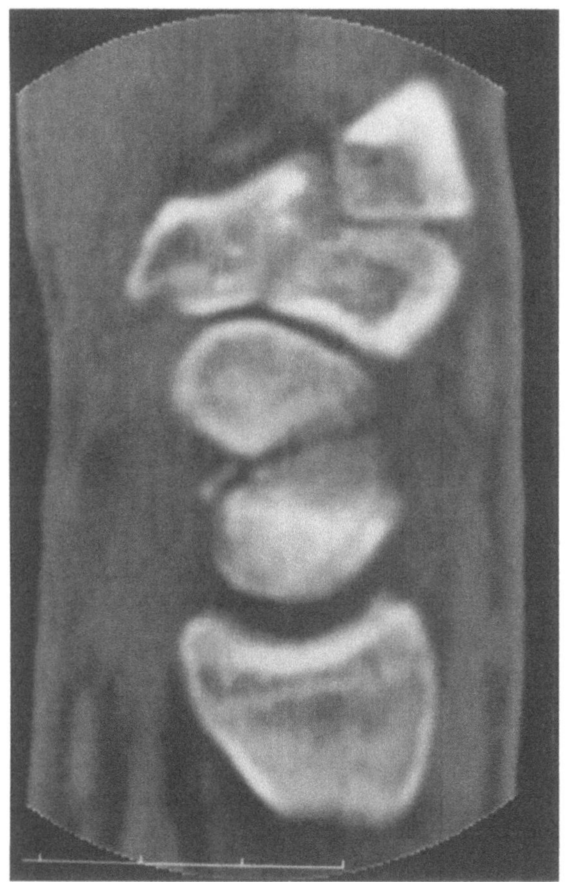

B

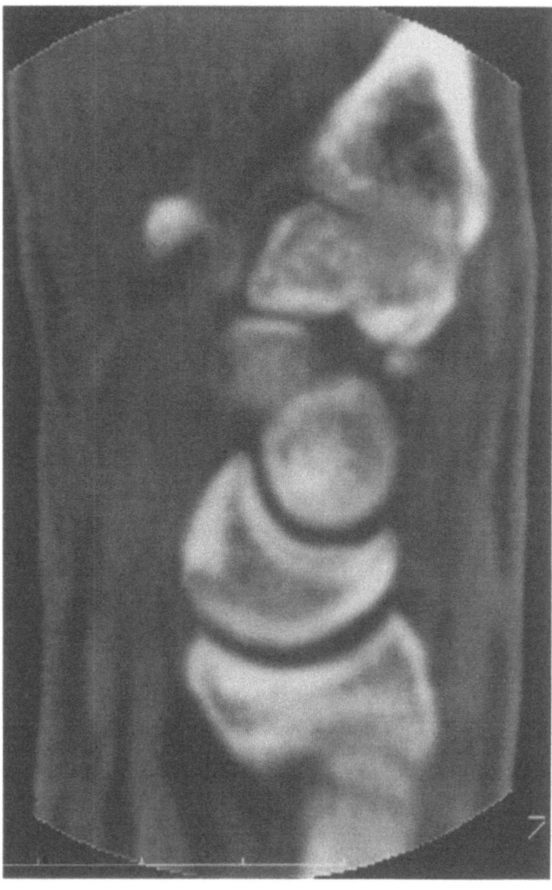

C

Fig. 7.8A–C. Scaphoid nonunion and avascular necroses of the proximal pole of the scaphoid. PA view (**A**) shows pseudoarthrosis and sclerotic proximal scaphoid pole. Sagittal CT with volar flexion of the distal pole of the scaphoid (**B**) and dorsally tilted lunate (**C**) or DISI instability pattern. *CT,* computed tomography

7.4.2.3
Triquetrolunate Dissociation

Triquetrolunate dissociation is the result of injuries to the ulnar side of the wrist with a tear of the lunotriquetral interosseous ligament. Often, the TFC is also torn. As mentioned earlier, the volar radiocarpal and/or dorsal radiocarpal ligaments also must be disrupted to allow the lunate to volarflex. The scaphoid and lunate are volarflexed; the lunate follows the tendency of the scaphoid to volarflex via the intact SL interosseous ligament, which is no longer counterbalanced by the tendency of the triquetrum to dorsiflex. This produces the "ring sign" and VISI pattern, respectively. The smooth wrist arc 1 is disrupted by a step-off between the lunate and the triquetrum; usually, the triquetrum is displaced proximally. The triquetrolunate angle is zero or positive, but this is difficult to assess because the triquetrum is difficult to identify on the lateral view. Unlike scapholunate dissociation, the capitate has no tendency to intrude between the lunate and triquetrum, resulting in a better healing potential.

7.4.2.4
Ulnar Translocation

The carpus slides down the slope of the radius, usually as a result of rheumatoid arthritis, but may be seen as an isolated traumatic sequela. Often, there is a VISI. There are two types of ulnar translocation. Generally, the whole proximal carpal row translates ulnarly, and the distance between scaphoid and radial styloid process increases. In the second type of translocation, the distance between radial styloid process and scaphoid remains normal, and thus the scapholunate space widens.

7.4.2.5
Dynamic Instability

The most common dynamic instability is the midcarpal (triquetrohamate) instability, which always is a dynamic instability. The volar capitato-triquetral and triquetrohamate ligaments are disrupted, which stabilizes the midcarpal joint on the ulnar side of the wrist. Dynamic instability may also result from malunited extraarticular distal radius fractures. There is a painful snap of the wrist. Radiographs are usually normal, and sometimes a VISI or DISI pattern exists. The abnormal motion is noted

during fluoroscopy with the forearm pronated as the wrist moves under axial loading from radial deviation to ulnar deviation (or vice versa). During deviation motion the proximal carpal row at a certain point suddenly (mostly with a snap or click) rotates from volarflexion in radial deviation to dorsiflexion in ulnar deviation (or vice versa). Since the SL and LT interosseous ligaments are intact, the proximal carpal row moves as a unit (Fig. 7.9).

Dynamic scapholunate instability (rotatory subluxation) ranges from clinical asymptomatic minor ligament tears to significant symptomatic ligament tears and rotatory subluxation with stress. In dynamic SL dissociation (Fig. 7.10), the standard PA view is normal; during certain motions the SL joint widens and then suddenly becomes normal with a painful snap. Sometimes the scaphoid has become immobile from synovitis and secondary fibrosis; the only sign in such a case is a positive Watson test.

7.5
Elbow Anatomy

The elbow is composed of three bony articulations contained within a common joint cavity. The radial head rotates within the radial notch of the ulna, allowing supination and pronation distally. The radial head is surrounded by the annular ligament, which is seen best on axial MR images (Fig. 7.11). Disruption of the annular ligament results in proximal radioulnar joint instability (Fig. 7.12). The radius articulates with the capitellum and the ulna articulates with the trochlea in a hinge fashion. The anterior and posterior portions of the joint capsule are relatively thin, whereas the medial and lateral portions are thickened to form the collateral ligaments. The medial collateral ligament (MCL) complex consists of anterior and posterior bundles as well as an oblique band that is also known as the transverse ligament. The functionally important anterior bundle of the MCL extends from the medial epicondyle to the medial aspect of the coronoid process. The anterior bundle is well seen on coronal MR images. It provides the primary constraint to valgus stress and commonly is damaged in throwing athletes (Fig. 7.13).

The lateral collateral ligament complex is more variable and less well understood than the medial collateral ligament. It is primarily composed of the radial collateral ligament, the annular ligament and the lateral ulnar collateral ligament (LUCL). The radial collateral ligament proper arises from the lateral

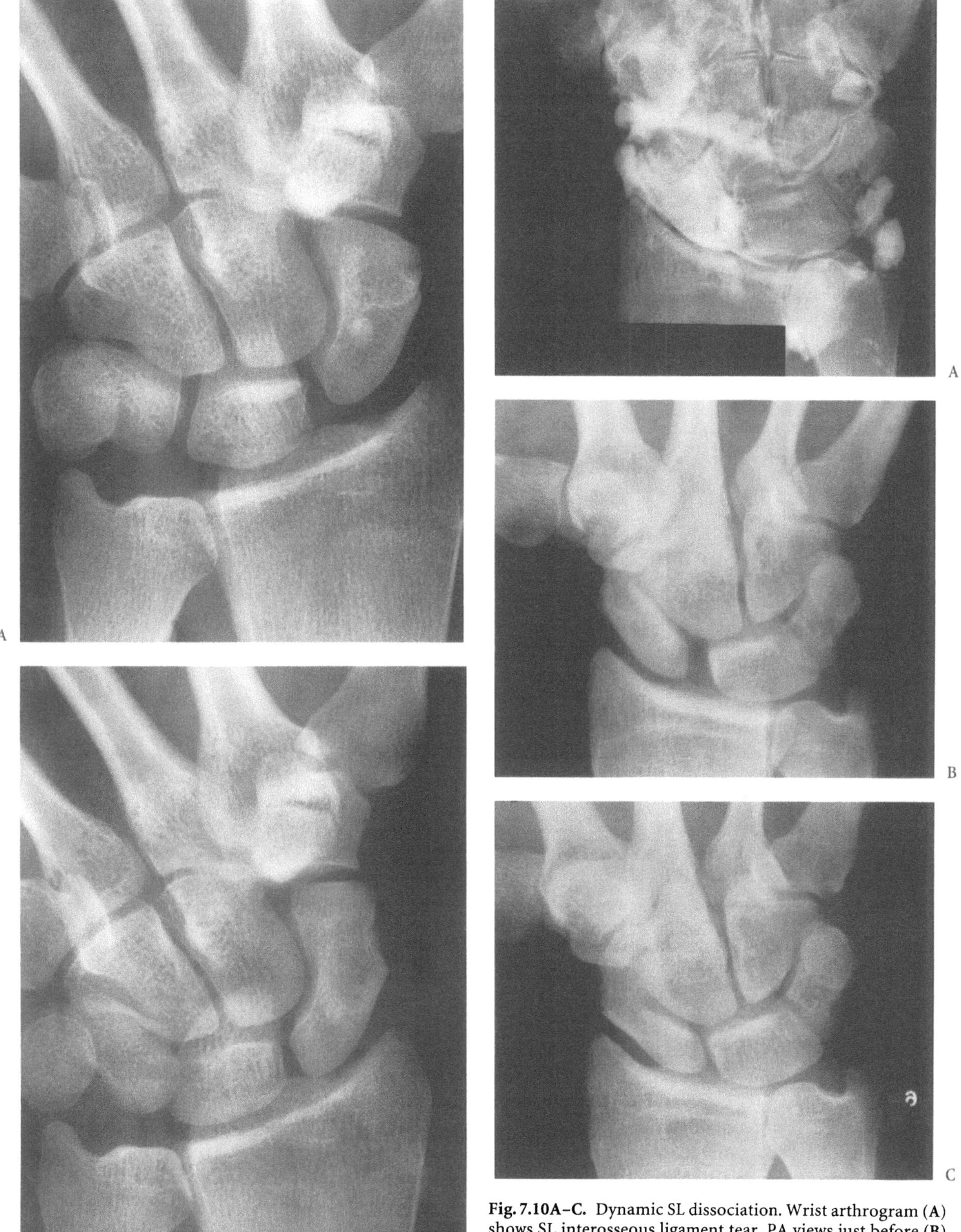

Fig. 7.9A,B. Midcarpal instability. PA views just before (**A**) and after (**B**) the painful snap with ulnar deviation. Before the sudden snap the proximal carpal row is volarflexed (**A**), with further ulnar deviation the proximal row suddenly extends (**B**), thereby producing the symptoms

Fig. 7.10A–C. Dynamic SL dissociation. Wrist arthrogram (**A**) shows SL interosseous ligament tear. PA views just before (**B**) and after (**C**) the symptomatic pop with dorsiflexion. The neutral PA view was normal (not shown); with dorsiflexion the SL joint space widened (**B**) to a certain point when suddenly it again became normal in width (**C**), producing a pop

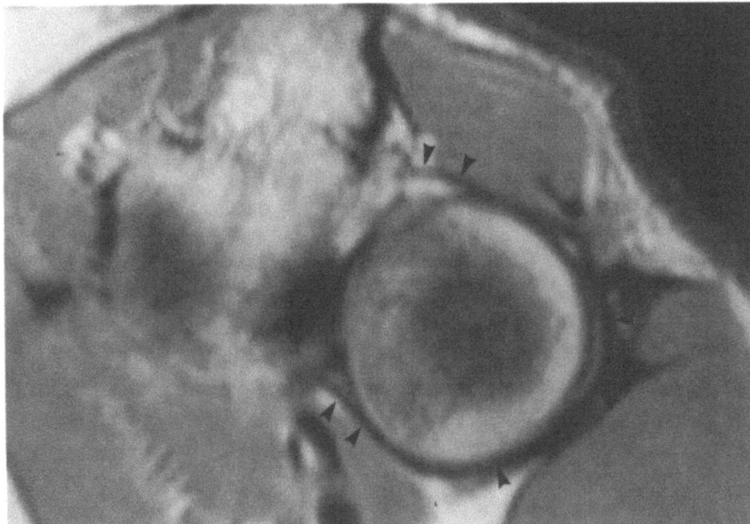

Fig. 7.11. Normal annular ligament. A proton density axial image shows the thin low-signal intensity ligament (*arrowheads*) surrounding the radial head

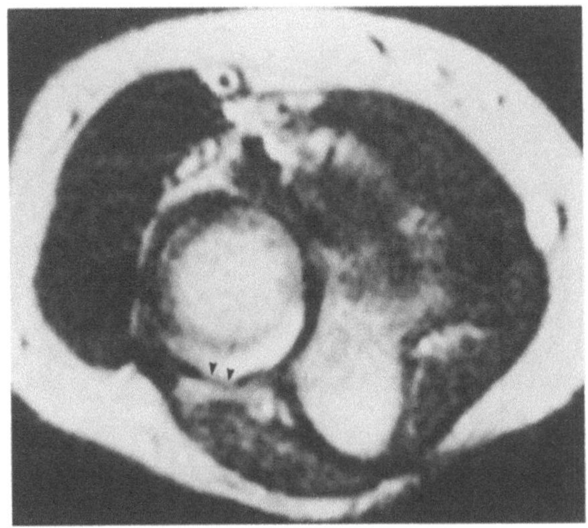

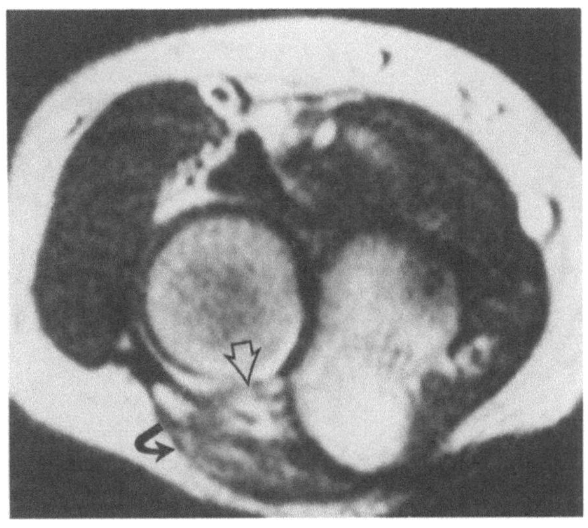

Fig. 7.12A,B. Annular ligament sprain in a 16-year-old gymnast after a fall. **A** T2-weighted axial images reveal a somewhat lax appearance of the annular ligament (*arrowheads*) **B** as well as increased signal and poor definition of the posterior fibers of the ligament (*open arrow*). Increased signal is also seen within the adjacent anconeus (*curved arrow*), compatible with muscle strain injury

epicondyle anteriorly and blends with the fibers of the annular ligament which surrounds the radial head. A more posterior bundle, known as the lateral ulnar collateral ligament (LUCL) or the ulnar part of the lateral collateral ligament, arises from the lateral epicondyle and extends along the posterior aspect of the radius to insert on the supinator crest of the ulna. The LUCL acts as a sling or guy-wire that provides the primary ligamentous constraint to varus stress. Disruption of the LUCL also results in the pivot-shift phenomenon and posterolateral rotatory instability of the elbow that was described by O'DRISCOLL et al.

in 1991. Both the radial collateral ligament anteriorly and the LUCL further posteriorly are well seen on coronal MR images.

The muscles of the elbow are divided into anterior, posterior, medial and lateral compartments. The anterior compartment contains the biceps and brachialis muscles that are evaluated best on sagittal and axial images. The brachialis extends along the anterior joint capsule and inserts on the ulnar tuberosity. The brachialis is commonly strained along with tearing of the adjacent anterior capsule after posterior elbow dislocation. The biceps lies superfi-

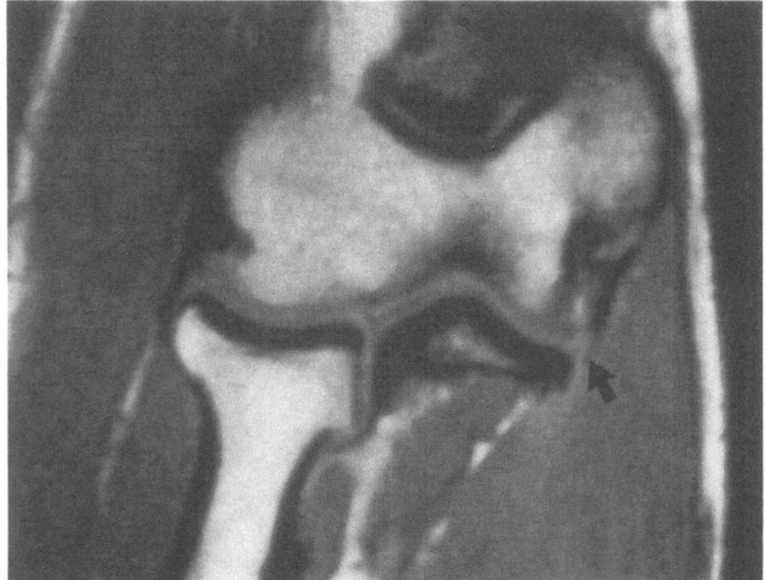

A

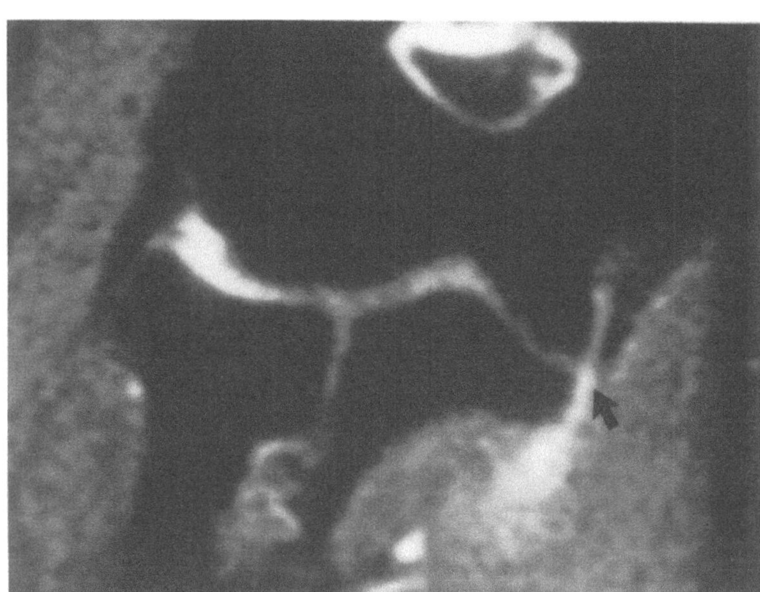

B

Fig. 7.13A,B. Acute MCL tear in a professional baseball player. T1-weighted (A) and STIR (B) coronal images reveal complete detachment of the anterior bundle of the MCL from the medial margin of the coronoid (*arrows*). *MCL*, medial collateral ligament; *STIR*, short tan inversion recovery

cial to the brachialis and inserts on the radial tuberosity. The posterior compartment contains the triceps and anconeus muscles, which are evaluated best on sagittal and axial images. The triceps inserts on the proximal aspect of the olecranon. The anconeus arises from the posterior aspect of the lateral epicondyle and inserts more distally on the olecranon. The anconeus provides dynamic support to the lateral collateral ligament in resisting varus stress. The medial and lateral compartment muscles are seen best on coronal and axial images. The medial compartment structures include the pronator teres and the flexors of the hand and wrist that arise from the medial epicondyle as the common flexor tendon. The common flexor tendon provides dynamic support to the MCL in resisting valgus stress. The lateral compartment structures include the supinator, the brachioradialis, and the extensors of the hand and wrist that arise from the lateral epicondyle as the common extensor tendon.

7.6
Elbow Pathology

7.6.1
Medial Collateral Ligament Injury

Degeneration and tearing of the MCL with or without concomitant injury of the common flexor tendon commonly occurs in throwing athletes. Injury of these medial stabilizing structures is due to chronic microtrauma from repetitive valgus stress during the acceleration phase of throwing.

Acute injury of the MCL can be detected, localized and graded with MR imaging. The status of the functionally important anterior bundle of the MCL complex may be determined by assessing the coronal and axial images. Acute ruptures of the MCL are well seen with standard MR imaging (Fig. 7.13). Partial detachment of the deep undersurface fibers of the anterior bundle may also occur in pitchers with medial elbow pain and are more difficult to diagnose with standard MR imaging. These partial tears of the MCL characteristically spare the superficial fibers of the anterior bundle and are therefore not visible from an open surgical approach unless the ligament is incised to inspect the torn capsular fibers. As a result, MR imaging is important to localize these partial tears, which are treated with repair or reconstruction. Detection of these undersurface partial tears is improved when intraarticular contrast is administered and CT-arthrography or MR-arthrography is performed. The capsular fibers of the anterior bundle of the MCL normally insert on the medial margin of the coronoid process. Undersurface partial tears of the anterior bundle are characterized by distal extension of fluid or contrast along the medial margin of the coronoid process (Fig. 7.14).

Midsubstance MCL ruptures can be differentiated from proximal avulsions or distal avulsions with MR imaging (Fig. 7.15). Midsubstance ruptures of the MCL accounted for 87% of cases, whereas distal and proximal avulsions were found in 10% and 3%, respectively, in a large series of surgically treated throwing athletes. Other investigators have found a lesser percentage of midsubstance ruptures. The fibers of the flexor digitorum superficialis muscle blend with the anterior bundle of the MCL. A strain of the flexor digitorum superficialis muscle commonly is seen when the MCL is injured (Figs. 7.14, 7.15). Chronic degeneration of the MCL is characterized by thickening of the ligament secondary to scarring often accompanied by foci of calcification or heterotopic bone. Patients with symptomatic MCL insufficiency usually are treated with reconstruction using a palmaris tendon graft. Graft failure is unusual but also may be evaluated with MR imaging (Fig. 7.16). Lateral compartment bone contusions may be seen in association with acute MCL tears and may provide useful

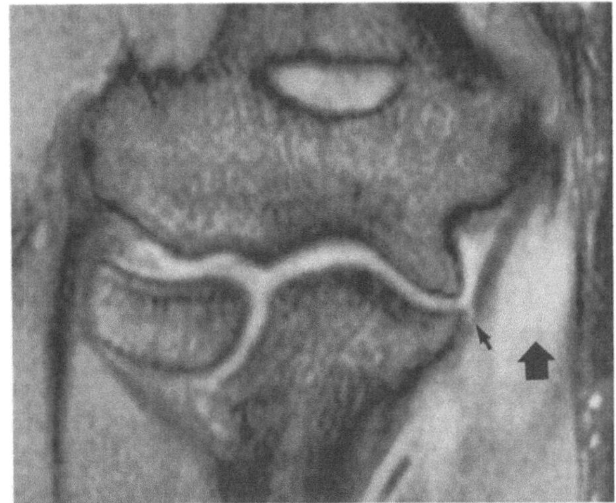
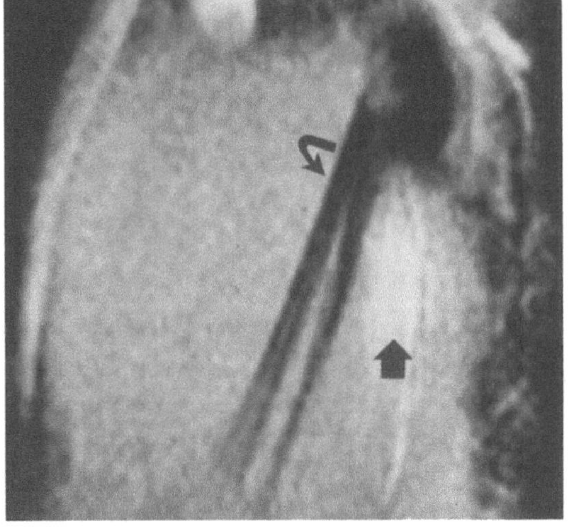

Fig. 7.14A,B. Partial tear of the MCL. A gradient-echo T2*-weighted coronal image (**A**) reveals partial detachment of the deep undersurface fibers of the anterior bundle of the MCL (*small arrow*). A strain of the adjacent flexor digitorum superficialis muscle is also noted (*large arrow*). A gradient-echo T2*-weighted sagittal image (**B**) also shows the muscle strain (*large arrow*) as well as the normal common flexor tendon (*curved arrow*)

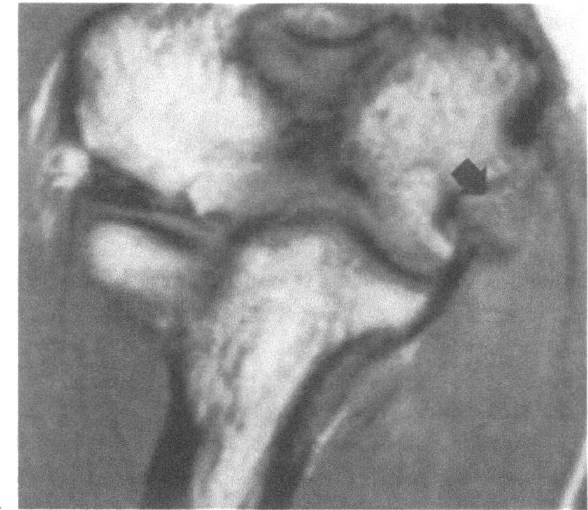 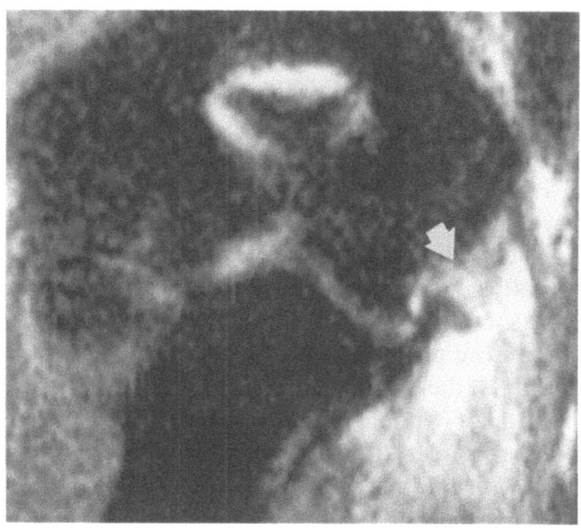

Fig. 7.15A,B. MCL tear in a professional baseball player. T1-weighted (A) and STIR (B) coronal images reveal rupture of the mid to proximal fibers of the anterior bundle of the MCL (*arrows*). Strain of the adjacent flexor digitorum superficialis muscle is also noted

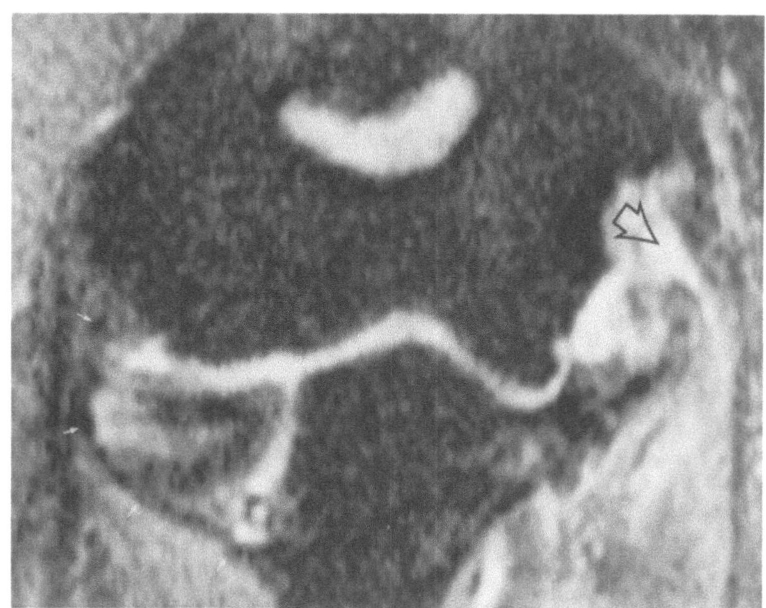

Fig. 7.16. MCL graft rupture and contusion of the radial head in a professional baseball player. A STIR coronal image reveals increased signal at the site of a ruptured MCL graft (*open arrow*). Increased signal is also seen within the lateral portion of the radial head secondary to impaction from valgus insufficiency. The normal LUCL is also well seen (*small white arrows*). *LUCL*, lateral ulnar collateral ligament

confirmation of recent lateral compartment impaction secondary to valgus instability (Fig. 7.16).

A number of different conditions may occur secondary to the repeated valgus stress to the elbow that occurs with throwing. Medial tension overload typically produces extraarticular injury such as flexor/pronator strain, MCL sprain, ulnar traction spurring and ulnar neuropathy. Lateral compression overload typically produces intraarticular injury such as osteochondritis dissecans of the capitellum or radial head, degenerative arthritis and loose body formation. MR imaging can assess for each of these related pathologic processes associated with repeated valgus stress. The additional information provided by MR imaging can be helpful in formulating a logical treatment plan, especially when surgery is being considered.

7.6.2
Elbow Dislocation and Subluxation: The Spectrum of Instability

Rupture of the MCL is also commonly encountered as a result of posterior dislocation of the elbow. The mechanism of posterior elbow dislocation usually involves falling on an outstretched arm. There is typically rupture of the medial and lateral collateral ligaments as well as the anterior and posterior capsule during posterior elbow dislocation. Associated rupture of the common extensor tendon or the common flexor tendon may also occur. The extent of injury secondary to elbow dislocation is well delineated with MR imaging.

Posterior dislocation of the elbow is an unusual event; however, it is the second most common major joint dislocation (after the shoulder) in adults and it is the most common dislocation in children under 10 years old. Children are predisposed to elbow dislocation due to the relative lack of congruity of the im-

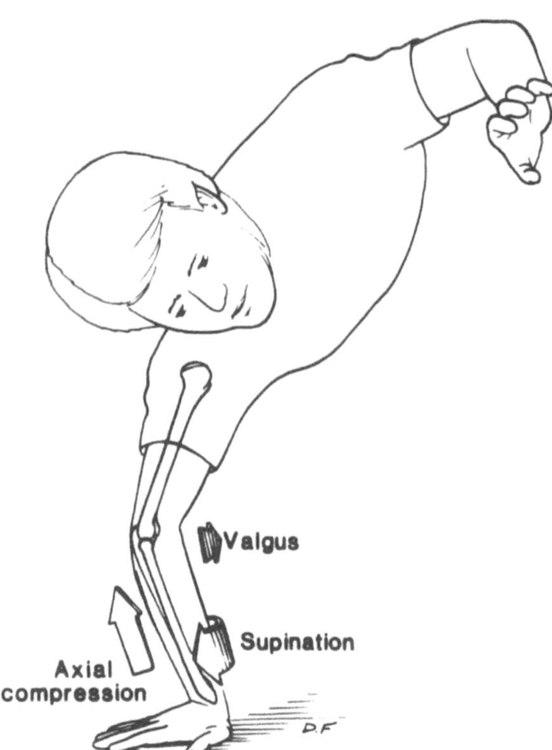

Fig. 7.17. Mechanism of elbow dislocation. A fall on the outstretched hand with the shoulder abducted produces an axial force on the elbow as it flexes. As the body internally rotates on the hand and approaches the ground, external rotation and valgus moments are applied to the elbow. (From O'DRISCOLL et al. 1992)

mature cartilaginous articulation compared with the constrained bony articulation of adults. Recurrent complete dislocation of the elbow is unusual but is more common in children and adolescents than adults. Many of the dislocations that occur in children go unrecognized because of spontaneous reduction, with the only finding a swollen tender elbow. MR imaging in such cases usually shows an effusion as well as a contusion or strain of the brachialis muscle. Bone contusions, from impaction during dislocation or relocation, may be seen at the posterior margin of the capitellum as well as the radial head and coronoid process.

The usual mechanism of dislocation involves a fall on the outstretched hand. A hyperextension force has been classically proposed to explain posterior dislocation of the elbow. More recent investigations by O'DRISCOLL and associates (1991) have resulted in a clearer understanding of how the flexed elbow may subluxate posterolaterally and may then dislocate. This mechanism involves hypersupination, valgus stress and axial compressive loading of the elbow that may occur during a fall on the outstretched hand (Fig. 7.17).

Elbow instability occurs as a spectrum from subluxation to dislocation that has been divided into three stages (Fig. 7.18). Each of these stages is associated with progressive soft tissue injury that extends from lateral to medial (Fig. 7.19). In stage 1, there is posterolateral subluxation of the ulna and radius relative to the humerus with disruption of the ulnar part of the lateral collateral ligament, which has been termed the "lateral ulnar collateral ligament" (LUCL). Rupture of the LUCL is considered the essential lesion of posterolateral rotatory instability. In stage 2, there is incomplete dislocation so that the coronoid appears perched on the trochlea (Fig. 7.20). There is further disruption of the lateral ligamentous structures in stage 2 as well as tearing of the anterior and posterior joint capsule. In stage 3, there is complete posterior dislocation with progressive disruption of the medial collateral ligament (MCL) complex. There may be disruption of the posterior bundle of the MCL only (stage 3A), in which case the elbow is stable to valgus stress. Stage 3B is characterized by additional disruption of the anterior bundle of the MCL so that the elbow is unstable in all directions. Complete disruption of the MCL (stage 3B) is the most common clinical situation after complete dislocation (Fig. 7.21). The common flexor and extensor tendons are often disrupted when there is complete posterior dislocation of the elbow (Fig. 7.22).

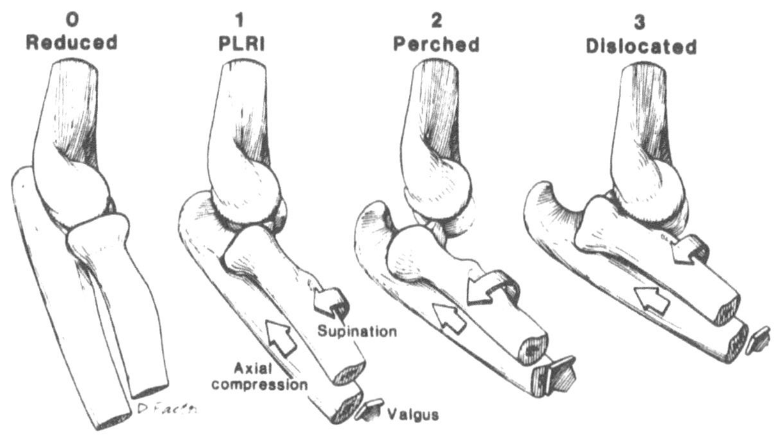

Fig. 7.18. Elbow instability occurs in a spectrum from subluxation to dislocation. The three stages shown correspond with the pathoanatomic stages of capsuloligamentous disruption illustrated in Fig. 7.19. Forces and moments responsible for displacements are also illustrated. *PLRI*, posterolateral rotatory instability. (From O'Driscoll et al. 1992)

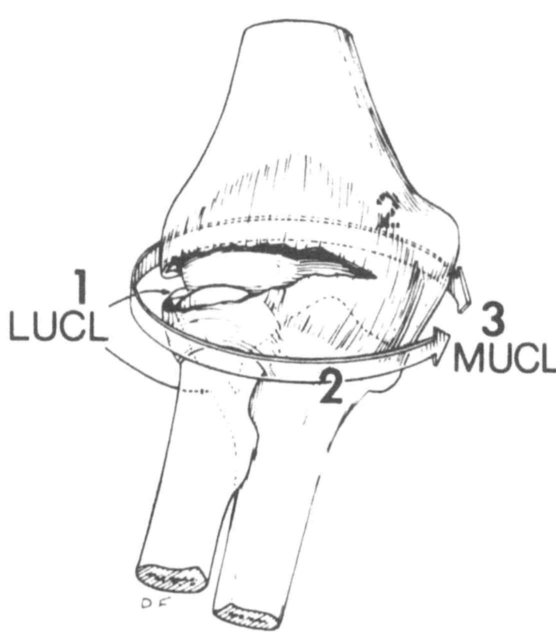

Fig. 7.19. Soft tissue injury progresses in a "circle" from lateral to medial in three stages correlating with those in Fig. 7.18. In stage 1, the ulnar part of the lateral collateral ligament, the lateral ulnar collateral ligament (*LUCL*), is disrupted. In stage 2, the other lateral ligamentous structures and the anterior and posterior capsule are disrupted. In stage 3, disruption of the medial ulnar collateral ligament (*MUCL*) can be partial with disruption of the posterior MUCL only (stage 3A) or complete (stage 3B). The common flexor and extensor origins are often disrupted as well. (From O'Driscoll et al. 1992)

The clinical assessment of elbow instability is difficult as the physical examination is often compromised by guarding and pain. The pivot-shift test of the elbow has recently been described as a clinical test for posterolateral rotatory instability of the elbow due to insufficiency of the LUCL. The pivot-shift test of the elbow is analogous to the widely known pivot-shift test of the knee to determine the integrity of the anterior cruciate ligament. This subluxation/reduction maneuver creates apprehension, however, and is usually not performable in the awake patient. Thus, clinical confirmation of recurrent instability of the elbow may require examination under anesthesia to elicit a pivot-shift maneuver.

We have found MR imaging to be quite reliable in detecting rupture of the LUCL. This ligament usually tears proximally at the lateral margin of the capitellum and is best evaluated on coronal and axial images. The LUCL may tear as an isolated finding on MR imaging in patients with posterolateral rotatory instability in stage 1 (Fig. 7.23). Tears of the LUCL also may be detected in association with rupture of the MCL in stage 3B (Fig. 7.24). Disruption of the LUCL is commonly seen in patients with severe tennis elbow who have tears of the common extensor tendon on MR imaging. Iatrogenic causes of LUCL disruption resulting in posterolateral rotatory instability include radial head excision for comminuted fractures of the radial head and overaggressive extensor tendon release for lateral epicondylitis (common extensor tendinosis). Indeed, Morrey in 1992 reported a series of 13 patients who underwent reoperation for failed lateral epicondylitis surgery. Stabilization procedures were required in four patients with either iatrogenic or unrecognized lateral ligament insufficiency. Iatrogenic tears of the LUCL were thought to occur secondary to a previous release of the common extensor tendon. Operative release of the extensor tendon may further destabilize the elbow when rupture of the LUCL and subtle associated instability are not recognized clinically and the patient is misdiagnosed with a primary abnormality of the common extensor tendon (Fig. 7.23).

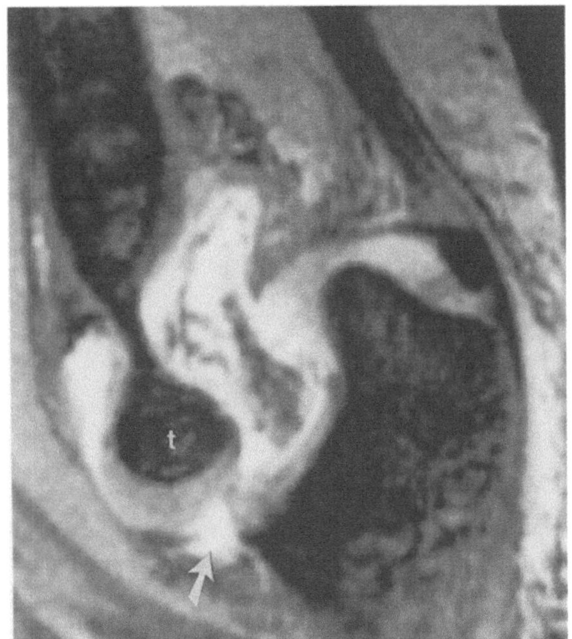

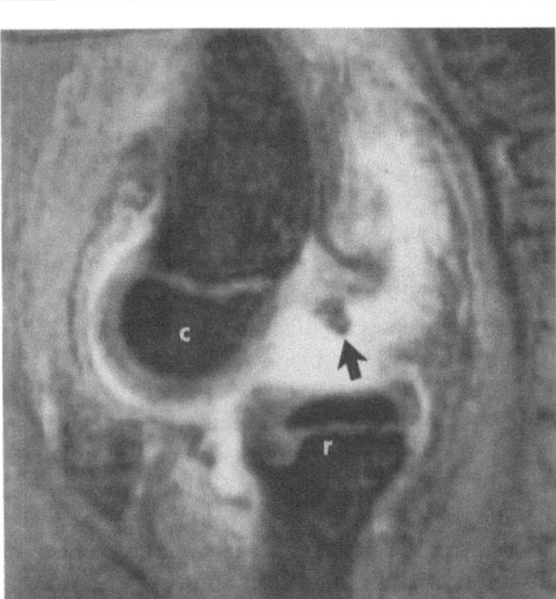

Fig. 7.20A,B. Torn lateral ulnar collateral ligament (LUCL) in an 11-year-old child with prior elbow dislocations and recurrent instability. **A** Gradient-echo T2*-weighted sagittal images reveal posterior subluxation of the radius and ulna as well as a redundant torn LUCL (*black arrow*). **B** The anterior capsule is also torn from the ulna (*white arrow*). *c*, capitellum; *r*, radius; *t*, trochlea

MR imaging can reveal concurrent tears of the LUCL and common extensor tendon in patients with lateral epicondylitis as well as isolated LUCL tears in patients with posterolateral rotatory instability.

Recurrent instability of the elbow involves a common pathway of posterolateral rotatory subluxation due to insufficiency of the LUCL. Surgical correction is performed by reattaching the avulsed LUCL to the humerus or reconstructing it with a tendon graft placed isometrically through tunnels in the ulna and the humerus as described by NESTOR et al. in 1992.

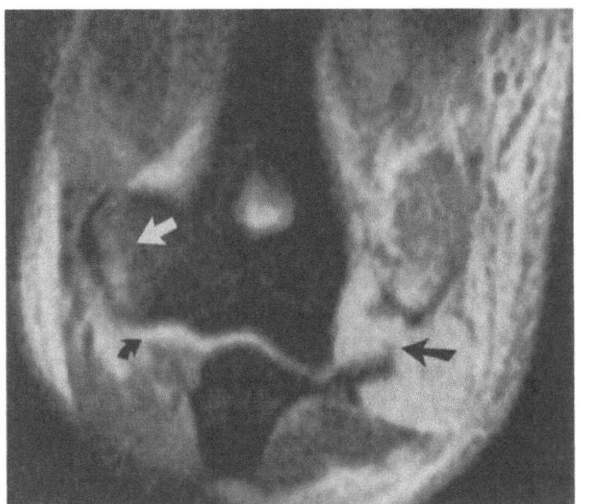

Fig. 7.21A,B. Acute elbow dislocation in a 17-year-old wrestler. A STIR coronal image (**A**) in a flexed elbow reveals detachment of the posterior bundle of the MCL from the medial epicondyle (*black arrow*). A STIR coronal image (**B**) further anteriorly reveals tearing of the proximal fibers of the anterior bundle of the MCL (*black arrow*) as well as tearing of the LUCL (*curved arrow*). A contusion of the capitellum is also noted (*white arrow*)

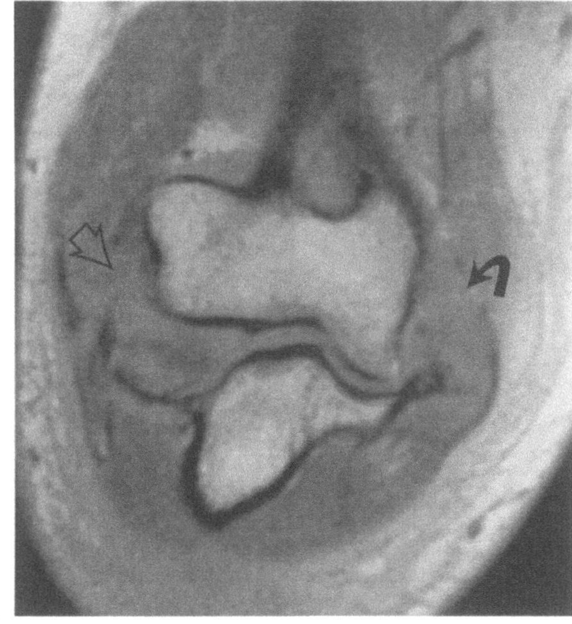

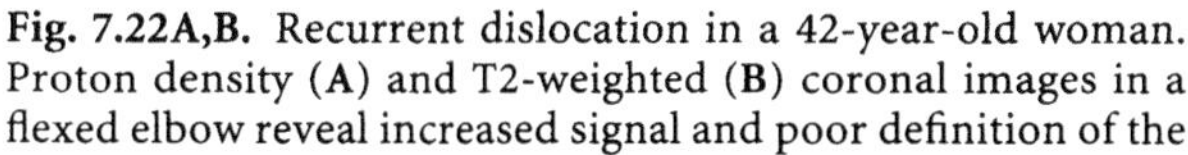

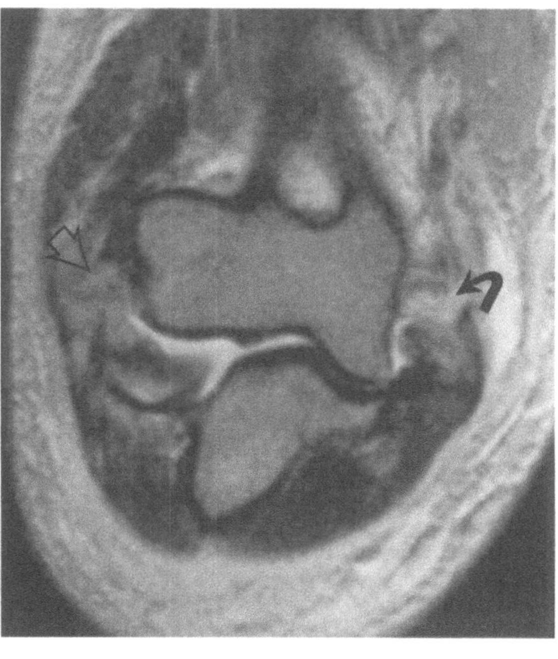

Fig. 7.22A,B. Recurrent dislocation in a 42-year-old woman. Proton density (**A**) and T2-weighted (**B**) coronal images in a flexed elbow reveal increased signal and poor definition of the fibers of the common flexor tendon (*curved arrows*) and the common extensor tendon (*open arrows*), compatible with tendon rupture

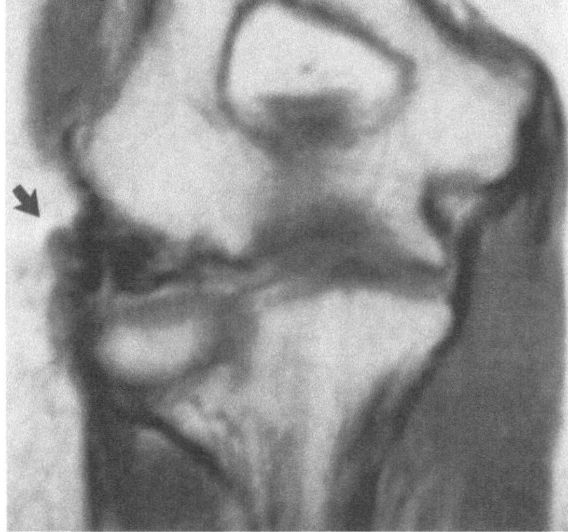

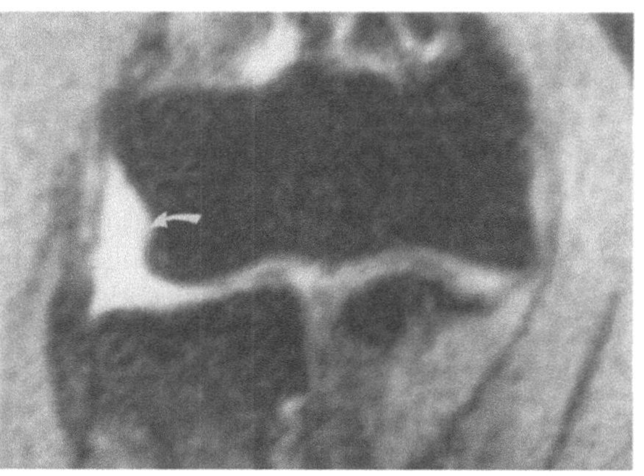

Fig. 7.23A,B. Torn lateral ulnar collateral ligament (LUCL) in a patient who developed posterolateral rotatory instability after extensor tendon release. T1-weighted (**A**) and STIR (**B**) coronal images reveal complete absence of the common extensor tendon and LUCL adjacent to the lateral epicondyle (*curved white arrow*). Micrometallic artifact is noted from prior surgical release (*black arrow*)

Elbow dislocations may be complicated by fractures that may further destabilize the joint. A fracture of the coronoid process is highly characteristic of a previous posterior dislocation or subluxation of the elbow. These fractures may be subtle on standard radiographs, especially when small or nondisplaced. Fractures of the coronoid process may predispose to recurrent posterior instability depending on the size of the fracture fragment and the presence of associated collateral ligament rupture. Coronoid process

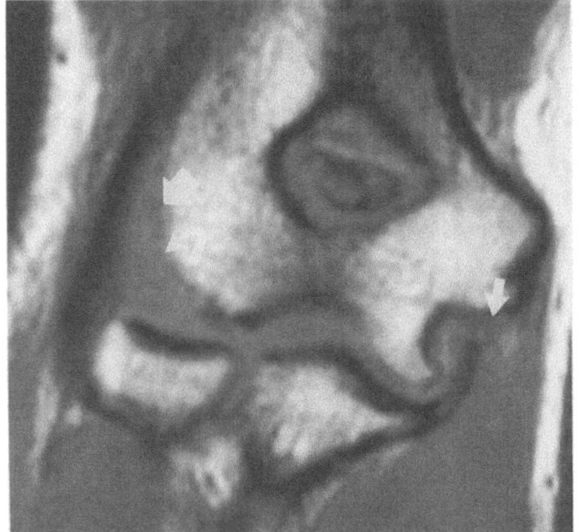

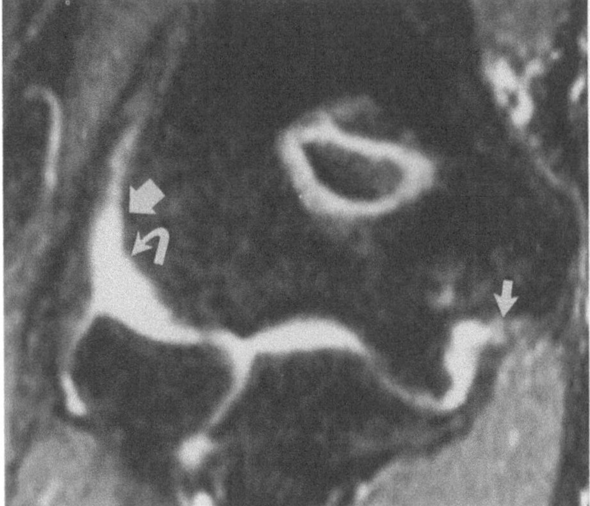

Fig. 7.24A,B. Professional football player with symptoms of instability 8 months after posterior dislocation. T1-weighted (**A**) and STIR (**B**) coronal images reveal complete detachment of the common extensor tendon (*large arrows*) and the LUCL (*curved arrows*) from the lateral epicondyle. The anterior bundle of the MCL is detached from the medial epicondyle (*small arrows*)

fractures occur as a result of direct shear injury by the trochlea during posterior dislocation or subluxation (Fig. 7.25). These fractures are not hyperextension avulsion injuries, as the tip of the coronoid is an intraarticular structure that does not have a capsular attachment (Fig. 7.26). The anterior capsule and the brachialis muscle insert further distally on the ulna. Anterior capsular injury and contusion or strain of the adjacent brachialis muscle are commonly seen after posterior elbow dislocation. MR imaging can depict these characteristic injuries in the acute setting when the diagnosis of dislocation or subluxation of the elbow is uncertain (Fig. 7.27). The joint capsule can also be assessed with MR imaging in patients who develop flexion contractures of the elbow as a complication of posterior dislocation injury (Fig. 7.28). Fortier et al. in 1995 reported their experience with MR imaging in 12 patients with post-traumatic contractures of the elbow. They found anterior capsular thickening in three cases and posterior capsular thickening in four cases on the sagittal MR images.

The coronoid is an important structure for stability of the elbow. Fractures of the coronoid process were classified by Regan and Morrey in 1992. Type I fractures are small shear fractures that do not destabilize the joint (Fig. 7.26). They should be recognized, however, as an indicator of posterior elbow dislocation/subluxation injury that may be associated with significant soft tissue disruption. Type II

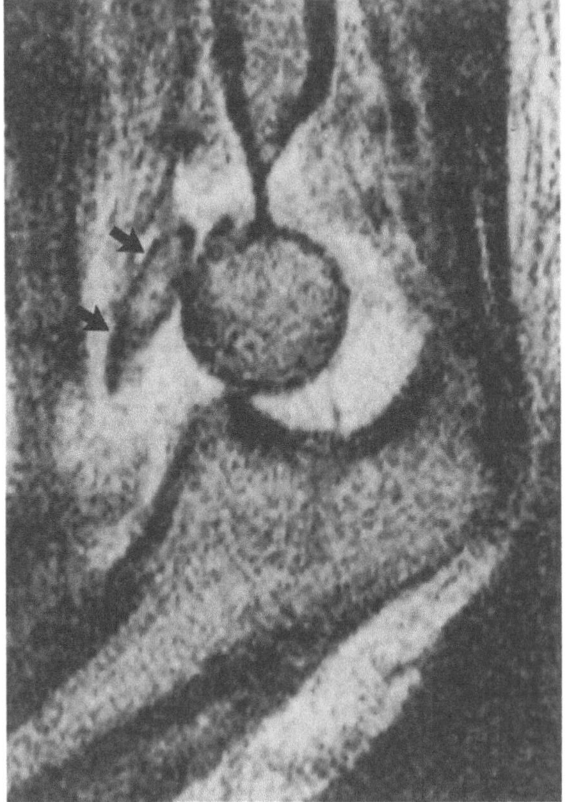

Fig. 7.25. Large coronoid process fracture secondary to a posterior elbow dislocation. A T2-weighted sagittal image reveals an anteriorly displaced fracture of the coronoid (*arrows*). Anterior capsular tearing, brachialis strain injury and posterior subluxation of the ulna relative to the trochlea are also noted

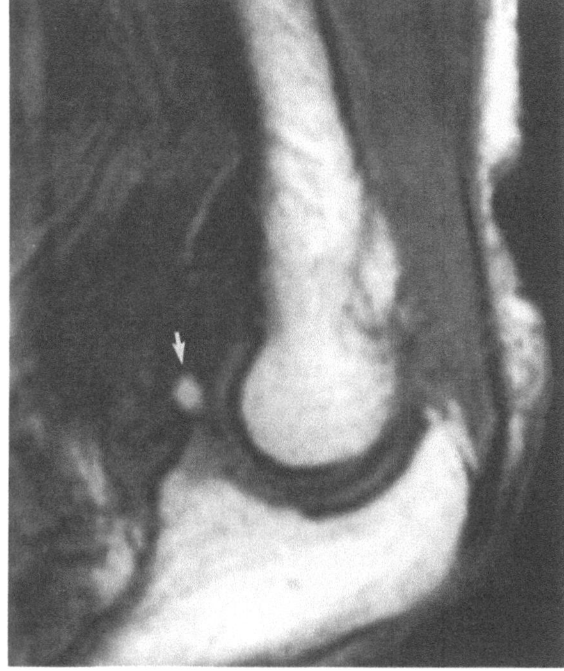

A

Fig. 7.26A,B. Radiographically subtle fracture of the superior margin of the coronoid in a 25-year-old man who fell while jogging. T1-weighted (**A**) and gradient-echo T2*-weighted (**B**) sagittal images reveal a small shear fracture of the coronoid (*small solid arrows*) as well as tearing of the anterior capsule (*open arrow*)

B

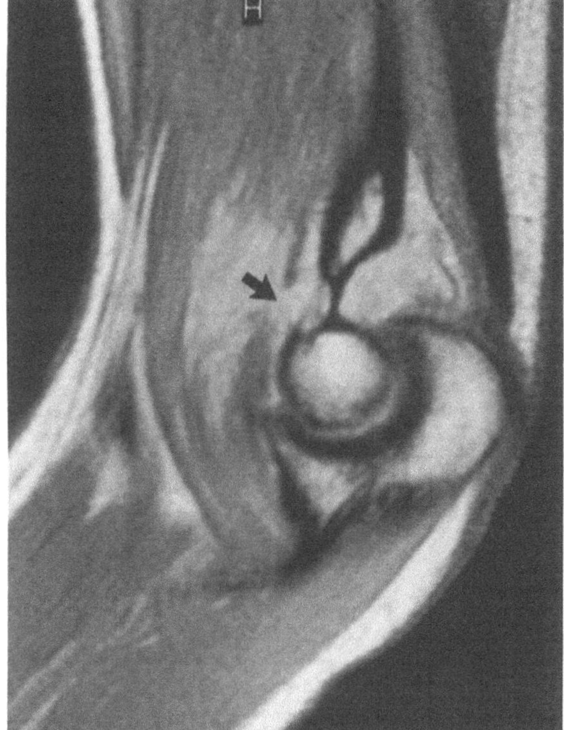

A

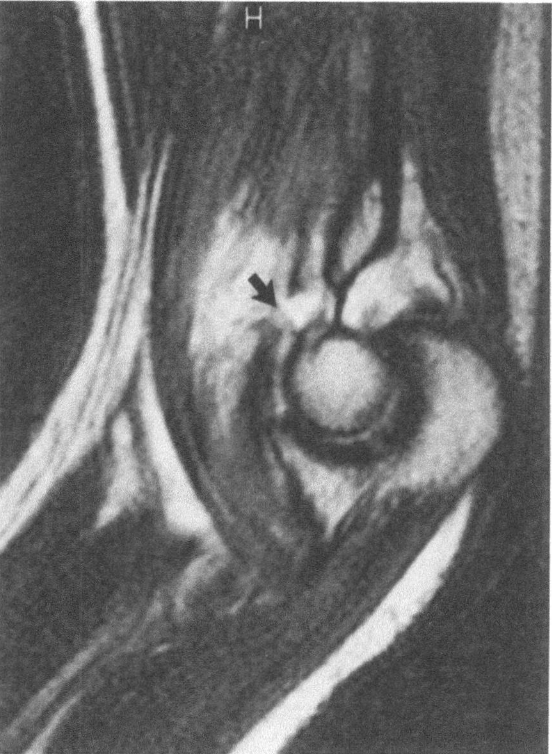

B

Fig. 7.27A,B. Characteristic findings of posterior subluxation or dislocation in a 25-year-old woman who was unable to extend her elbow after an acute injury. Proton density (**A**) and T2-weighted (**B**) sagittal images in a flexed elbow reveal a strain of the brachialis and tear of the anterior joint capsule (*arrows*). The LUCL and MCL were torn on other images (not shown)

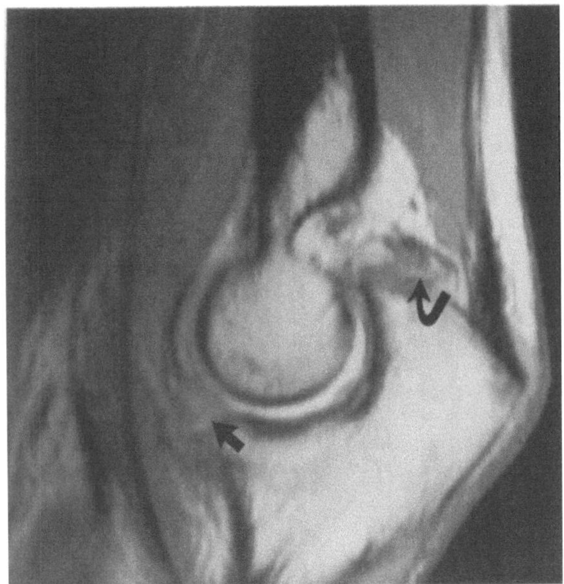

Fig. 7.28. Flexion contracture 6 months after a posterior subluxation injury of the elbow. A proton density sagittal image in a flexed elbow reveals thickening of the anterior (*straight arrow*) and posterior (*curved arrow*) joint capsule compatible with fibrosis that limits full extension of the elbow

fractures involve less than 50% of the coronoid. They should be fixed if the joint remains dislocated or subluxed. Type III fractures involve more than 50% of the coronoid and have a poor prognosis. Type III fractures as well as malunions and nonunions of the coronoid in patients with instability also require fixation.

Approximately 10% of elbow dislocations result in fractures of the radial head; conversely, about 10% of patients with a radial head fracture have an elbow dislocation. Displaced fractures of the radial head are best treated with internal fixation when there is ligamentous disruption and instability. CT is the technique of choice when additional information about the fracture morphology or degree of comminution is needed. MR imaging may detect and characterize radial head fractures and is useful for excluding associated collateral ligament injury that may contribute to instability. The integrity of the MCL is especially important if excision of the radial head is being considered.

The median or ulnar nerves may rarely become entrapped within the elbow joint after a posterior dislocation. This complication is typically seen when the common flexor tendon is torn or the medial epicondyle is avulsed. These structures should be carefully evaluated when the findings on

MR imaging are indicative of dislocation injury and there is clinical evidence of median or ulnar neuropathy.

7.6.3
Instability of the Proximal Radioulnar Joint

The radial head may dislocate in association with fractures of the ulnar shaft. Isolated traumatic dislocation of the radial head is uncommon, however. This diagnosis has probably been confused in the past with the more common but previously unrecognized diagnosis of posterolateral rotatory instability of the elbow. Most traumatic dislocations of the proximal radioulnar joint are associated with anterior dislocation of the radial head whereas most congenital dislocations occur posteriorly. In congenital dislocation of the radial head there is usually neuromuscular dysfunction and dysplasia of the radial head and capitellum.

WEISS and HASTINGS determined in 1992 that the annular ligament and the central band of the interosseous membrane are the main stabilizers of the proximal radioulnar joint in pronation and that the central band is the significant stabilizer in supination. Both the annular ligament and the central band of the interosseous membrane are well seen with MR imaging and can be assessed on axial T2-weighted images (Fig. 7.12).

References

Amadio PC (1991) Carpal kinematics and instability: a clinical and anatomic primer. Clin Anat 4:1–12

Berger RA, Landsmeer JMF (1990) The palmar radiocarpal ligaments: a study of adult and fetal human wrist joints. J Hand Surg [Am] 15:847–854

Berger RA, Blair WF, Crowninshield RD, Flatt AE (1982) The scapholunate ligament. J Hand Surg [Am] 1:87–91

Burgess RC (1987) The effect of rotatory subluxation of the scaphoid on radioscaphoid contact. J Hand Surg [Am] 12:771–774

Cautilli GP, Wehbe MA (1991) Scapho-lunate distance and cortical ring sign. J Hand Surg [Am] 16:501–503

Conway JE, Jobe FW, Glousman RE, Pink M (1992) Medial instability of the elbow in throwing athletes. Treatment by repair or reconstruction of the ulnar collateral ligament. J Bone Joint Surg [Am] 74:67–83

Fortier MV, Forster BB, Pinney S, Regan W (1995) MR assessment of posttraumatic flexion contracture of the elbow. J Magn Reson Imaging 4:473–477

Fritz RC (1995) MR imaging of the elbow. Semin Roentgenol 30:241–264

Horii E, Garcia-Elias M, An KN, et al. (1991) A kinematic study of luno-triquetral dissociations. J Hand Surg [Am] 16:355–362

Kauer JMG (1979) The collateral ligament function in the wrist joint. Acta Morphol Neerl Scand 17:252–253

Kauer JMG (1986) The mechanism of the carpal joint. Clin Orthop 202:16–26

Kauer JMG (1996) The wrist joint: anatomic and functional considerations. In: Gilula LA (ed) Imaging of the wrist and hand. Saunders, Philadelphia, pp 43–55

Levinsohn EM, Rosen ID, Palmer AK (1991) Wrist arthrography: value of the three-compartment injection method. Radiology 179:231–239

Lichtman DM, Martin RA (1988) Introduction to the carpal instabilities. In: Lichtman DM (ed) The wrist and its disorders. Saunders, Philadelphia, pp 244–250

Lichtman DM, Schneider JR, Swafford AR, Mack GR (1981) Ulnar midcarpal instability. Clinical and laboratory analysis. J Hand Surg [Am] 6:515–523

Linscheid RL, Dobyns JH, Beabout JW, Bryan RS (1972) Traumatic instability of the wrist. J Bone Joint Surg [Am] 54:1612–1632

Linscheid RL, Dobyns JH, Beckenbaugh RD, Cooney WP, Wood MB (1983) Instability patterns of the wrist. J Hand Surg [Am] 8:682–686

Manaster BJ (1991) The clinical efficacy of triple-injection wrist arthrography. Radiology 178:267–270

Mayfield JK, Johnson RP, Kilcoyne RF (1976) The ligaments of the human wrist and their functional significance. Anat Rec 186:417–428

Metz VM, Mann FA, Gilula LA (1993) Tree-compartment wrist arthrography: correlation of pain site with location of uni- and bidirectional communications. AJR Am J Roentgenol 160:819–822

Mirowitz SA, London SL (1992) Ulnar collateral ligament injury in baseball pitchers: MR imaging evaluation. Radiology 185:573–576

Morrey BF (1992) Reoperation for failed surgical treatment of refractory lateral epicondylitis. J Shoulder Elbow Surg 1:47–55

Nestor BJ, O'Driscoll SW, Morrey BF (1992) Ligamentous reconstruction for posterolateral rotatory instability of the elbow. J Bone Joint Surg [Am] 74:1235–1241

Obermann WR (1994) Radiology of carpal instability: a practical approach. Elsevier, Amsterdam

O'Driscoll SW, Bell DF, Morrey BF (1991) Posterolateral rotatory instability of the elbow. J Bone Joint Surg [Am] 73:440–446

O'Driscoll SW, Morrey BF, Korinek S, An KN (1992) Elbow subluxation and dislocation. A spectrum of instability. Clin Orthop 280:186–197

Palmer AK, Werner FW (1981) The triangular fibrocartilage complex of the wrist – anatomy and function. J Hand Surg [Am] 6:153–162

Regan W, Morrey BF (1992) Classification and treatment of coronoid process fractures. Orthopedics 15:845–848

Rominger MB, Bernreuter WK, Kenney PJ, Lee DH (1993) MR imaging of anatomy and tears of wrist ligaments. Radiographics 13:1233–1246

Ruby LK, An KN, Linscheid RL, Cooney WP, Chao EYS (1987) The effect of scapholunate ligament section on scapholunate motion. J Hand Surg [Am] 12:767–771

Ruby LK, Cooney WP, An KN, et al. (1988) Relative motion of selected carpal bones: a kinematic analysis of the normal wrist. J Hand Surg [Am] 13:1–10

Smith DK (1993) Volar carpal ligaments of the wrist: normal appearance on multiplanar reconstructions of three-dimensional Fourier transform MR imaging. AJR Am J Roentgenol 161:353–357

Taleisnik J (1976) The ligaments of the wrist. J Hand Surg [Am] 1:110–118

Taleisnik J (1985) Carpal kinematics. In: Taleisnik J (ed) The wrist. Churchill Livingstone, New York, pp 39–49

Timmerman LA, Andrews JR (1994) Undersurface tear of the ulnar collateral ligament in baseball players. A newly recognized lesion. Am J Sports Med 22:33–36

Timmerman LA, McBride DG (1995) Elbow dislocations in sports. Sports Med Arthrosc Rev 3:210–218

Tjin A Ton ER, Pattynama PMT, Bloem JL, Obermann WR (1995) Interosseous ligaments: device for applying stress in wrist MR imaging. Radiology 196:863–864

Totterman SMS, Miller R, Wasserman B, Blebea JS, Rubens DJ (1993) Intrinsic and extrinsic carpal ligaments: evaluation by three-dimensional Fourier transform MR imaging. AJR Am J Roentgenol 160:117–123

Viegas SF, Patterson RM, Peterson PD, et al. (1990) Ulnar-sided perilunate instability: an anatomic and biomechanic study. J Hand Surg [Am] 15:268–278

Weber ER (1988) Wrist mechanics and its association with ligamentous instability. In: Lichtman DM (ed) The wrist and its disorders. Saunders, Philadelphia, pp 41–52

Weiss APC, Hastings H (1992) The anatomy of the proximal radioulnar joint. J Shoulder Elbow Surg 1:193–199

8 Instability of the Knee

M. Steinborn[1] and M. Reiser[2]

CONTENTS

8.1
Introduction

Of all the joints of the human body, the knee is the one most often affected by injuries. According to Cotta and Dreyer (1967), about 7% of all traumatic injuries involve the knee. The continuing development of broad sports, particularly alpine skiing, together with the increasing number of motor vehicle accidents has resulted in an enhanced incidence of injuries to various structures of the knee joint, which represent an increasingly significant cost factor to the public health system.

Injuries to the anterior cruciate ligament (ACL) make up 47.6% of all ligamentous injuries to the knee. Injury to the medial collateral ligament occurs as an isolated entity in 28.8% of cases, while in another 12.8% of patients it is associated with lesions of the ACL. Less commonly affected are the posterior cruciate ligament (PCL; 3.6%), the lateral collateral ligament (2.0%) and combined injuries to the medial

collateral ligament and the PCL (1.6%) or to the lateral collateral ligament and the ACL (1.2%).

The following chapter considers the various aspects of instability of the knee joint. First, we will discuss the anatomical and functional aspects, followed by differentiation of the various types of instability. The main part of this chapter deals with diagnostic procedures, with particular emphasis on diagnostic imaging techniques.

8.2
Anatomy

In the knee joint, the *articulatio genus*, the cartilage-clad surfaces of the two femoral condyles articulate with the tibial plateau, the *facies articularis superior* of the tibia. This joint architecture allows both flexional and extensional movements, while, with flexion, some rotational movements are additionally possible. The incongruency of the articular surfaces is reduced by the interposed menisci which simultaneously form a flexible socket for the femoral condyles. The lateral meniscus forms an almost closed ring, while the medial meniscus assumes a more C-like shape.

The joint capsule is attached to the tibia along the bone-cartilage border. On the fibula, the insertional line of the synovial layer only partially corresponds to the more distal insertion of the fibrous portion of the capsule. At the anterior surface of the femur, the synovial layer folds back proximal to the patella by about a finger-width, forming the suprapatellar recess. Laterally, the insertional line leaves the femoral epicondyles uncovered, while along the dorsal aspect it follows the bone-cartilage border. The anterior wall of the capsule is reinforced anteriorly by the patellar ligament and anteromedially and anterolaterally by the retinacula of the patella. The dorsal wall is reinforced by the tendinous segments of the semimembranosus, popliteal and gastrocnemius muscles and by fibrous elements of the tibiofibular joint. Regulation of motion in the knee joint is ac-

[1] M. Steinborn, MD, Department of Radiology, Klinikum Grosshadern, Ludwig-Maximilians-Universität, Marchioninistrasse 15, 81377 Munich, Germany
[2] M. Reiser, MD, Department of Radiology, Klinikum Grosshadern, Ludwig-Maximilians-Universität, Marchioninistrasse 15, 81377 Munich, Germany

complished mainly by the ligaments since bony and muscular regulation is minimal.

According to NICHOLAS et al. (1973) the active and passive elements of joint stability in the knee can be divided into a medial, central and lateral complex. These three complexes are primarily dorsal; ventral stability is achieved by the action of the extensor apparatus of the knee joint.

8.2.1
Medial Complex

The medial complex prevents valgus and lateral rotational instability of the knee. It consists of the medial collateral ligament, the dorsomedial capsule, the semimembranosus muscle and the pes anserinus.

The medial collateral ligament consists of a superficial layer, a deep layer and a posteromedial capsule reinforcement with diagonal arrangement of fibers, which is also known as the "posterior oblique ligament." The deep layer blends with the joint capsule and thus with the medial meniscus. The deep and superficial layers are separated from one another by a narrow bursa and a peribursal layer of fat. The dorsomedial capsule is reinforced by the oblique popliteal ligament, a segment of the terminal tendon of the semimembranosus muscle which extends to the lateral femoral condyle.

The semimembranosus muscle inserts proximal to the pes anserinus group on the dorsomedial aspect of the head of the tibia, and a portion of its fibers reinforces the posterior wall of the knee joint capsule.

8.2.2
Central Complex

The central complex assures stability in the sagittal plane and is formed by the cruciate ligaments and the menisci. The ACL extends from the anterior intercondylar area of the tibia to the medial surface of the lateral femoral condyle. The PCL arises fan-shaped from the anterior third of the inner surface of the medial femoral condyle and extends to the posterior intercondylar area of the tibia. The cruciate ligaments project from the posterior capsule into the joint space. They are surrounded on all sides by synovial lining: hence, they are intraarticular but extrasynovial. The menisci bind crescent-shaped to the joint capsule and are wedge-shaped in cross section. The anterior and posterior horns of the menisci are fixed to the anterior and posterior intercondylar areas, respectively. The medial meniscus, additionally, is attached to the medial collateral ligament and is thus less mobile than its mate. The transverse ligament binds both menisci along their anterior rims. The posterior horn of the lateral meniscus is also joined to the medial femoral condyle by the variable anterior and posterior meniscofemoral ligaments.

8.2.3
Lateral Complex

The lateral complex prevents varus and internal rotational instability. It is made up of the lateral collateral ligament, the iliotibial tract, the biceps femoris muscle, the popliteal muscle and the dorsolateral joint capsule. In contrast to the medial collateral ligament, the lateral collateral ligament has no contact with the joint capsule. The space between the capsule and ligament is traversed by the tendon of the popliteal muscle and a strand of fibers branching off from the tendon of the biceps femoris.

The iliotibial tract inserts laterally on the femur above the intermuscular septum and sends out fibers to the head of the fibula and to the lateral retinaculum of the patella. It serves as both an active and a passive stabilizer. The biceps femoris effects lateral stabilization in extension, while, during flexion, it causes lateral rotation of the tibia. The popliteal muscle, whose tendon penetrates the dorsal capsule and extends from the lateral condyle of the femur to the posterior aspect of the tibia, is a medial rotator and, together with the arcuate popliteal ligament, reinforces the dorsolateral portions of the capsule. A large tendinous segment inserts at the posterior horn of the lateral meniscus and dorsal joint capsule and translocates the posterior horn of the lateral meniscus and the joint capsule during the dorsal gliding phase of the femoral condyle.

8.3
Functional Anatomy

The motion of the knee joint in the sagittal plane corresponds to a rocking-gliding motion. During the first phase of flexion, there is primarily a rocking motion of the femoral condyles, which continues to an angle of flexion of 10°–15° medially and 25°–

30° laterally before shifting increasingly to a gliding motion.

The passive stabilizers of the knee joint are exposed to varying degrees of tension during the changing functional condition of the joint. The fibrous bundles of the ACL can be divided into two main components: a longer, more powerful anteromedial and a shorter posterolateral bundle. During extension, the fibers of the posterolateral bundle are taut. With increasing flexion, the fibers of the anteromedial bundle become tense, while those of the posterolateral bundle relax. Thus, portions of the ACL are taut in every position of the knee joint. The posterior cruciate ligament similarly exhibits a well-developed anterolateral and a weaker posteromedial bundle. The anterolateral bundle is taut during flexion, while the posteromedial bundle reaches its maximum tension upon extension. The lateral collateral ligament is tense only in extreme extension. The medial collateral ligament is completely taut upon hyperextension in the knee joint; during extension, the posterior longitudinal and capsule-reinforcing fibers are tense, while during flexion only the anterior longitudinal fibers are taut.

8.4
Pathophysiology

Most injuries to internal structures of the knee are the result of indirect application of force to the joint. Basically, depending on the degree of injury, it is possible to differentiate simple and complex instability. Instability is said to be simple in cases in which pathological motion in the joint is limited to a single plane. Fresh, simple instabilities secondary to isolated tearing of a ligament, however, are rare. More often, complex instabilities are found in which loss of stability extends to two or more planes of motion.

8.4.1
Complex Instabilities

The classification of complex instabilities is based on the rotational dislocation of the head of the tibia upon flexion of the knee joint. The rotational movement is divided analogous to the displacement of the axis of rotation into a medial and lateral direction. In the sagittal plane, instability is described as anterior or posterior.

8.4.1.1
Anteromedial Instability

Anteromedial instability is the most commonly encountered complex instability. In this form of instability, the medial tibial plateau rotates excessively anteriorly and the joint space opens medially. The fundamental mechanism of injury consists of valgus and lateral rotational stress during flexion of the knee. This leads to injury of parts of the medial complex, particularly the collateral ligaments and the dorsomedial capsule, and to a lesion of the ACL and medial meniscus. In 1950, O'DONOGHUE referred to this combined injury to the medial collateral ligament, the ACL and the medial meniscus as the "unhappy triad."

8.4.1.2
Anterolateral Instability

Anterolateral instability is characterized by excessive forward rotation of the tibial plateau with lateral opening of the joint space. It is caused by adduction or medial rotational trauma to the flexed knee. This leads to injury to structures of the lateral complex, particularly the lateral collateral ligament and the posterolateral capsule wall, as well as to injury of the ACL and the anterior horn of the lateral meniscus.

8.4.1.3
Posterolateral Instability

In posterolateral instability, there is excessive posterior rotation of the lateral tibial plateau with lateral gaping of the joint space. It is most commonly caused by direct trauma to the head of the tibia when slightly rotated medially and is accompanied by injury to the PCL, the lateral collateral ligament and the posterolateral section of the joint capsule.

8.4.1.4
Posteromedial Instability

In posteromedial instability, the tibial plateau rotates posteriorly and medially, with medial gaping of the joint space. It is due to a hyperextensional mechanism or to direct application of force to the laterally rotated lower leg during flexion in the knee joint. It is characterized by injury to the PCL and to the medial section of the joint capsule.

8.5
Clinical Signs

Clinical diagnosis begins with adequate historical questioning of the patient regarding the traumatic event and his subjective complaints. Partial ruptures of the capsule ligament structures often produce enhanced pain during active or passive motion in the joint, while complete ruptures are often accompanied by pain only upon passive manipulation into a pathologic joint position. Injuries to the medial collateral ligament are often associated with acute stabbing pain during the accident event itself.

A subjective sign of ligamentous instability is the giving way of the joint, occurring primarily on uneven ground or during unexpected motions.

Joint blockage is mostly the result of a ruptured meniscus being caught between the opposing articular surfaces. A reflex inhibition of extension and flexion, however, can also be observed in cases of rupture of the cruciate ligaments. Furthermore, effusions and soft tissue swelling may also restrict joint motion.

Joint effusion apparent immediately after an accident suggests hemarthrosis. Clinical examination reveals a visible bulging of the upper joint recess and fluctuating patella. Every post-traumatic effusion must be tapped for diagnostic and therapeutic reasons. Bloody effusion is suggestive of internal injury to the knee with vascular involvement and usually represents an indication for arthroscopy.

Hemarthrosis may also occur in cases of intraarticular fractures. At arthroscopy, NEUMANN et al. (1991) found fresh ruptures of the cruciate ligaments in 84.5% of patients with hemarthrosis and clinical suspicion of isolated rupture of the ACL. In cases in which hemarthrosis was believed to be an isolated diagnosis (stable hemarthrosis), a fresh injury to the cruciate ligaments was found in 35% of patients.

In a study of 620 patients, hemarthrosis was accompanied in 90% of cases with intraarticular lesions that required operative treatment. In 51% of cases, fresh ruptures of the ACL were observed (BENEDETTO et al. 1990).

Recent reports on the use of magnetic resonance imaging (MRI) in the literature, however, suggest that about 50% of arthroscopies in patients with hemarthrosis secondary to internal knee injuries can be avoided by subjecting patients to MRI (RUWE et al. 1992).

As a rule, the degree of injury to the capsule ligament structures stands in inverse correlation to the amount of intraarticular effusion since large defects allow drainage of the fluid into surrounding soft tissues.

8.6
Diagnostics

8.6.1
Clinical Diagnosis

Clinical diagnosis is based on various examinations to identify simple and complex instabilities. First, there is a comparison with the uninjured extremity in order to determine the individual degree of ligament laxity. With all tests, the quality of the strike upon reaching the end point of motion is important. A hard strike tends to exclude a complete tear of the ligaments, while a soft strike is typical of rupture or is typically a residual of an older, more extensive instability.

8.6.1.1
Tests for Varus- and Valgus Instability

The collateral ligaments are first palpated from proximal to distal. Pressure pain over the medial femoral condyle (ski point) may suggest a proximal lesion of the collateral ligament, which most commonly occurs at this point. Lesions of the lateral collateral ligament near its proximal insertion are rare, but a lesion of this ligament should be ruled out by careful palpation of the lateral femoral condyle.

Testing for medial and lateral instability takes place in extension and at 20° flexion of the knee joint. Pathological mobility at 20° flexion suggests isolated injury to the collateral ligaments since the posterior sections of the capsule are relaxed and do not contribute to joint stability. Pathological mobility at full extension points to injury of posterior and lateral capsular structures. In cases with significant pathological mobility, simultaneous injury to the cruciate ligaments must also be suspected. The importance of the posterior sections of the capsule for stability of the knee joint in extension becomes apparent from the fact that even complete dissection of both the medial collateral and anterior cruciate ligament does not result in medial instability of the knee joint in extension as long as the posterior parts of the capsule are intact (ABBOT et al. 1944).

8.6.1.2
Anterior Instability

There are a number of clinical methods for evaluating anterior instability. Routinely, the anterior drawer test, the Lachman test and the pivot-shift test are used. Clinical studies have shown that the Lachman test yields the most reliable results (KIM et al. 1995).

8.6.1.2.1
LACHMAN TEST

Diagnosis of ACL lesions is most reliably done using the Lachman sign. The Lachman test evaluates the anterior drawer phenomenon of the tibia in near-complete extension (20° flexion) by anterior subluxation of the tibia opposite the stationary femur. The dislocation is estimated in millimeters, and the result is evaluated as normal (0–2 mm), nearly normal (3–5 mm), abnormal (6–10 mm) or very abnormal (>10 mm). Strike quality is determined as hard or soft.

8.6.1.2.2
PIVOT-SHIFT PHENOMENON

The pivot-shift sign is pathognomonic for isolated or combined ACL insufficiency. The pivot-shift phenomenon is a painful anterior subluxation of the tibia occuring when the extended knee joint is suddenly flexed during valgus stress, slight medial rotation or axial pressure. The joint is particularly dislocated in the lateral compartment, and the dislocation reaches its maximum at 20°–30° flexion.

The pivot-shift test tends to be positive more frequently in older rather than in fresh injuries.

8.6.1.3
Posterior Instability

The evaluation of posterior instability is based on the posterior drawer test in flexion and near-extension at neutral, medial and lateral rotational position of the foot. The most important test is the posterior sag. Here, both knee joints are held parallel at 90° flexion. The affected knee exhibits a "posterior sag" of the head of the tibia upon inspection of the silhouette of the structure. This resting position in the posterior

drawer is due to gravity and represents useful evidence of a PCL lesion.

The reversed pivot-shift test can be used to demonstrate posterolateral instability. Here, the tibial plateau is dislocated dorsally by lateral rotation and valgus stress, only to be reduced ventrally by increasing extension, which takes place with a palpable and audible snap.

8.6.2
Radiologic Procedures

8.6.2.1
Conventional Radiography

Radiographic plainfilms in anterior-posterior and lateral projection represent the primary imaging technique in every patient presenting with trauma to the knee joint in order to exclude injuries to osseous structures. Avulsion ruptures of the cruciate ligaments occur mostly at the anterior or posterior intercondylar areas (Fig. 8.1); femoral lesions are only rarely observed. Evaluation of a bony avulsion of the intercondylar eminence should include projections according to Frik, in which the central projection runs parallel to the tibial plateau.

Avulsion ruptures of the collateral ligaments are also rare. Most common is an avulsion rupture of the lateral collateral ligament at the head of the fibula.

As early as 1934, FELSENREICH described a number of radiologic changes of the intercondylar eminence secondary to older ruptures of the cruciate ligaments. These include the widening and heightening of the medial intercondylar tubercle, the deepening of the groove between the tubercles, changes in the lateral intercondylar tubercle as well as formation of grooves and tubercles at the level of the origin and insertion especially of the ACL. Evidence of an old proximal lesion of the medial collateral ligament is the Stieda-Pellegrini shadow, a calcification or ossification at the level of the medial condyle.

Tomography has been widely replaced by high-resolution computed tomography (CT) as a method for visualizing fractures of the head of the tibia or of the condyles. Similarly, stress radiographs have become less important since the introduction of computed and magnetic resonance tomography.

An effusion in the knee joint recognizable on lateral radiographs cannot be seen as a sensitive sign of a capsule ligament lesion. In about 25% of cases with injuries to the cruciate ligaments, meniscus lesions

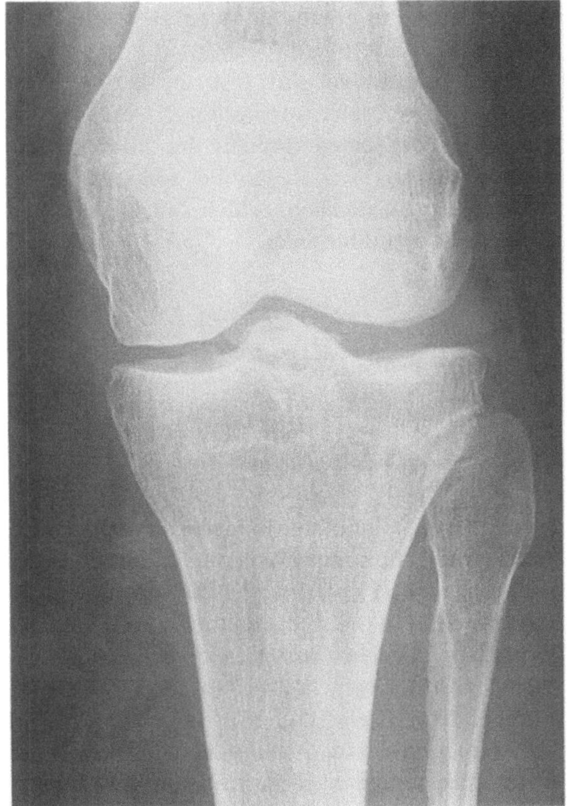

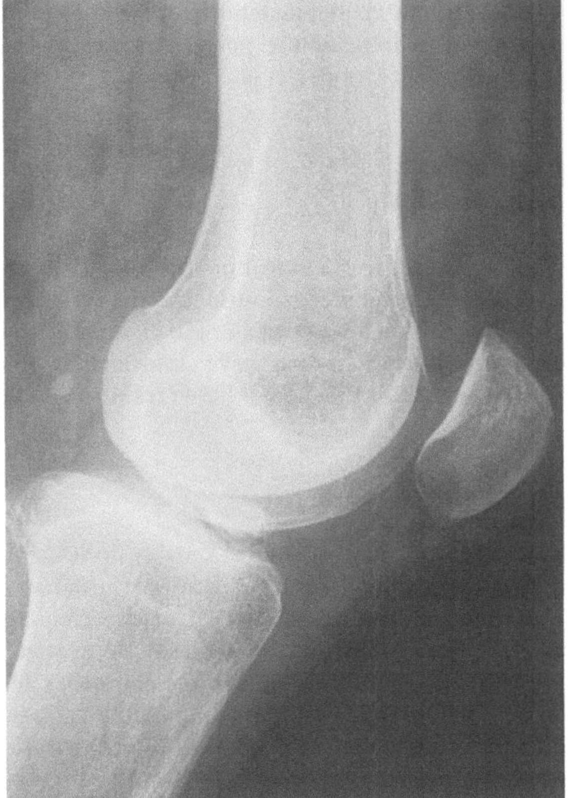

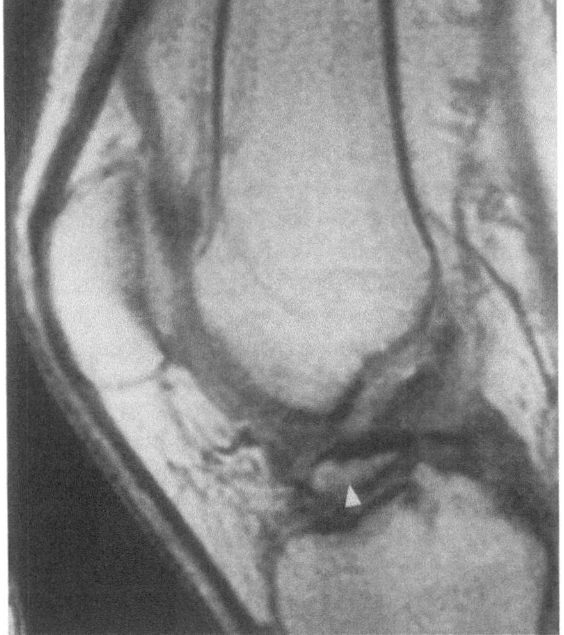

Fig. 8.1a–c. Chronic avulsion rupture of the ACL. The conventional radiographs in anteroposterior (a) and lateral (b) view demonstrate an avulsion of the intercondylar eminence. The sagittal T1-w SE image (c; TR 600/TE 24) demonstrates the avulsion fracture of the insertion of the ACL. The displaced intercondylar eminence presents a normal bone marrow signal (*arrowhead*). *W*, Weighted

or osteochondral fractures, there is no radiologic evidence of joint effusion (FISHWICK et al. 1994).

Special Projections for Instabilities. The stress radiograph can determine and document the degree of

instability. The radiograph should be taken using appropriate equipment since manual techniques possess inadequate precision of measurement and expose the examiner to unnecessary radiation. Lateral instability is documented in anterior-posterior projection with knee joint flexion of circa 20° and in comparison with the unaffected extremity. For suspected lesions of the posteromedial or posterolateral capsule ligament structures, radiographs with full extension (0° flexion) of the knee joint are performed.

Radiologic documentation of an anterior or posterior drawer phenomenon is obtained by lateral views with 30° or 90° flexion of the knee, respectively. The interpretation of these findings requires comparison with the unaffected limb. A difference of more than 3 mm between the two limbs is considered pathologic.

Stress radiographs have gradually lost their importance since the introduction of computed and magnetic resonance tomography. Furthermore, studies have shown that stress radiographs are not associated with higher diagnostic reliability than careful clinical examination (RUNKEL et al. 1993).

Since introduction of modern imaging techniques, the method of arthrography has lost its place in the clinical diagnosis of knee joint injuries.

8.6.2.2
Computed Tomography

CT enables good visualization and evaluation of both the ligamentous structures and the menisci (ARCHER et al. 1978; PAVLOV et al. 1979). Gas arthrographic CT for the first time has permitted adequate evaluation of the cruciate ligaments (REISER et al. 1982) (Fig. 8.2). With improved CT techniques, both cruciate and collateral ligaments can be imaged without intraarticular contrast enhancement. With the help of multiplanar reconstruction techniques in sagittal projection, the cruciate ligaments can be visualized along their entire course. Injured ligaments can be identified at CT by recognition of thickening, their failure to be imaged in one slice and by their inhomogeneous, hypodense structure. The ACL normally exhibits an attenuation at CT between 50–70 HU, while values of 80–100 HU have been reported for the PCL. The collateral ligaments exhibit physiologic densities of 50–70 HU (PASSARIELLO et al. 1986).

8.6.2.3
Ultrasonography

Ultrasonography (US) is a noninvasive method for visualization of soft tissue structures, whose applica-

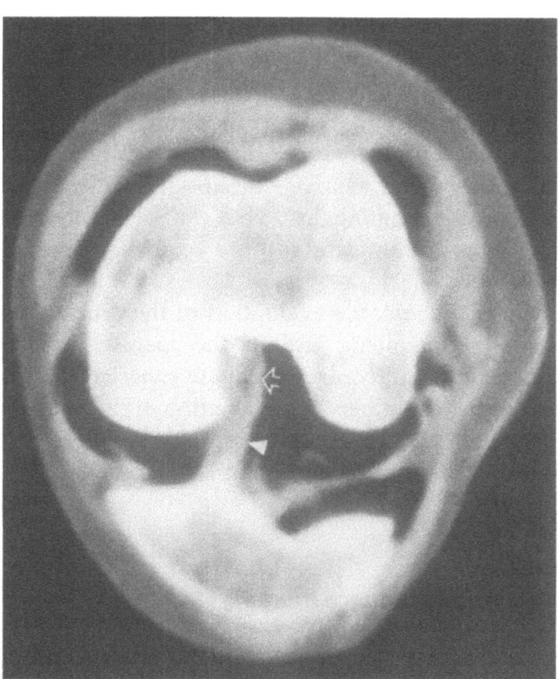

Fig. 8.2. Complete rupture of the ACL. CT arthrography with air shows a normal distal portion of the ACL (*arrowhead*). There is a complete rupture in the proximal portion of the ligament with the thin and irregular stump (*open arrow*) lying on the PCL (*curved arrow*)

tion to imaging of the knee joint has been the subject of increasing interest. In anatomically accessible regions, US has proven a sensitive method for detecting pathologic changes and for differentiating solid and liquid processes. In contrast, visualization of the anatomically less accessible regions of the interior of the joint, particularly the cruciate ligaments and the menisci, though possible with this method, must be considered critically regarding their diagnostic worth.

Because of their poor delineability from surrounding structures, ruptures of the collateral ligaments can only be detected indirectly. There may be a unilateral difference in soft tissue attenuation and an associated hypoechoic hematoma. Lateral and medial instability may be demonstrated by gaping of the lateral or medial osseous borders of the joint space. Direct sonographic evaluation of the cruciate ligaments is hampered by the fact that they cannot be visualized along their entire length, and a perpendicular sound wave projection is impossible due to their anatomic situation. In cases of fresh ruptures, a unilateral, irregular, hypoechoic thickening or only partial visualization of the ligament may be obtained using an infrapatellar approach. More commonly, indirect evidence is obtained using a popliteal approach: unilateral, hypoechoic areas at the dorsal insertions of the cruciate ligaments suggest hematomas secondary to fresh injuries.

Similarly problematic is the imaging of tears, partial rupture and synovial bleeding since they also yield positive findings at US but cannot be differentiated from a complete rupture requiring operative therapy.

On the whole, the evaluation of the cruciate and collateral ligaments and of the menisci is time-consuming and requires adequate experience on the part of the examiner. For evaluation of the collateral ligaments, US represents a primary supplement to clinical examination and plain radiography.

8.6.2.4
Magnetic Resonance Imaging

Because of its capacities for direct visualization of pathologic changes of the ligaments, menisci, and cartilaginous and osseous structures in multiplanar projection, MRI has quickly become the method of choice in the work-up of internal lesions of the knee. Technical advances in the coil and sequence areas have led to a significant improvement in the quality of the examination with concomitant reduction in examination times.

Reasonably priced MRI units dedicated to the examination of peripheral joints may lead to the stage in which MRI will represent the primary diagnostic modality for evaluation of injuries of the knee joint. Since arthroscopy is an invasive technique with the usual associated operative risks, its diagnostic application should be critically reconsidered in the age of MRI.

Of decisive importance for the correct diagnosis of ligamentous lesions is knowledge of the types of injuries and their characteristic appearance at MRI. The following sections therefore are dedicated to both the technical aspects and the signs and staging of lesions of individual ligaments.

8.6.2.4.1
ANTERIOR CRUCIATE LIGAMENT

For examination of the ACL, the knee should be positioned at 10°–15° lateral rotation in order to orient the ligament in a sagittal plane. In sagittal slices of ≤5 mm thickness, the normal ligament is visualized along its entire length in about 90% of cases (MINK 1987). The ACL is about 35 mm in length and about 11 mm thick (KENNEDY et al. 1974). In cases in which

sagittal projection does not visualize the ligament as an uninterrupted structure, oblique sagittal or oblique coronal planes can be alternatively obtained along the course of the ligament. Ligaments and tendons usually show low signal intensities at MRI. The ACL, however, shows streak-like areas of signal intensity in the proximity of its tibial insertion. These are due to adipose and synovial elements which are interposed between individual fiber bundles near the insertion of the ligament (Fig. 8.3).

MRI is a reliable method for evaluation of the ACL. In several large studies, the sensitivity and specificity for the evaluation of ruptures of the ACL have been reported to be between 90% and 95% (FISCHER et al. 1991; LEE et al. 1988; MINK et al. 1988).

There are a number of direct and indirect signs of rupture of the ACL visualized at MRI, knowledge of which is essential for exact diagnosis and differentiation of acute and chronic ruptures of the ligament.

Acute Ruptures. Rupture of the anterior cruciate ligament is said to be acute when the causative event

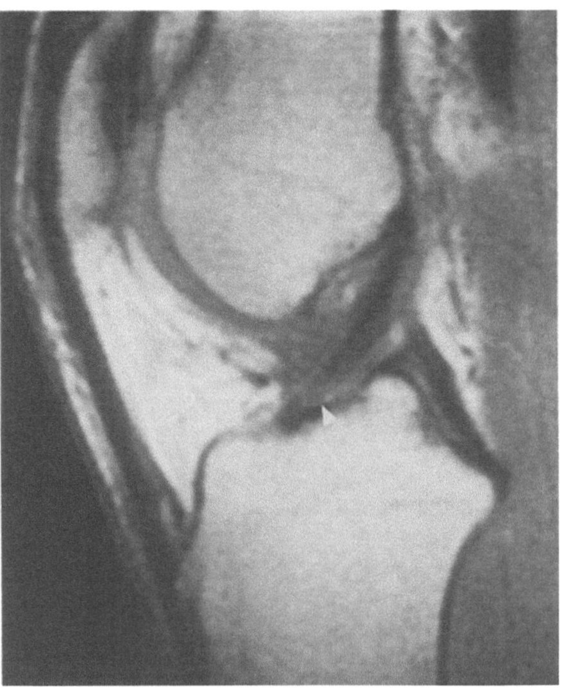

Fig. 8.3. Nornal appearance of the ACL on sagittal T1-w SE image (TR 600/TE 24). The ACL is seen as a band of low signal intensity. In the distal part, areas of intermediate signal intensity can be seen, secondary to an interposition of fat in the distal fibers (*arrowhead*)

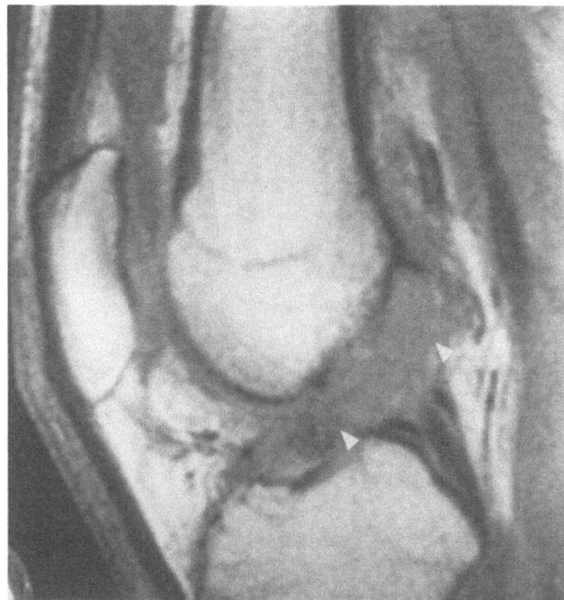

Fig. 8.4. Acute interstitial rupture of the ACL. The sagittal T1-w SE image (TR 600/TE 24) shows replacement of the normal ACL by a poorly defined mass. The ACL shows a high signal intensity over its entire course (*arrowheads*), representing torn and edematous ligament fibers

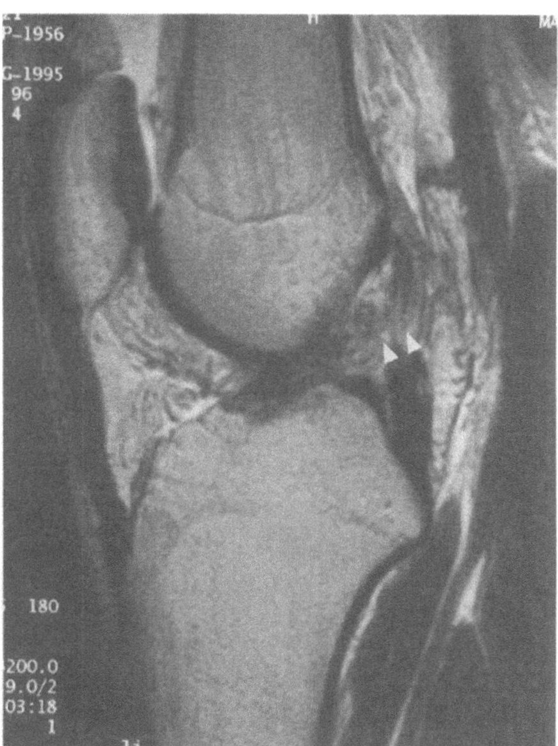

Fig. 8.5. Acute proximal rupture of the ACL. Sagittal T2-w TSE image (TR 4200/TE 119) shows a soft tissue mass proximally (*arrowheads*) representing a hematoma and torn ligamentous fibers, indicating a complete rupture near the femoral insertion site. *TSE*, turbo spin echo

has taken place no more than 2 weeks prior to examination. The most reliable sign of complete rupture of the cruciate ligament is visualization of discontinuity with retraction of the proximal and distal stumps. Often, however, there are only intraligamental increases in signal intensity which can be followed along the entire length of the ligament, but no apparent interruption of its continuity. The ligament is thickened along its entire length (Fig. 8.4). About 50% of acute ACL lesions show this signal pattern. Classifying the various ruptures based on their direct sings, it has been found that this type of lesion is associated with the lowest diagnostic sensitivity since diffuse changes of signal intensity in the ligament may be due to hematoma or to edematous changes and do not automatically indicate complete rupture of the ligament (BARRY et al. 1996).

Ruptures in the proximal femoral segment of the ACL often show a poorly defined soft tissue mass in the proximal segment of the ligament, which represents the hematoma forming around the retracted stump (Fig. 8.5). Ruptures in the mid part of the ligament are most often visualized as an interruption of the low signal intensity ligament (Fig. 8.6). The normal course of the proximal and distal stumps may be maintained since the ends may be held to-

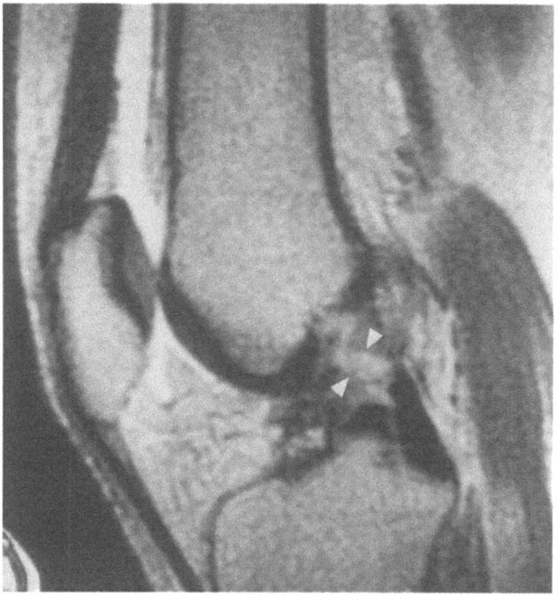

Fig. 8.6. Acute ACL rupture in the mid portion of the ligament. The sagittal T2-w SE image (TR 3000/TE 80) shows a complete interruption of the ligament with high signal intensity representing fluid (*arrowheads*)

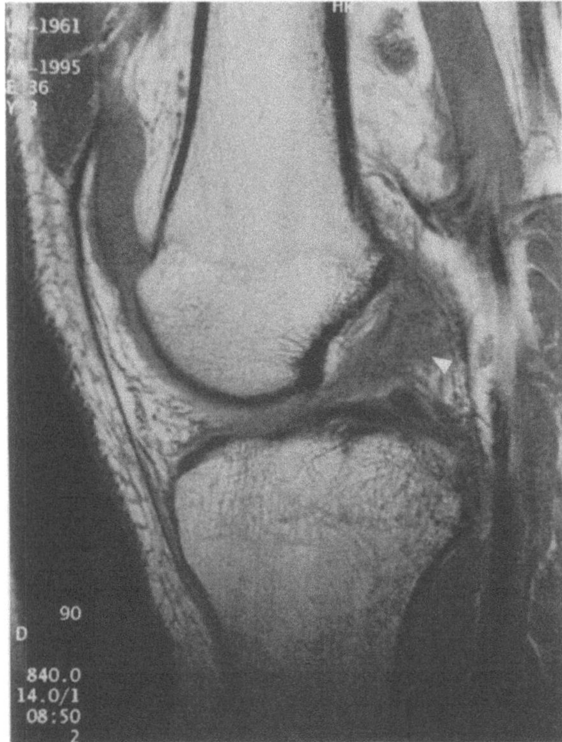

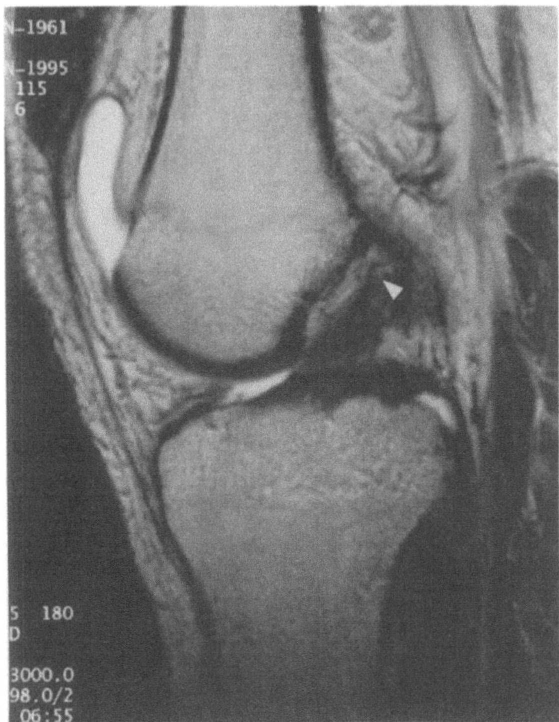

Fig. 8.7a,b. Partial rupture of the ACL. The sagittal T1-w SE image (**a**; TR 840/TE 14) shows a signal increase of the ACL and a soft tissue mass at the proximal end of the ACL (*arrowhead*). No continuous dark fibers can be identified. The corresponding T2-w TSE image (**b**; TR 3000/TE 99) shows some thickening and focal signal increase of the proximal ligament (*arrowhead*). Continuous ligamentous structures can be identified, indicating that part of the ligament is still intact

gether by the synovia and components of the blood in the vicinity of the rupture. Avulsive ruptures of the intercondylar eminence are seen in less than 5% of cases.

Diagnosis of these types of injuries might be difficult, particularly when there is no significant dislocation of the osseous fragment.

In some instances, differentiation of complete and partial ACL tear may become extremely difficult. Between 10% and 28% of injuries represent partial ruptures: most frequently there is tearing of the anterior bundle, while the posterior bundle remains intact. Partial ruptures may heal spontaneously, but, in the course of time, may progress to complete ruptures. Signs suggestive of partial rupture of the ACL at MRI include areas of high intraligamentous signal intensity in the presence of normal segments of ligament, wavy course of the ligament and the failure to delineate normal segments of ligament on T1-weighted sequences, while normal segments can be visualized on T2-weighted and STIR sequences (ULMANS et al. 1995) (Fig. 8.7).

The low sensitivity and specificity of MRI in the diagnosis of partial ruptures of the ACL as compared to arthroscopy can be explained partially by arthroscopy's inability to visualize intraligamentous changes apparent at MRI and by the superposition of intact ligamentous structures by synovia and components of blood at MRI.

MRI exhibits high sensitivity in the visualization of osseous injuries. Especially the radiographically occult bone contusion found in ACL injuries presents a very specific sign suggestive of rupture of the ACL. The contusion is caused by an anterior subluxation of the tibia during which a collision of the posterior tibial plateau with the femoral condyle takes place (KAPLAN et al. 1992). STIR sequences are particularly sensitive in the imaging of such changes. The exact localization of changes in signal intensity on the lateral femoral condyle is dependent on the degree of flexion in the knee joint at the time of subluxation. Usually, these changes are observed on the anterior or medial portion of the lateral femoral condyle, while they consistently appear on the dorsal portion of the lateral tibial plateau (MURPHY et al. 1992) (Figs. 8.8, 8.9).

While the sensitivity of bone marrow changes associated with ruptures of the ACL has been reported in various studies as ranging between 56% and 94% (MINK et al. 1989; KAPLAN et al. 1992; MURPHY et al. 1992), the specificity of these changes is consistently reported in the range of 97%–100% (MURPHY et al.

1992; GENTILI et al. 1994; MCCAULEY et al. 1994; ROBERTSON et al. 1994).

A definitive differentiation between a partial and complete rupture on the basis of the presence of such a bone bruise is, however, not possible (MCCAULEY et al. 1994).

In a study published by SNAERLY et al. (1996), it has been shown that the generally accepted high specificity of bone marrow changes associated with ruptures of the ACL cannot be applied to pediatric patients. Subluxations with resulting contusions of the bone may occur without ruptures of the ligament due to the higher elasticity of the entire ligamentous apparatus in this age group.

Besides osseous contusions to the lateral femoral condyle and to the tibial plateau, other osseous lesions have been reported in association with ruptures of the ACL. A bony avulsion of the lateral capsule immediately below the lateral tibial plateau (Segond fracture) is a reliable indicator of a meniscoligamentous injury to the knee joint, particularly to the ACL. MRI is a sensitive method for detection of a Segond fracture, which presents with bone marrow edema at the lateral tibial margin (DE LEE et al. 1983; JOHNSON 1979; SEEBACHER et al. 1986). In contrast, the often very small bony fragments are not reliably visualized at MRI and may require radiographic or computed tomographic imaging (WEBER et al. 1991).

The evaluation of indirect signs of rupture of the ACL is particularly important in cases in which the direct imaging of the ligament does not substantiate a definitive diagnosis. Reports in the literature have described a number of indirect signs whose diagnostic reliability remains the subject of controversy. Besides the above-mentioned bone marrow edema at the lateral tibial plateau and lateral femoral condyle, the indirect signs of rupture of the ACL include changes in the course of the ACL and PCL, the sulcus sign on the lateral femoral condyle, anterior subluxation of the tibia and posterior displacement of the posterior horn of the lateral meniscus (KAPLAN et al. 1992; LEE et al. 1988; FITZGERALD et al. 1993; ROBERTSON et al. 1994).

Since these secondary signs depend in part upon the instability of the joint, they may be of use in differentiating complete and partial ruptures of the ACL.

As a rule, these indirect signs exhibit high specificity but low sensitivity. Only the evaluation of the course of the ACL, which can be performed in relation to either the tibial plateau or the posterior margin of the femoral condyles (Blumensaat line), is said to possess both high specificity and sensitivity (GENTILI et al. 1994).

Subacute Ruptures. During the acute phase, an exact evaluation of the ligament is often hampered by post-traumatic hematoma and synovial reactions. After 2 to 8 weeks, however, the retracted stumps are usually more easily delineated (Fig. 8.10). Often, there may be a secondary effusion which, in T2-weighted sequences, can produce an arthrographic effect.

Chronic Ruptures. In the course of time, following rupture of the ACL, the absent blood supply leads to atrophy, which may be so pronounced that no residual ligamentous tissue can be seen. By apposition of the proximal stump to the PCL, revascularization is possible and is visualized as a dark band-like proximal structure being attached to the PCL (Fig. 8.11).

Often, MRI may show indirect signs of joint instability that point to an old rupture of the ACL. These

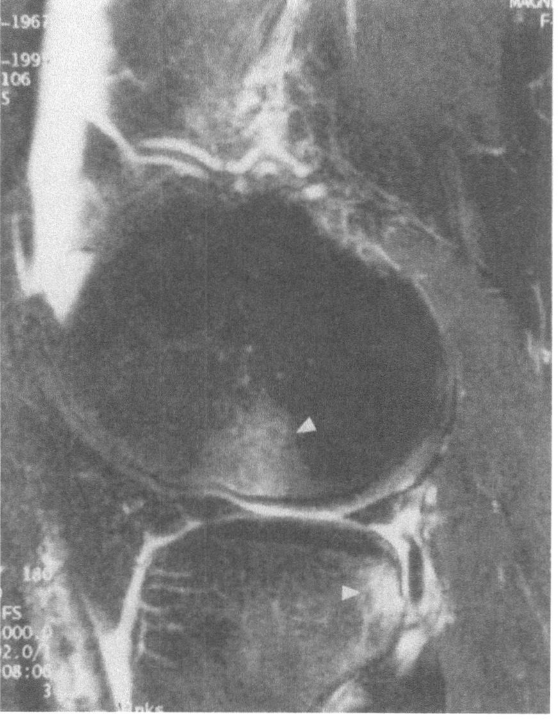

Fig. 8.8. Bone marrow edema in ACL tear: sagittal STIR image (TR 4000/TE 42/TI 130) shows high signal intensity of subchondral bone marrow (*arrowheads*) at the posterolateral tibial plateau and lateral femoral condyle in association with complete rupture of the ACL. *STIR,* short tau inversion recovery

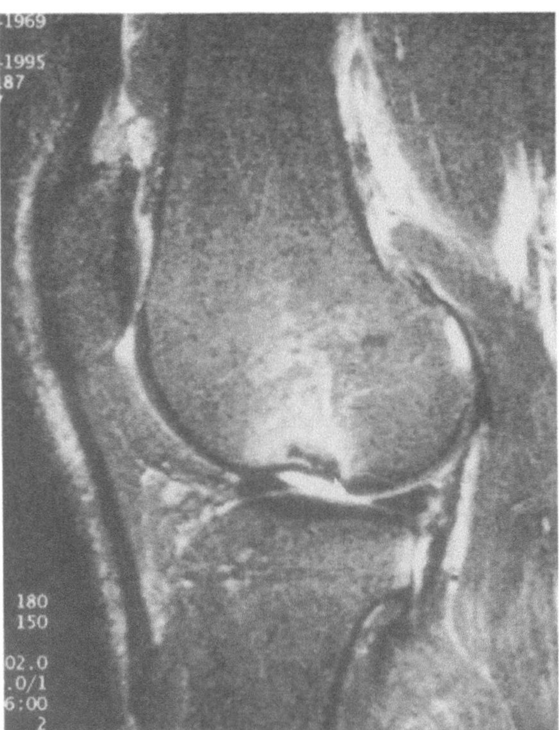

Fig. 8.9. Bone injury in acute ACL tear. Sagittal STIR image (TR 4300/TE 50/TI 150) shows an impaction fracture at the mid portion of the lateral femoral condyle (*arrowhead*) surrounded by a subchondral bone marrow edema

obtained from the patellar ligament or from the tendon of the semitendinosus muscle.

The value of MRI in the postoperative follow-up of ACL reconstruction has been the subject of contradictory statements in the literature (ALLGAYER et al. 1991; CHEUNG et al. 1992; MOESER et al. 1989; RAK et al. 1991; YAMATO and YAMAGISHI 1992). This is due primarily to the fact that different criteria must be applied for the evaluation of a transplant than for that of an original ligament. For example, significant alterations in signal intensity with pronounced contour irregularities may be observed at MRI in transplanted patients with absolutely no clinical evidence of joint instability. The causes of these extensive changes in signal intensity relate to processes of revitalization that lead to a sprouting of vessels and to synovial proliferation along the entire length of the ligament (ARNOUZKY et al. 1986).

Finally, such changes in signal intensity cannot be definitively differentiated from degenerative changes in the implant, e.g., secondary to an impingement.

signs include the anterior subluxation of the tibia against the femur, the resulting posterior displacement of the posterior horn of the lateral meniscus and the increased buckling of the PCL (Fig. 8.12).

Reconstruction. As a rule, ruptures of the ACL require operative therapy, since instability of the knee joint results in accelerated degeneration of the menisci and the joint cartilage and in secondary early knee joint arthrosis.

A number of operative techniques have been proposed (KNAEPLER et al. 1994). The reinsertion of the ACL represents the form of operative revision that is anatomically most correct. This, however, is only possible if the ACL has torn directly at its physiologic point of insertion, which is observed in only about 5% of all cases.

Long-term studies have shown that primary suturing of the ligament does not produce functionally adequate healing of the ACL (FEAGIN et al. 1976). In the majority of cases, therefore, replacement of the ACL represents the method of choice. This may be done by autologous grafting of a portion of tissue

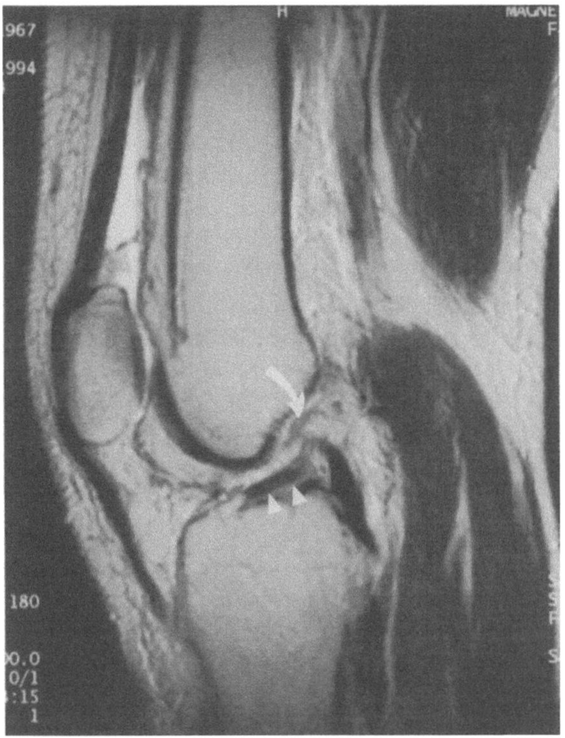

Fig. 8.10. Subacute tear of the ACL: the sagittal T2-w TSE image (TR 3500/TE 99) shows a horizontally oriented distal ACL (*arrowheads*). Of the proximal part, only some serpiginous, discontinuous fibers can be identified (*curved arrow*)

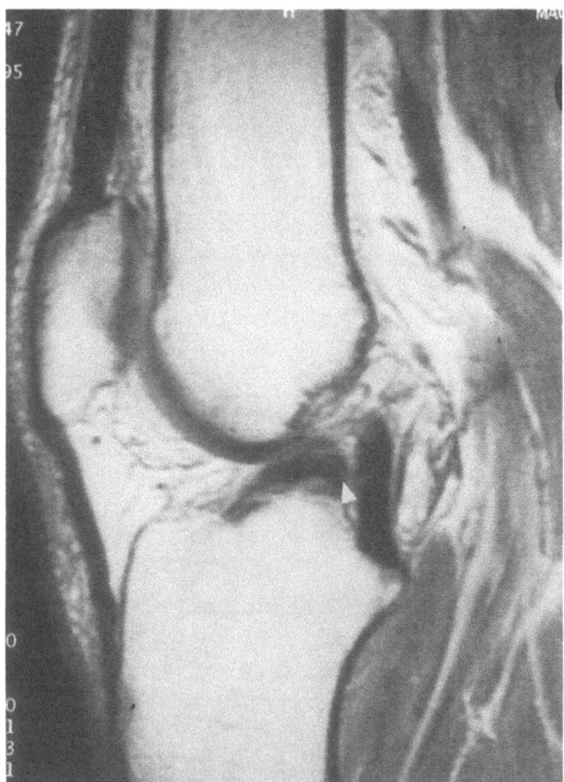

Fig. 8.11. Chronic tear of the ACL. Sagittal T2-w TSE image shows a horizontal orientation of the distal half of the ACL. The ACL extends proximally to the level of the PCL (*arrowhead*). The femoral part of the ligament cannot be identified. Arthroscopically, the distal part of the ACL was attached to the anterior surface of the PCL

In summary, the finding at MRI of a transplant with low signal intensity in all segments correlates, in a high percentage of patients, with a clinically stable ligament (Fig. 8.13). Increased signal intensity or wavy contours of the neoligament at MRT, however, preclude a reliable evaluation of the stability of the ligament (Figs. 8.14, 8.15).

In contrast, MRI is well suited for determining whether the transplant has been inserted at a biomechanically adequate position.

8.6.2.4.2

POSTERIOR CRUCIATE LIGAMENT

As is the case with the ACL, the PCL is invested with a synovial sheath and is thus intraarticular but extrasynovial. With a length of about 38 mm and a width of about 13 mm, it is thicker and longer than the ACL. Its width is the reason for its greater stability, such that ruptures of the PCL are among the less common knee joint injuries. Clinical examination is associated with low diagnostic reliability, so a large

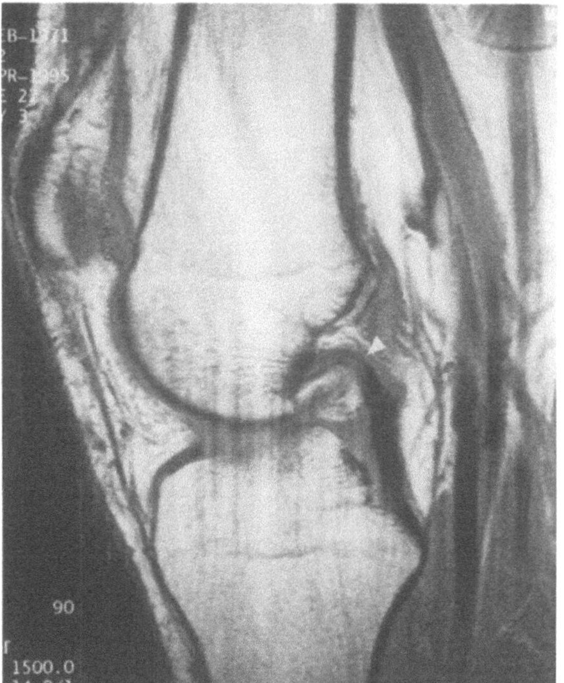

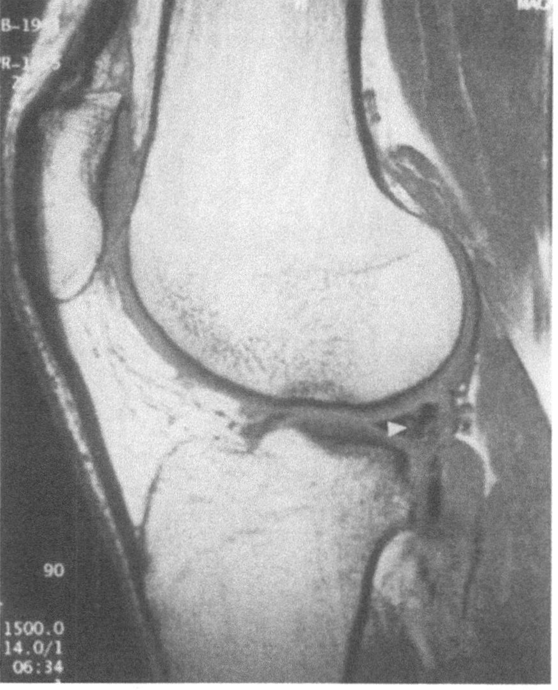

Fig. 8.12a,b. Instability in a patient with chronic tear of the ACL. The sagittal proton density-w TSE image (a) shows an abnormal contour of the PCL (*arrowhead*). Buckling of the PCL can be found in chronic dysfunction of the ACL with anterior subluxation of the tibia. On lateral views (b), the anterior subluxation of the tibia and the posterior dislocation of the posterior horn of the lateral meniscus can be seen. In addition, there is a vertical tear of the posterior horn of the lateral meniscus (*arrowhead*)

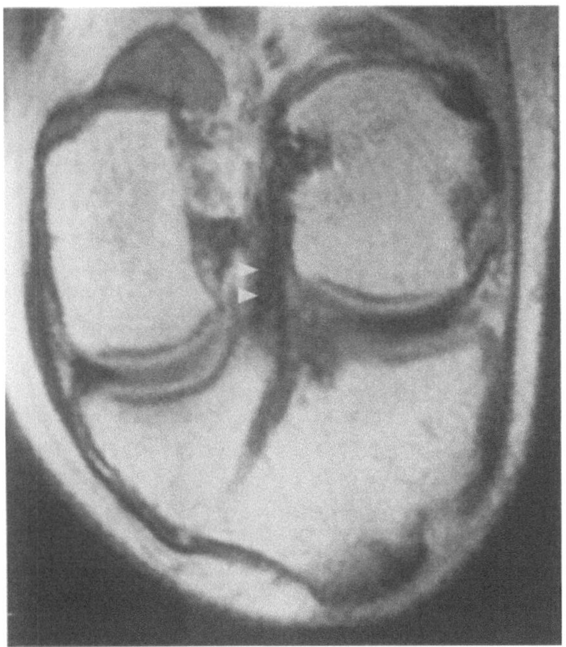

Fig. 8.13. Stable ACL reconstruction. The paracoronal T1-w SE image (TR 600/TE 24) which is oriented along the course of the ligament demonstrates a continuous semitendinosus graft. The intact tendon fibers demonstrate a low signal intensity (*arrowheads*)

proportion of injuries to the PCL go undetected (HUGHSTON 1988). A chronic rupture of the PCL with its resulting instability leads primarily to increased stress in the femoropatellar joint with early development of femoropatellar arthrosis. The appropriate therapy for rupture of the PCL is controversial. While the need for operative revision of combined injuries is generally accepted, there is a divergence of opinion regarding the treatment of isolated ruptures of the PCL (TORG et al. 1989).

Because of its caliber and its homogeneous low signal intensity, the PCL is visualized in sagittal projections throughout its entire length in about 95% of cases. The midsection often appears thickened due to its close proximity to the meniscofemoral ligaments (Fig. 8.16).

Acute Rupture. Injuries to the PCL are reported to amount to 2%–23% of all injuries to the knee (TORG et al. 1989; Loos et al. 1981). In about 30% of these cases injury to the PCL is an isolated entity, but in the majority of cases it is associated with other injuries.

In a study reported by SONIN et al. (1995), 42% of patients with rupture of the PCL exhibited additional

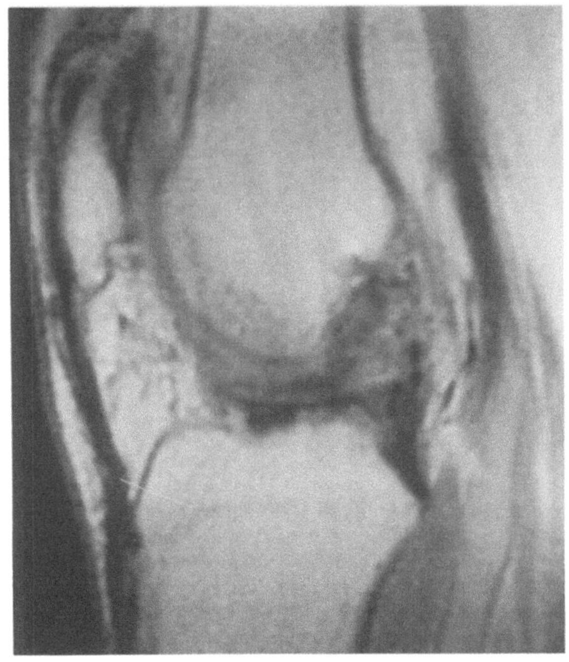

a

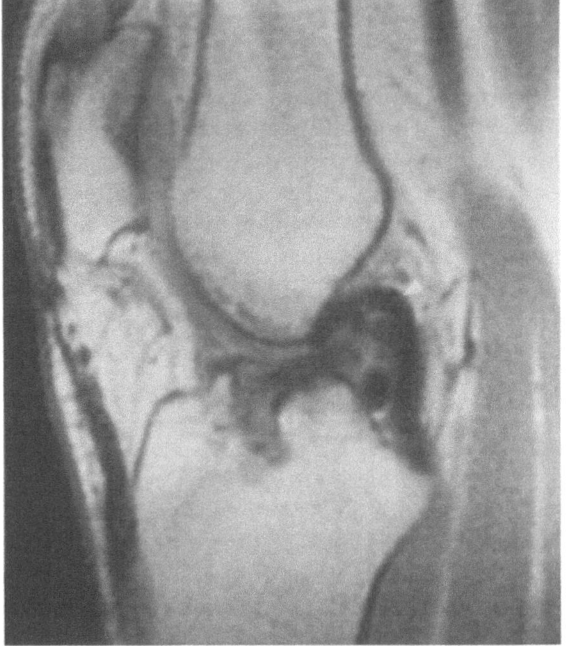

b

Fig. 8.14a,b. Unstable ACL reconstruction. On sagittal T1-w SE images (a; TR 600/TE 24), no continuous ligamentous structure can be identified. As an indirect sign of ligamentous instability, the posterior cruciate ligament shows a buckled configuration (*arrowhead*; b)

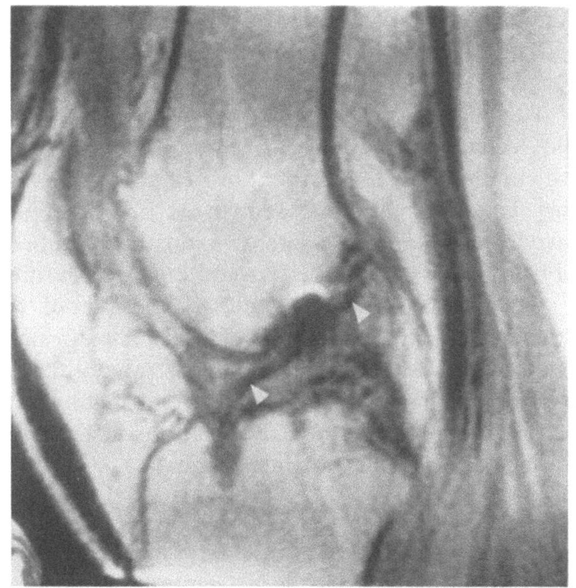

Fig. 8.15. Patient with unstable ACL reconstruction. On a sagittal T1-w SE image (TR 600/TE 24), the graft appears to be very thin throughout its course (*arrowheads*). There are areas of intermediate signal intensity but no signs of complete discontinuity. The instrumented measurements of knee stability with an arthrometer showed severe anterior instability

ligament injuries (27% ACL, 20% MCL, 7% LCL), 52% suffered meniscus tears (35% medial, 28% lateral), while in 35% there were also osseous lesions. Osseous lesions such as contusions of the bone occur primarily in the anterior parts of both the tibial plateau and the lateral femoral condyle. This is explained by the accident mechanism, either hyperextensional trauma or collisional trauma with dorsal dislocation of the tibia.

Signs of complete rupture of the PCL at MRI include the inability to delineate regular ligamentous structure, a diffuse increase in soft tissue with increased signal intensity in T1- and T2-weighted sequences localized in the normal course of the ligament, or a focal interruption of the ligament (Fig. 8.17). Partial or intraligamentous rupture is characterized by intraligamentous increases in signal intensity in the presence of delineated continuous ligament segments.

An avulsion rupture of the ligament is most commonly encountered at the point of its tibial insertion. In comparison with the avulsion rupture of the ACL, there is more often a dislocation of the fragment, which facilitates diagnosis.

Chronic Rupture. Because the continuity of the ligament is often maintained and atrophic processes, as observed in the case of ruptures of the ACL, occur

more rarely, chronic ruptures of the PCL often show merely residual changes in signal intensity throughout the course of the ligament. Since scar tissue is also of low signal intensity, post-traumatic cicatrix formation often cannot be differentiated from intact ligamentous structures at MRI.

8.6.2.4.3
MEDIAL COLLATERAL LIGAMENT

The medial collateral ligament (MCL) consists of a superficial and a deep layer. The superficial layer arises from the medial femoral condyle and inserts into the medial tibial margin about 5 cm distal to the joint space. The deep layer tightly blends with the base of the meniscus and is differentiated into the meniscofemoral and meniscotibial ligaments. Between the two layers, there is a narrow bursa and loose connective tissue which, due to its high content of adipose tissue, exhibits relatively high signal intensity at MRI and is not to be confused with a meniscocapsular separation.

The MCL is best visualized in a coronal plane. In its femoral and tibial insertional areas, its dark su-

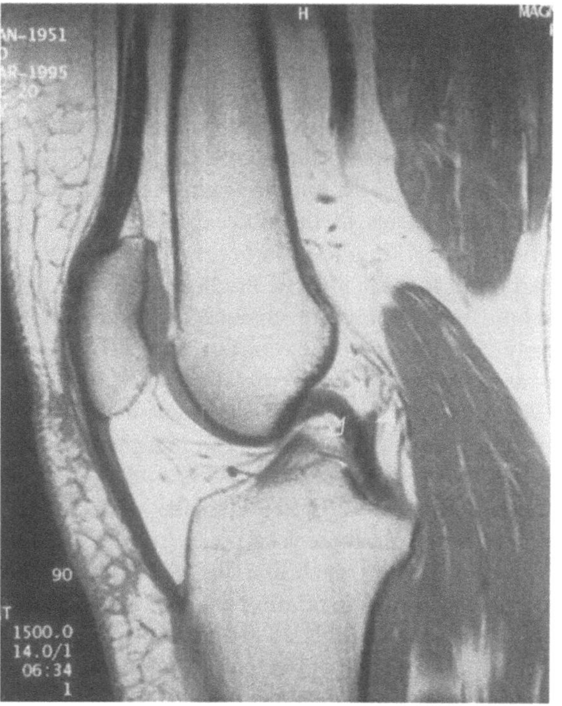

Fig. 8.16. Normal appearance of the PCL. On a sagittal PD-w TSE image (TR 1500/TE 14), the ligament is seen as a uniform dark band. Anterior and posterior to the PCL, low signal intensity structures can be identified in up to 60% of the MR examinations representing the anterior (Humphyrey; *open arrow*) and posterior (Wrisberg; *arrowhead*) meniscofemoral ligaments

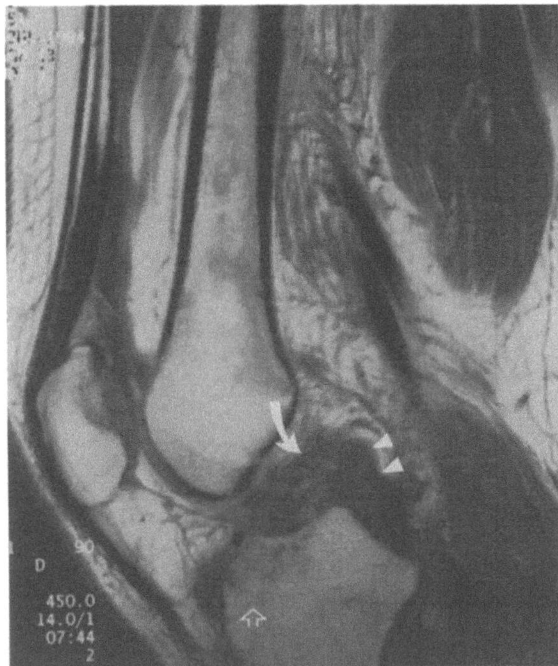

Fig. 8.17. Complete rupture of the PCL: sagittal T1-w SE image (TR 450/TE 14) shows widening and signal increase of the PCL (*arrowheads*). The femoral insertion cannot be identified. There is a bone contusion at the anterior tibial plateau (*open arrow*). In adjunction, the ACL is ruptured, too (*curved arrow*), and the tibia is displaced posteriorly

perficial component is difficult to differentiate from the adjacent dark cortical bone.

Based on severity and analogous to clinical classification, injuries to the MCL can be divided into three classes. In grade I injury, which clinically corresponds to stretching of the ligament with microscopic tears, there are changes in signal intensity only in the periligamentous connective tissue, caused by soft-tissue edema or by small hematomas (Fig. 8.18). Grade II and grade III lesions, which correspond clinically to partial and complete ruptures, respectively, are associated with a thickened ligament with altered signal intensity (Fig. 8.19). In grade III lesions, there is complete rupture with pronounced medial instability (Fig. 8.20). Often, however, an exact differentiation of grade II and grade III lesions is not possible at MRI. Extensive edema or hematoma in the connective tissue space between the superficial and deep portions of the ligament often results in the superficial layer being raised from the underlying bone.

The evaluation of the deep layer of the MCL is based only on indirect signs. Rupture of the meniscofemoral or meniscotibial ligaments may result in leaking of synovial fluid from the joint space into the area of the interligamentous bursa. A further

sign suggestive of a lesion of the deep layer of the MCL is the dislocation of the meniscus from the joint space.

The healing process in ligamentous injuries usually leads to formation of bradytrophic scar tissue which, due to its low content of free protons, shows low signal intensity in all sequences. It is differentiated from the uninjured ligament mostly on the basis of its thickness and wave-like contour irregularities.

Calcifications, which are the substrate of the Stieda-Pellegrini shadows visualized on plain radiography and which indicate older lesions of the internal ligaments, are hardly distinguishable from scar tissue at MRI, since calcifications also exhibit low signal intensities in all sequences.

8.6.2.4.4
LATERAL COLLATERAL LIGAMENT

Injuries in the area of the lateral complex are seldom encountered. Nevertheless, exact diagnosis is important, especially because lesions of the posterolateral capsule ligament structures may produce extreme degrees of instability.

Analogous to the MCL, pathological changes to the LCL can be grouped in three classes based on

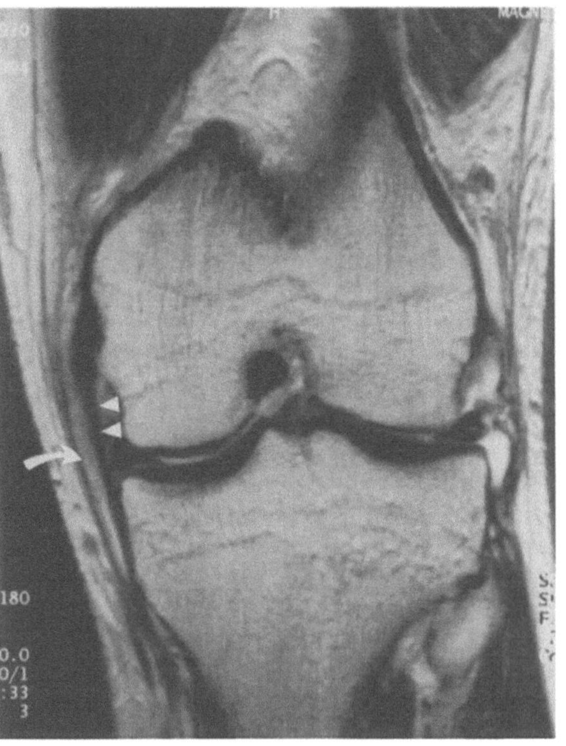

Fig. 8.18. MCL tear grade 1: Coronal T2-w TSE image (TR 3500/TE 99) shows fluid (*curved arrow*) superficial to the dark MCL (*arrowheads*). The ligament itself shows no signal increase and no displacement from the bone. *MCL*, medial collateral ligament

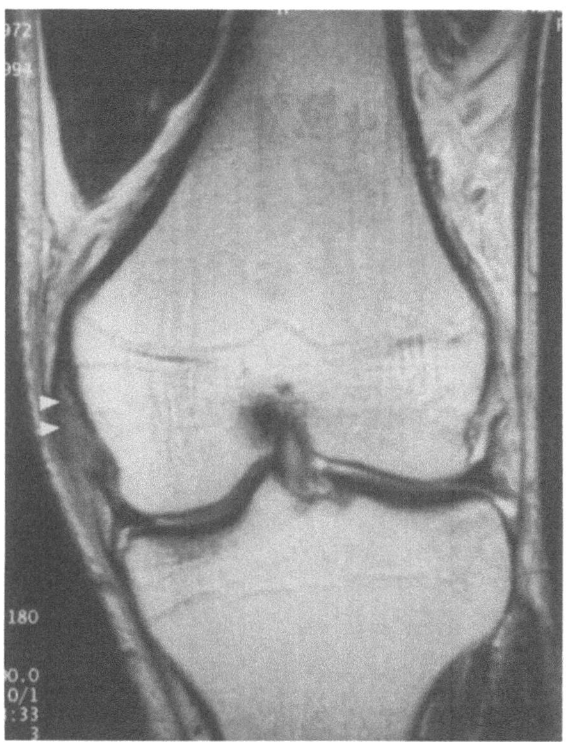

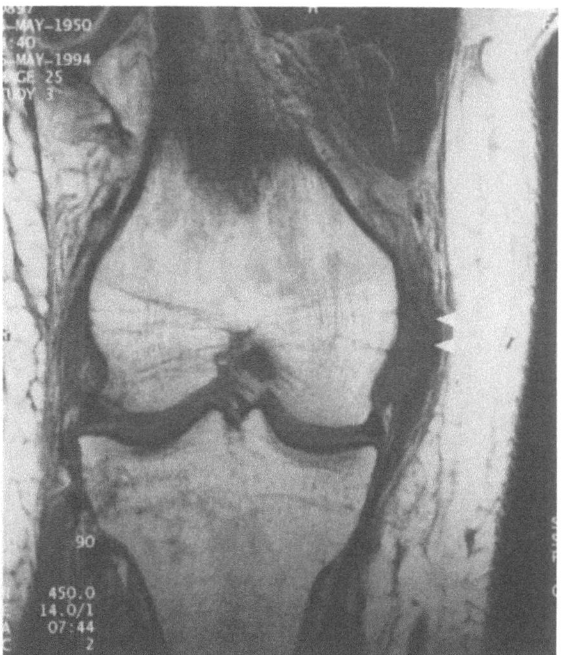

Fig. 8.19. MCL tear grade II/III: coronal T2-w TSE image (TR 3500/TE 99) shows displacement of the proximal MCL from the femur. The proximal MCL is thickened and shows a diffuse signal increase representing torn ligamentous fibers and acute hemorrhage (*arrowheads*)

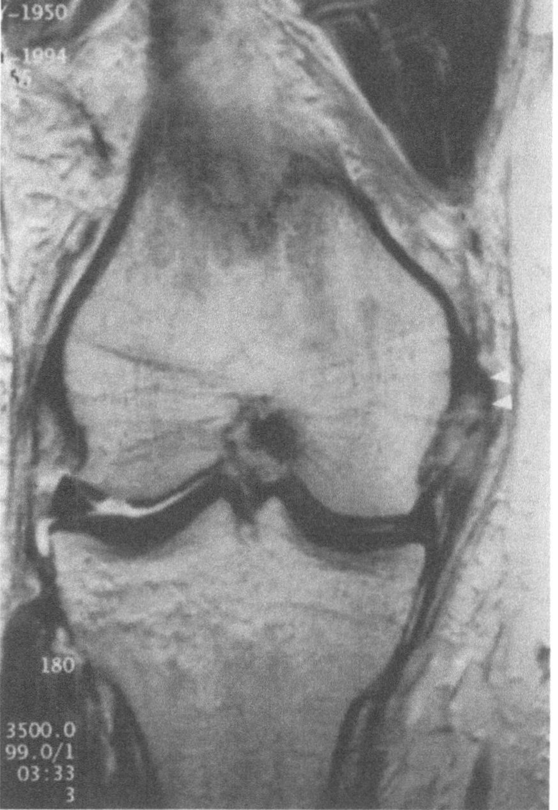

severity. A grade I lesion corresponds to microscopic tears, visualized at MRI as increased intra- and periligamentous signal intensity in T2-weighted sequences. Partial rupture (grade II) is characterized by increased signal intensity and thickening of the affected structure, while grade III shows complete discontinuity or absence of the structure in question (Fig. 8.21).

Ruptures on the LCL occur either in the midsection of the ligament or as bony avulsion ruptures at the fibular insertion. Since the course of the ligament is diagonal and extends from the lateral epicondyle posteriorly, inferiorly and laterally to the head of the fibula, it is often difficult to visualize it along its entire length in coronal projections. Therefore, axial and, if necessary, sagittal projections should be obtained.

8.7
Conclusion

The reliability of clinical examination in cases of acute trauma to the knee joint depends to a great

Fig. 8.20a,b. MCL tear grade III: coronal T1-w SE image (a; TR 450/TE 14) shows diffuse thickening and signal increase of the proximal portion of the MCL (*arrowheads*). The continuity of the ligament is lost. Coronal T2-w TSE image (b; TR 3500/TE 99) shows high signal intensity of the proximal mass representing edema and/or hemorrhage. At the femoral insertion site, the retracted proximal end of the ligament can be seen (*arrowheads*)

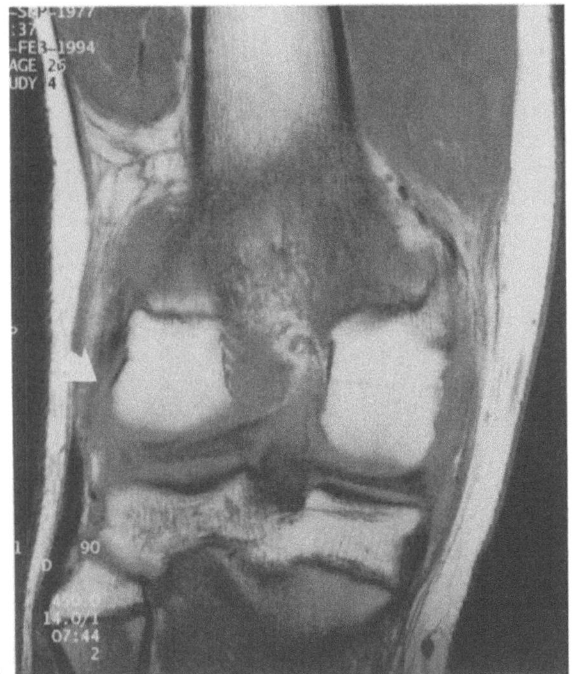

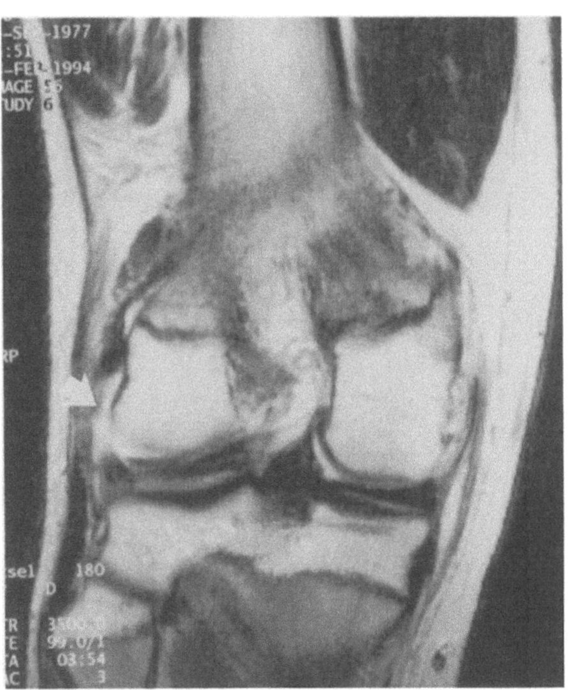

Fig. 8.21a,b. Grade III tear of the LCL in a 16-year-old boy. Coronal T1-w SE image (**a**; TR 450/TE 14) shows thickening and singal intensity increase of the LCL at the femoral insertion (*arrow*). Coronal T2-w TSE image (**b**; TR 3500/TE 99) shows the interruption of the LCL at the femoral insertion and high signal intensity fluid at the site of injury (*arrow*). *LCL*, lateral collateral ligament

part on the experience of the examiner and the cooperation of the patient, which often results in a discrepancy between clinical diagnosis and intraoperative findings (JOHNSON 1982; KATZ and FINGEROTH 1986; NOYES et al. 1991).

The correct diagnostic interpretation of the degree of injury determines the subsequent treatment of the injured knee. In order to optimize treatment, it is important that an exact diagnosis be made promptly since delay in beginning therapy may result in early development of secondary joint lesions.

Shortly after the introduction of tomographic imaging techniques, their possible applications in the preoperative diagnosis of meniscoligamentous injuries of the knee became apparent (ARCHER and YEAGER 1978; PAVLOV et al. 1979; REICHER et al. 1985; REISER et al. 1986). Because of the absence of radiation exposure and the capacity for multiplanar projection, MRI has established itself as the method of choice in the diagnosis of meniscus and ligament injuries of the knee joint. Major comparison studies have underscored the high reliability of MRI in the diagnosis of lesions of internal knee structures. The introduction of dedicated, low-field systems has led to questions regarding the importance of field strength for the method's diagnostic reliability. Early comparison studies of low-field (0.3 T) and high-field systems show no significant difference in the diagnosis of meniscus and ligament lesions (BARNETT 1993; BARRY et al. 1996).

RUWE et al. (1992) report that the use of MRI in patients with knee joint trauma could reduce the need for diagnostic arthroscopy by up to 50%. This would represent a significant reduction in costs and spare patients without lesions the treatment risks associated with surgery and anesthesia.

References

Abbot LC, Saunders JB, Bost FC, Anderson CE (1944) Injuries to the ligaments of the knee joint. J Bone Joint Surg 26: 503

Allgayer B, Gradinger R, Lehner K, Flock K, Gewalt Y (1991) Die Kernspintomographie zur Beurteilung des vorderen Kreuzbandersatzes mit Sehnentransplantaten. ROFO 155:294–298

Archer CR, Yeager V (1978) Internal structures of the knee visualized by CT. J Comput Assist Tomogr 2:181

Arnouzky SP, Warren RF, Ashlock MA (1986) Replacement of the anterior cruciate ligament using a patellar tendon allograft. J Bone Joint Surg [Am] 68:376–385

Barnett J (1993) MR diagnosis of internal derangement of the knee: effect of field strength on efficacy. AJR 161:115–118

Barry KP, Mesgarzadeh M, Triolo J, Moyer R, Tehranzadeh J, Bonakdarpour A (1996) Accuracy of MRI patterns in evaluating anterior cruciate ligament tears. Skeletal Radiol 25:365–370

Benedetto KP, Sperner G, Gloetzer W (1990) Der Kniegelenkhämarthros – differentialdiagnostische Überlegungen zur Planung einer Operation. Orthopäde 19:69–76

Cheung Y, Magee TH, Rosenberg ZS, Rose DJ (1992) MRI of anterior cruciate ligament reconstruction. J Comput Assist Tomogr 16:134–137

Cotta H, Dreyer J (1967) Zur Diagnostik und Therapie der Kniebinnenverletzungen. Dtsch Med J 18:153

De Lee JC, Riley MB, Rockwood CA (1983) Acute straight lateral instability of the knee. Am J Sports Med 11:404–411

Feagin JA, Curl WC (1976) Isolated tear of the anterior cruciate ligament: 5 years follow-up study. Am J Sports Med 4:95–100

Felsenreich F (1934) Die Röntegendiagnose der veralteten Kreuzbandläsion des Kniegelenks. Fortschr Röntgenstr 49:341

Fischer SP, Fox JM, Del Pizzo W, Friedman MJ, Snyder SJ, Ferkel RD (1991) Accuracy of diagnoses from magnetic resonance imaging of the knee. J Bone Joint Surg [Am] 73:1–10

Fishwick NG, Learmonth DJA, Finlay DB (1994) Knee effusions, radiology and acute knee trauma. Br J Radiol 67:934–937

Fitzgerald SW, Remer EM, Friedman H, Rogers LF, Hendrix RW, Schafer MF (1993) MR evaluation of the anterior cruciate ligament: value of sagittal images with coronal and axial images. AJR 160:1233–1237

Gentili A, Seeger LL, Yao L, Do HM (1994) Anterior cruciate ligament tear: indirect signs at MR imaging. Radiology 193:835–840

Hughston JC (1988) The absent posterior drawer sign in some acute posterior ligament tears of the knee. Am J Sports Med 16:39–43

Johnson LL (1979) Lateral capsular ligament complex: anatomical and surgical considerations. Am J Sports Med 7:156–160

Johnson LL (1982) Impact of diagnostic arthroscopy on the clinical judgement of an experienced arthroscopist. Clin Orthop 167:75–83

Kaplan PA, Walker CW, Kilcoyne RF, Brown DE, Tusek D, Dussault RG (1992) Occult fracture patterns of the knee associated with anterior cruciate ligament tears: assessment with MR imaging. Radiology 183:835–838

Katz JW, Fingeroth RJ (1986) The diagnostic accuracy of ruptures of the anterior cruciate ligament comparing the Lachman test, the anterior drawer sign, and the pivot shift test in acute and chronic knee injuries. Am J Sports Med 14:88–91

Kennedy JC, Weinberg HW, Wilson AS (1974) The anatomy and function of the anterior cruciate ligament. J Bone Joint Surg 56:223–235

Kim SJ, Kim HK (1995) Reliability of the anterior drawer test, the pivot shift test, and the Lachman test. Clin Orthop 317:237–242

Knaepler H, Krudwig W, Witzel U (1994) Überlegungen zur differenzierten Therapie bei Insuffizienz des vorderen Kreuzbandes. Akt Traumatol 24:188–194

Lee JK, Yao L, Phelps CT, Wirth CR, Czajka J, Lozman J (1988) Anterior cruciate ligament tears: MR imaging compared with arthroscopy and clinical tests. Radiology 166:861–864

Loos WC, Fox JM, Blazina ME, Del Pizzo W, Friedman MJ (1981) Acute PCL injuries. Am J Sports Med 9:86–92

Mc Cauley TR, Moses M, Kier R, Lynch JK, Barton JW, Jokl P (1994) MR diagnsosis of tears of anterior cruciate ligament of the knee: importance of ancillary findings. AJR 162:115–119

Mink JH (1987) The ligaments of the knee. In: Mink JH, Reicher MA, Crues JV (eds) Magnetic resonance imaging of the knee. Raven Press, New York, p 93–111

Mink JH, Levy T, Crues JV (1988) Tears of the anterior cruciate ligament and menisci of the knee: MR imaging evaluation. Radiology 167:769–774

Mink JH, Deutsch AL (1989) Occult cartilage and bone injuries of the knee: detection, classification, and assessment with MR imaging. Radiology 170:823–829

Moeser P, Bechtold RE, Clark T, Rovere G, Karstaedt N, Wolfman N (1989) MR imaging of anterior cruciate ligament repair. J Comput Assist Tomogr 13:105–109

Murphy BJ, Smith RL, Uribe JW, Janecki CJ, Hechtman KS, Mangasarian RA (1992) Bone signal abnormalities in the posterolateral tibia and lateral femoral condyle in complete tears of the anterior cruciate ligament: a specific sign? Radiology 182:221–224

Neumann A, Schiller K, Witt S, Betz A, Krueger P, Schweiberer L. (1991) Der Kniegelenkshämarthros. Absolute Indikation zur Operation? Unfallchirurg 94:560–564

Nicholas JA (1973) The five-one reconstruction for anteromedial instability of the knee. J Bone Joint Surg [Am] 55:899

Noyes FR, Cummings JF, Grood ES, Walz-Hassefeld KA, Wroble RR (1991) The diagnosis of knee motion limits, subluxations, and ligament injury. Am J Sports Med 19:163–170

O'Donoghue DH (1950) Surgical treatment of fresh injuries to the major ligaments of the knee. J Bone Joint Surg [Am] 32:721–737

Passariello R, Trecco F, De Paulis F, Masciocchi C, Bonanni G, Zobel BB (1986) CT demonstration of capsuloligamentous lesions of the knee joint. J Comput Assist Tomogr 10:450–456

Pavlov HJ, Hirschy JC, Torg JS (1979) Computed tomography of the cruciate ligaments. Radiology 132:389–393

Rak KM, Gillogly SD, Schaefer RA, Yakes WF, Liljedahl RR (1991) Anterior cruciate ligament reconstruction: evaluation with MR imaging. Radiology 178:553–556

Reicher MA, Bassett IW, Gold RH (1985) High resolution magnetic resonance imaging of the knee joint: normal anatomy. AJR 145:895–902

Reiser M, Rupp N, Karpf M, Feuerbach S, Paar O (1982) Erfahrungen mit der CT-Arthrographie der Kreuzbänder des Kniegelenkes. ROFO 137:372–379

Reiser M, Rupp N, Pfänder K, Schepp S, Lukas P (1986) Die Darstellung von Kreuzbandläsionen durch die MR-Tomographie. ROFO 145:193–198

Robertson PL, Schweitzer ME, Bartolozzi AR, Ugoni A (1994) Anterior cruciate ligament tears: evaluation of multiple signs with MR imaging. Radiology 193:829–834

Runkel M, Blum J, Roeder W, Ahlers J, Kreitner KF et al. (1993) Zur Wertigkeit des radiologischen Lachman-Tests bei vorderen Kreuzbandrupturen. Akt Traumatol 23:297–301

Ruwe P, Wright J, Randall L, Lynch JK, Jokl P, McCarthy S (1992) Can MR imaging effectively replace diagnostic arthroscopy? Radiology 183:335–339

Seebacher JR, Ingleis AF, Marshall DVM, Warren RS (1986) The structure of the posterolateral aspect of the knee. J Bone Joint Surg [Am] 64:467–469

Snaerly WN, Kaplan PA, Dussault RG (1996) Lateral-compartment bone contusions in adolescents with intact anterior cruciate ligaments. Radiology 198:205–208

Sonin AH, Fitzgerald SW, Hoff FL, Friedman H, Bresler ME (1995) MR imaging of the posterior cruciate ligament: normal, abnormal, and associated injury patterns. Radiographics 15:551–561

Torg JS, Barton TM, Pavlov H, Stine R (1989) Natural history of the posterior cruciate deficient knee. Clin Orthop 246:208–216

Ulmans H, Wimpfheimer O, Haramati N, Applbaum YH, Adler M, Bosco J (1995) Diagnosis of partial tears of the anterior cruciate ligament of the knee: value of MR imaging. AJR 165:893–897

Weber WN, Neumann CH, Barakos JA, Petersen SA, Steinbach LS, Genant HK (1991) Lateral tibial rim (Segond) fractures: MR imaging characteristics. Radiology 180:731–734

Yamato M, Yamagishi T (1992) MRI of patellar tendon anterior cruciate ligament autografts. J Comput Assist Tomogr 16:604–607

9 Instability of the Tibiotalar Joint

R. Passariello[1] and M. Mastantuono[2]

CONTENTS

9.1
Introduction

The skeletal framework of the ankle joint is formed by the tibiotalar articulation and the distal tibiofibular syndesmosis. For correct clinical recognition of ankle lesions, one must remember that the hindfoot is an extremely integrated structure. The central element of this structure is the talus, which closely related with the tibia, calcaneus, cuboid and navicular. These skeletal components are connected by the peritalar ligamentous system, supported by the musculotendinous structures that pass around the talus.

The high congruity between talus and tibiofibular joint and the close articular relationship created by the ligamentous complexes gives the tibiotarsal articulation a high degree of stability and often permits one to foresee, on the basis of the dynamics of trauma, the damage to the different bony and ligamentous structures involved (Crim 1989; Erickson 1990).

Although conventional X-ray examination permits correct evaluation of the bony lesions and clinical examination leads to appropriate therapy, nowadays CT and MRI are increasingly being used successfully (Figs. 9.1, 9.2), especially for evaluation of tibiotarsal lesions. These techniques give us the opportunity to understand and codify the different post-traumatic clinical syndromes and to identify the best surgical access route in a part of the body where arthroscopy is very often difficult or useless (Resnick 1974).

9.2
Capsuloligamentous Pathology

There are three main ligamentous structures in the ankle, each constituting several layers. These structures are the medial collateral ligament (deltoideus), the lateral ligamentous complex, and the distal tibiofibular syndesmotic complex.

The lateral ligamentous complex (Figs. 9.3, 9.4) is most frequently involved in ankle sprains (85%). For biomechanical reasons, correlated with the intrinsic articular structure, the stabilizing action of the extrinsic periarticular components, and the kinematic modalities of the deambulation system during inversion sprains, the various components of the lateral ligamentous complex are damaged according to an expected sequence related to the applied destructive force. The first component to be affected is the anterior fibulotalar ligament (Fig. 9.5), and the second, with greater force, is the fibulo-calcanear, ligament. Only in very particular cases in which inversion trauma causes significant derangement of the articular connections, is the posterior fibulotalar ligament damaged (Bleichrodt 1989; Cardone 1993; Keene 1989).

The tibio-tarsal joint is more frequently subject to inversion insufficiency after trauma. The deltoid ligament is rarely involved in distorsive traumas, and cases of eversion almost always involve minor involutive, tendinous, and capsulo-ligamentous pathology.

Often, a tear or sprain of the distal anterior tibiofibular ligament may be associated with major ligament injury or fracture; the occurrence of this lesion alone is a serious event as it leads to widening of the tibiofibular mortise, greatly reducing ankle articular stability. Tearing of the distal posterior

---

[1]R. Passariello, MD, Cattedra di Radiologia, Università La Sapienza, Policlinico Umberto 1, Viale Regina Elena 324, 00161 Rome, Italy
[2]M. Mastantuono, MD, Cattedra di Radiologia, Università La Sapienza, Policlinico Umberto 1, Viale Regina Elena 324, 00161 Rome, Italy

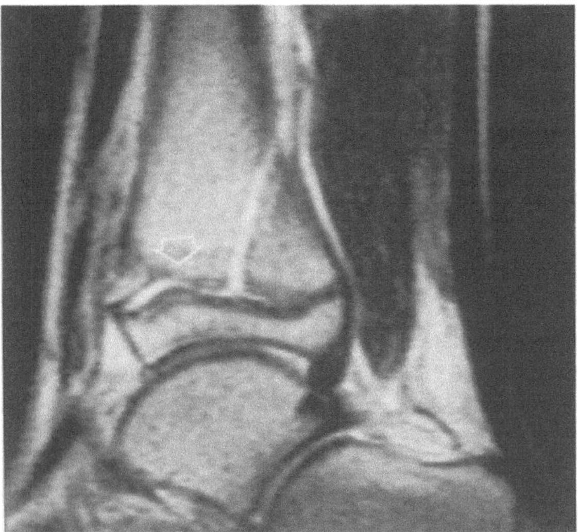

Fig. 9.1. T2-weighted MR image (SE). Epiphyseal detachment (*open arrow*). *SE*, spin echo

tibiofibular ligament is less common and produces a similar instability pattern.

As in other anatomic regions, distractive stress on the ligamentous structure of the tibiotarsal joint causes elastic distress which is followed by a return to normal length when the traction ceaser. Beyond a certain limit, the traction causes plastic deformation of the ligamentous structures which corresponds microscopically to an interruption of a variable contingent of fibers that may be more or less significant, according to the stress applied.

Functional and stress radiological examinations of the tibiotarsal joint may be useful for evaluating the syndromes of insufficiency of the hindfoot; their utility in acutely ill patients is doubtful and they should be avoided in the case of incomplete cicatrization of the capsuloligamentous structures because the imposed stress could interfere with the regular process of recovery.

The stress radiograms most often utilized are the posteroanterior projection, applying varus stress, and the lateral projection ("drawer sign"). In chronic relaxations, even minor articular widening is usually of diagnostic value, while in acute relaxation, even major articular openings are not. In congenital relaxations we often find a major opening of the articular rima even in the absence of previous trauma (FROST 1977).

Clinical and radiological examination of the contralateral tibiotarsal joint can help to differentiate post-traumatic relaxation from congenital relaxation.

After trauma, ankle stability may be compromised even in the absence of ligamentous injuries, as

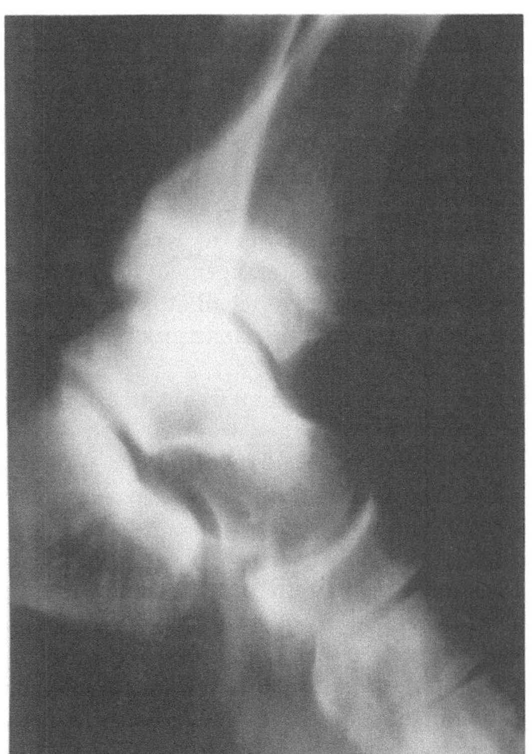

A

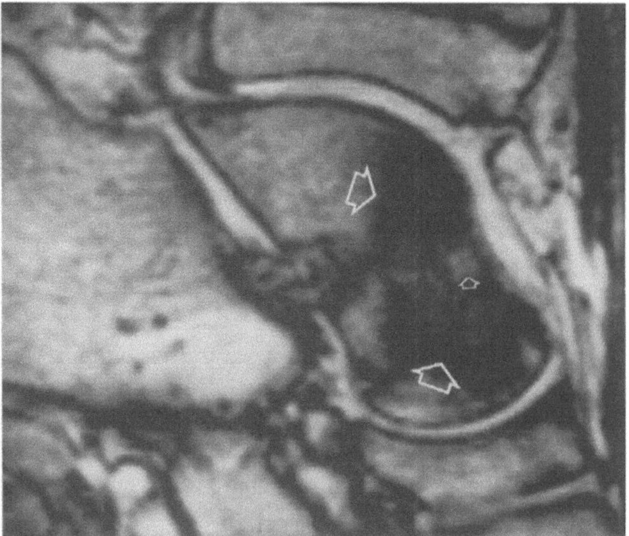

B

Fig. 9.2. A case of osteoid osteoma not clearly assessed by X-ray plainfilm or stratigraphy. **B** The superior capability of MRI (GE image) shows the nidus (*small open arrow*) and cancellous bone edema (*large open arrows*), permitting exact localization of the lesion; it makes specific treatment possible. *GE*, gradient echo

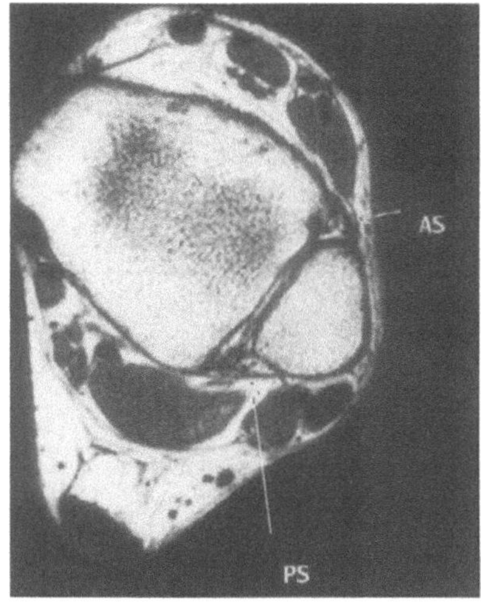
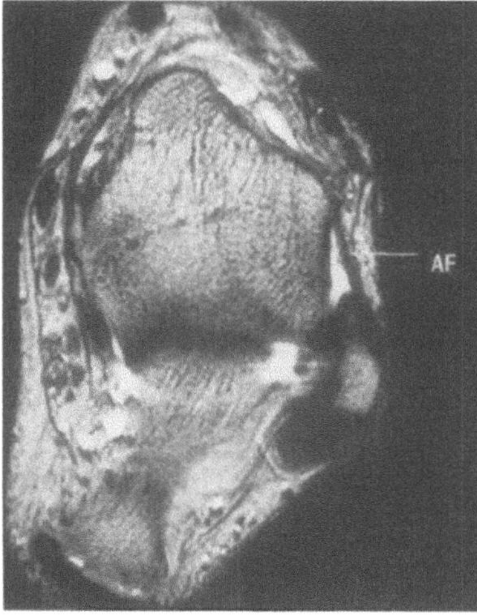
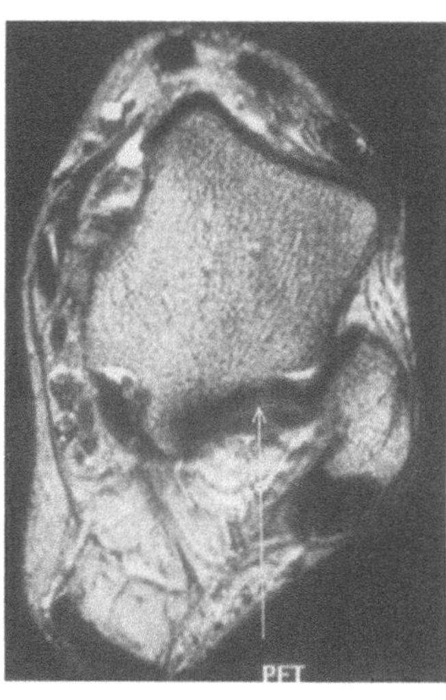

Fig. 9.3A–C. Normal anatomy. **A** Anterior tibiofibular (*AS*) and posterior tibiofibular (*PS*) syndesmotic ligaments are clearly visible in axial images. **B** Anterior talofibular ligament (*AF*) and **C** posterior talofibular ligament are well depicted in oblique axial plane; in MRI they appear as low signal intensity bands

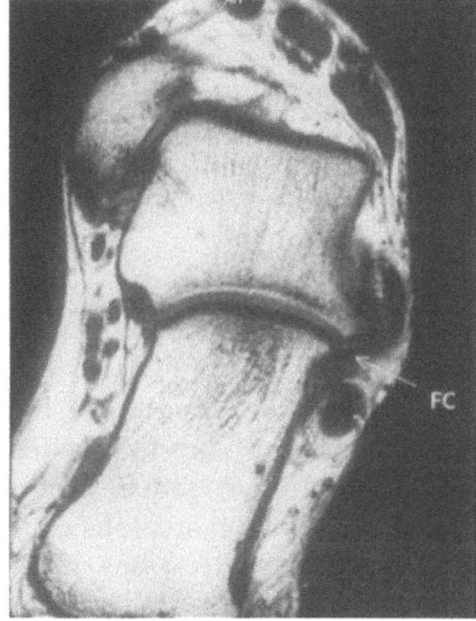

Fig. 9.4. The calcaneofibular ligament (*FC*) is best demonstrated in coronal MR images with the foot in plantar flexion

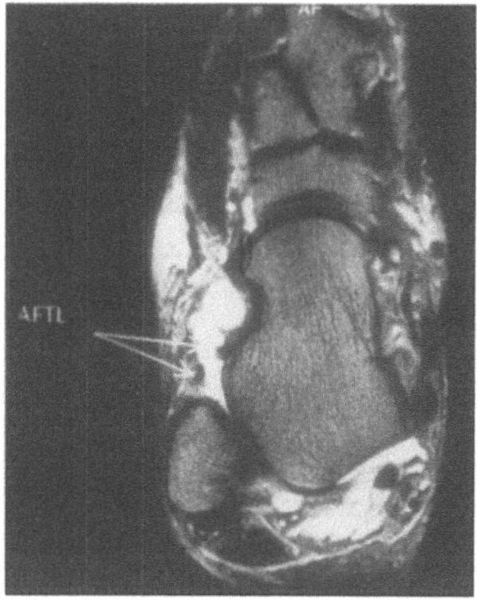

Fig. 9.5. Complete lesion of the anterior fibulotalar ligament (*AFTL*) after inversion stress

is the case in Pilon fracture, in which the integrity of the tibiofibular syndesmosis is preserved but a comminuted fracture of the distal tibia extends into the dome of the plafond; this fracture, even if well consolidated, leads to reduction of joint stability and early degenerative arthropathy because of the articular involvement (subtle alteration in the shape of the dome of the plafond and irregularity of the mortise surface). Of course, fracture of the talus, which is frequently associated with Pilon fracture, worsens clinical outcome (STEINBRONN 1994).

Less common is ankle instability following mono-, bi-, or trimalleolar fracture if well consolidated.

Plain film analysis of ankle bone fractures and the pattern of disruption of the ankle mortise may point towards specific ligament injuries; on the other hand, the particular site of fracture line may predict ligament integrity. For instance, the presence of medial malleolus transverse fracture is indicative of deltoid ligament integrity, while the deltoid ligament is usually torn if the medial malleolus is intact in the

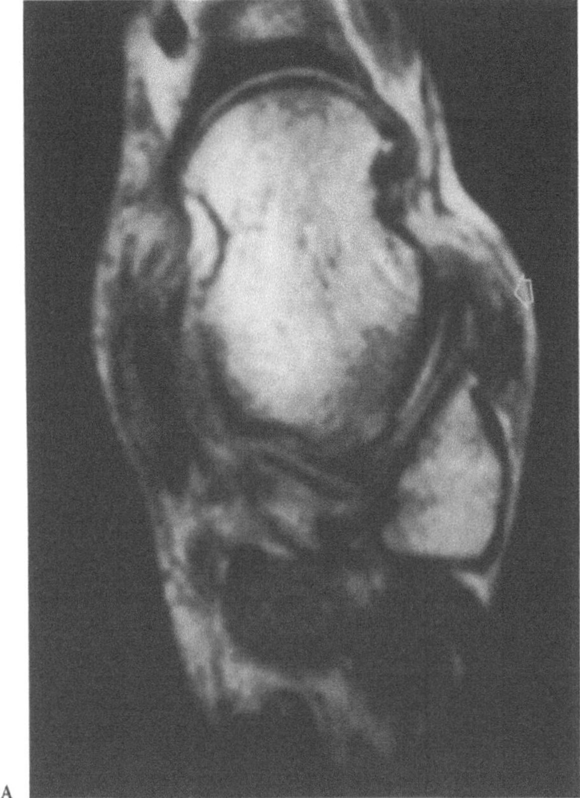

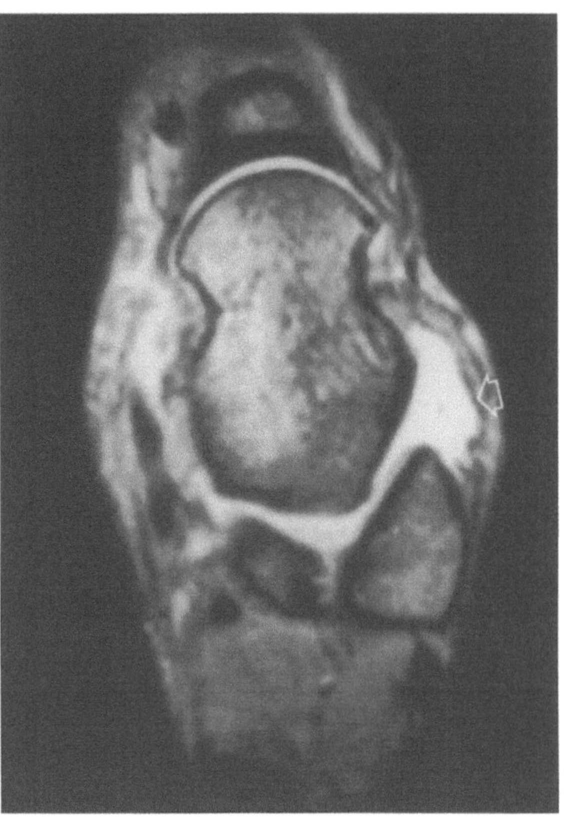

A   B

Fig. 9.6. A In this case the anterior fibulotalar ligament tear is less recognizable due to the presence of edema and synovial reaction (*open arrow*). **B** The ligamentous absence is evident on a T2-weighted image (*open arrow*)

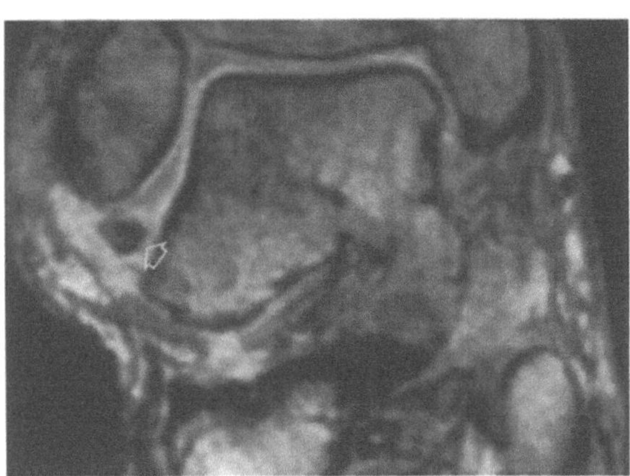

Fig. 9.7. Coronal MR, GE image. Below the fibular apex an osteochonadral fragment is evident (*open arrow*)

presence of a fracture of the fibula above the ankle joint.

Examinations with injection of contrast medium into the articulation could be useful in evaluating acute ligamentous lesions of the tibiotarsal joints. In acute ligamentous lesions, there is always an associated capsular lesion. Contrast examinations are not useful in the evaluation of chronic relaxations because in this phase there is always recicatrization of capsular lesions (FUSSEL 1973).

The lateral ligamentous lesions can also be evaluated with a tenogram of the fibular tendons, but these examinations are not frequently used.

In the acute phase of ligamentous distress, CT or MR imaging recognizes alterations of the ligamentous structures by virtue of their enlargement and inhomogeneity, which becomes more evident but less recognizable due to the presence of edema and synovial reactions (Fig. 9.6). As with all ligamentous structures closely connected to the capsular walls, trauma is followed by cicatrization and sclerosis which, though not an original anatomic structure, create a reinforcement area for the articular capsule, that is sufficient for future stabilization of the ankle. On CT and MRI, there is direct evidence of normal ligament structures, which have a ribbon-like aspect. These structures present homogeneous low signal intensity in all standard MRI sequences and homogeneous high density on CT. MRI offers greater potential for three-dimensional imaging and, with due regard to safety, permits a panoramic study of the

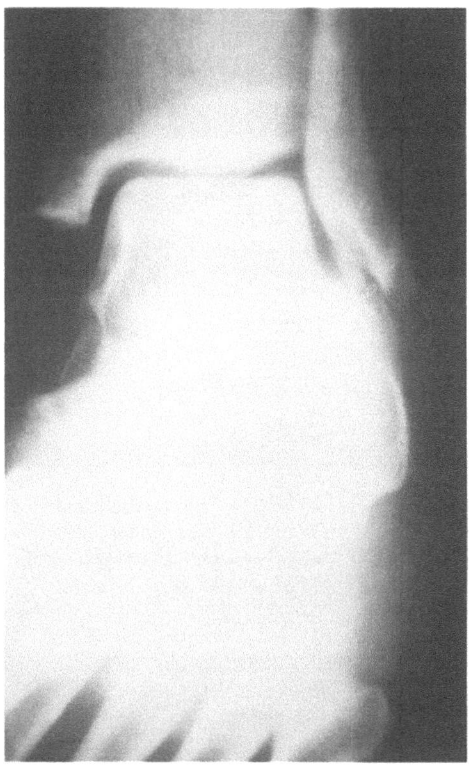

Fig. 9.8. X-ray demonstrates a calcified fragment in the tibiofibular recess (*open arrow*)

articulation using specific scanning planes for the individual ligamentous components.

In the case of bone avulsion or displacement of osteochondral fragments, MRI enables recognition of larger fragments, and in the acute phase the presence of spongious edema at the dislocation site documents the bone lesion (Fig. 9.7). X-ray and CT in such cases yield better visualization of small calcified fragments (Fig. 9.8) (TEHRANZADEH 1992, 1994; VOGLER 1994).

9.3
Particular Aspects of CT and MR Imaging

9.3.1
Osteochondral Lesions and Bone Damage

Although, from the theoretical point of view, conventional radiology may be considered sufficient for complete evaluation of the bone structures, experience has proved that MRI, with its high contrast resolution, can show osteochondral lesions and significant bone damage that are missed completely by other methods, especially in the early phase, even if

there are clear clinical manifestations. At the tibiotarsal joint, in particular at the talar dome, osteochondral lesions are very frequent and are usually evident after inversion or eversion traumas of the ankle.

Forced inversion and dorsiflexion usually produces a lesion on the lateral margin of the talar dome due to the impingement with the fibular styloid process; inversion stresses in plantar flexion with external rotation of the tibia cause medial lesions (impact between posteromedial tibia and medial talar margin).

Osteochondral lesions of the talus may be present even without a history of trauma, but in these cases it is often possible to relate the morphological patterns to a functional overload of the ankle with repeated mechanical strain (FALETTI 1995; FERKEL 1991; MIDDLETON 1987).

In the initial phases, after a distorting trauma, the osteochondral lesion of the talar dome is usually evident only in the bone component; in these cases the general term "transchondral fracture" is proposed. This term is now often used to describe morphological patterns that, until recently, were called "osteochondritis dissecans".

Although in some cases there may be isolated damage to the chondral component without significant involvement of the underlying sub-chondral bone, this kind of damage is infrequent and in our experience transitory, since the subchondral bone almost always rapidly becomes involved.

For accurate evaluation of these pathologies, the best technique is MRI (Figs. 9.9, 9.10, 9.11). Generally, for detection of spongious involvement, it is best to use gradient echo (GE) sequences. The best characterization of the lesion is given by the integration of GE T1- and T2-weighted sequences.

The possibility of documenting bone damage and its extent at an early stage is important from the clinical point of view, because it very often influences therapy and, consequently, the prognosis of the lesion. In selected cases, the use of intraarticular contrast medium is necessary for better MRI evaluation of cartilage damage; under these circumstances, CT and stratigraphic evaluations after the administration of contrast medium are still useful (MUNK 1992; ROSEMBERG 1988a,b).

Especially in the evaluation of the cancellous bone of the talus, analysis of the signal intensity of the different sequences makes it possible to differentiate the ischemic areas from the hyperemic reactive alterations or RSDS (reflex sympathetic dystrophic syndrome; Fig. 9.12). For this reason, it is necessary to

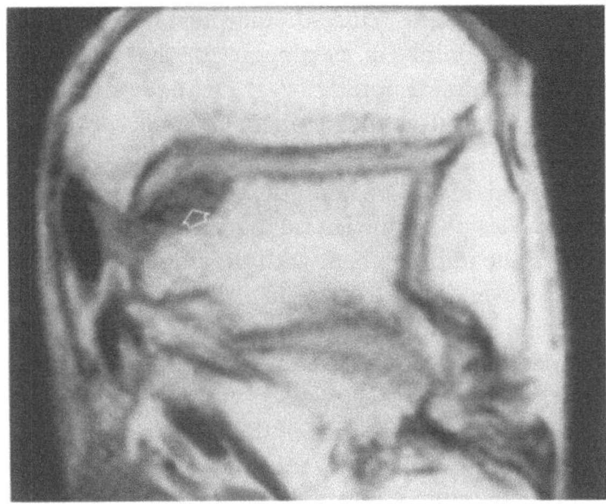

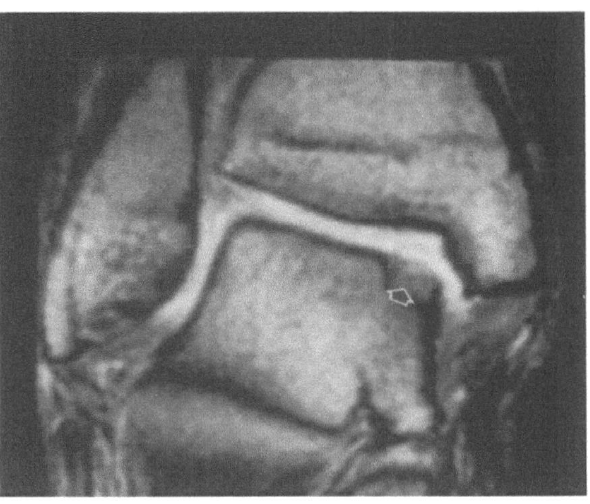

Fig. 9.9. A T1-weighted MR image: transchondral fracture (*open arrow*) of the medial talar dome. Low signal intensity in the subchondral bone component; initial damage to the chondral component with attenuated signal intensity and ar-

ticular cartilage evident only on the medial aspect of the defect. **B** GE sequence: a similar subchondral alteration (*open arrow*) with initial fragmentation of the cartilage of the talar dome

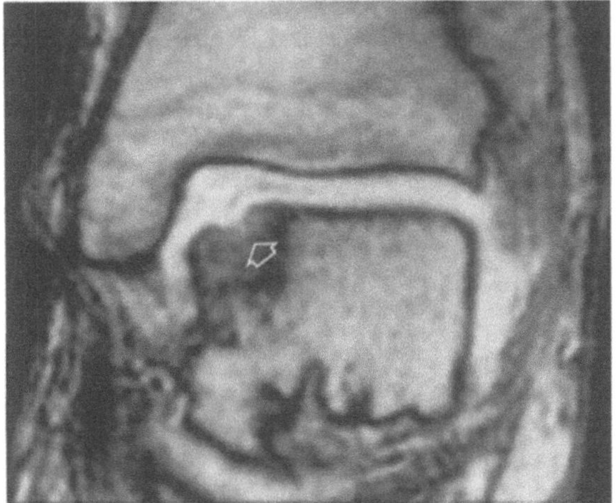

Fig. 9.10. Osteochondral lesion. Coronal MRI (GE) demonstrates severe subchondral and chondral irregularity of the medial talar dome (*open arrow*)

recall the existence of some complicated cases in which, in the context of a hyperemic alteration of the cancellous bone of the talus, a focal area with apparently normal signal is found (Fig. 9.13). Long-term follow-up often reveals ischemic bone lesions, such as osteonecrosis, in the nonhyperemic area.

9.4
Synovial Pathology of the Tibiotarsal Joint

Aspecific synovitides of the tibiotarsal joint are very frequent following trauma and are almost always found clinically in the acute phase. Persistent post-

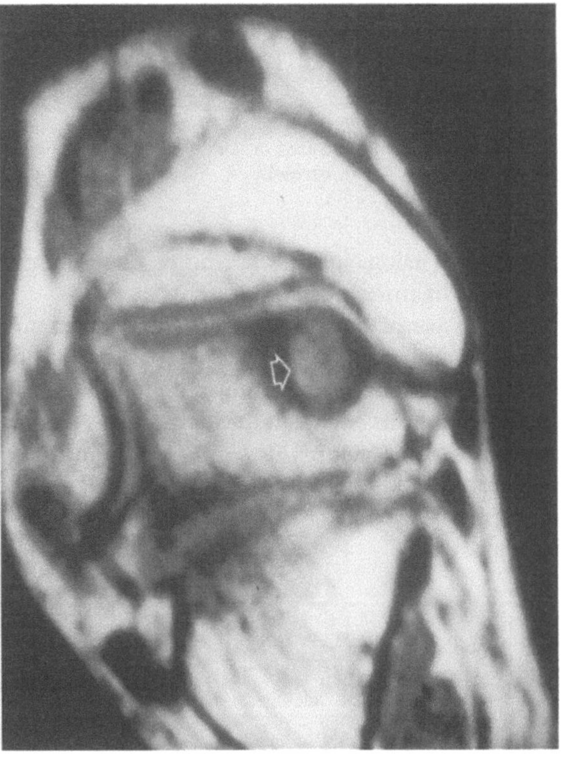

Fig. 9.11. Coronal T1-weighted MR image (SE) shows a medial talar osteochondral defect of intermediate signal intensity (*open arrow*) surrounded by reactive bone filled with synovial fluid. The overlying hyaline cartilage seems to be intact (asymptomatic patient with history of inversion stress)

traumatic synovitis is particularly significant because it often indicates a modification of articular biomechanics or the presence of osteochondral or hidden bone lesions. The prognosis is not always

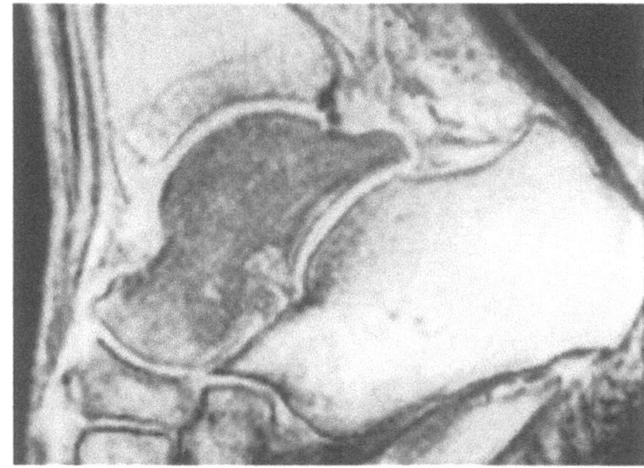

Fig. 9.12. Reflex sympathetic dystrophic syndrome (RSDS) of the talus: homogeneous alteration of the signal in GE

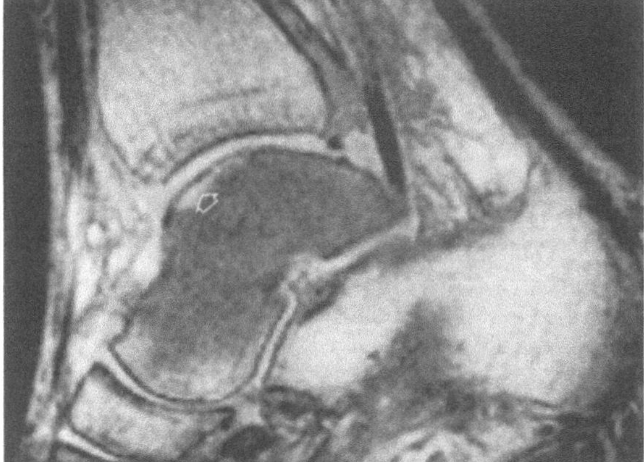

Fig. 9.13. In the context of hyperemic alteration of the cancellous bone of the talus, it is possible to find a focal area of apparently normal signal intensity (*open arrow*)

positive, delaying the recommencement of sporting activities.

In the aspecific synovitides, besides the presence of liquid is possible to discern villous and nodular structures; MRI yields important prognostic information distinguishing the hyperplastic character of synovitis and demonstrating the fibrous organizational phenomena.

In the early phases, hyperplastic synovitides are not well evaluated with MRI because the hyperplastic synovial villous and nodular formations are clearly hyperemic and have a signal intensity almost identical to that of the articular fluid (hyperintensity on T2). Venous administration of contrast medium, which can help to better define the hyperplastic synovitis in the early phase is rarely used after trauma; its use is restricted to patients with rheumatic pathologies. Persistent hyperplastic synovitis may follow fibrous cicatricial phenomena. If they worsen, these phenomena are well recognized on MRI, especially with T2-weighted sequences, where the decrease in signal intensity of the nodular and villous structures and the presence of scattered areas with low signal intensity permits their distinction on T2 from fluid hyperintensity (Fig. 9.14).

These findings are important because the sclerosis of the synovial tissue indicates the persistence of an inflammatory process and represents an obstacle to the functional healing of the articulation. It is also the main cause of pain. When fibrotic reactions cause a mechanical impediment, impingement ensues. The hyaline connective tissue localized in the recesses is currently termed "meniscoid lesion" after

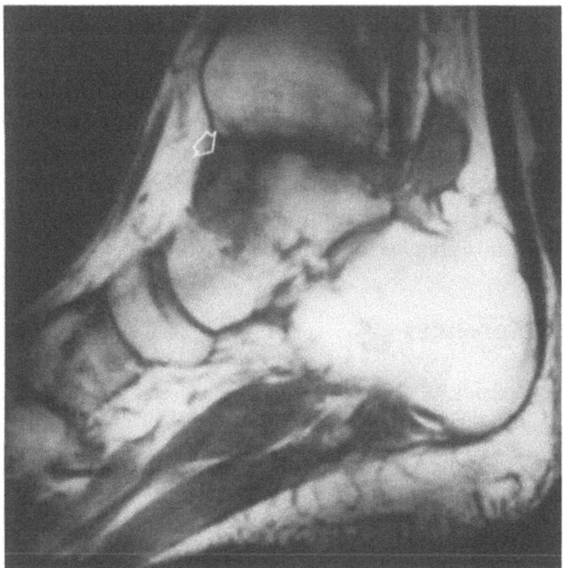

A

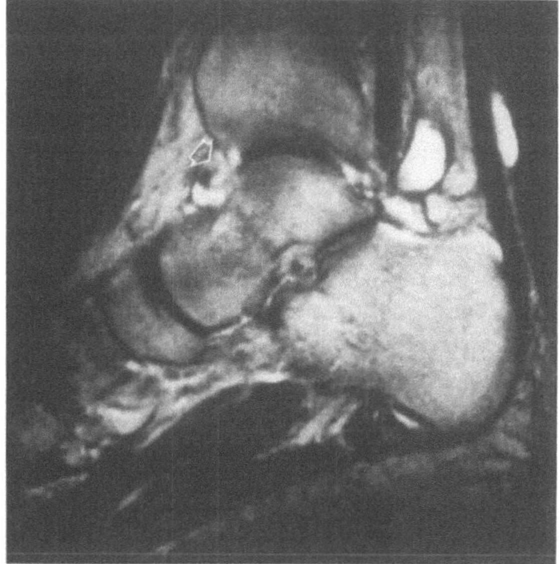

B

Fig. 9.14. A T1-weighted and **B** T2-weighted MR images of persistent synovitis of the ankle (*open arrows*)

its appearance. The impingement caused by this structure can lead to erosion of the talar dome or foci of chondromalacia. Therefore, accurate study of the articular recesses is important, particularly so in the case of persistent synovitides, which are very common in ankle instability, to differentiate aspecific hyperplastic synovitis from the hemorrhagic, metaplastic, and neoplastic forms.

With regard to the hemorragic synovitides, the most important differential diagnoses are pigmented villonodular synovitis (PVNS) and giant-cell tumors of the synovia. Its diagnosis in early phase is of capital importance for prognosis as there are no systemic symptoms to characterize it as in rheumatoid arthritis or secondary hemophilic conditions.

PVNS and giant-cell tumors of the synovia, though distinguished from one another in the literature, do not differ from the histologic (giant cells), clinical, or surgical point of view. Most likely, they constitute a single pathologic entity and the different designations simply emphasize the different nature of the synovial damage: PVNS is intraarticular, while the giant-cell tumors affect bursa and tendon sheaths. In both cases, there is severe inflammation, often accompanied by serohematic effusion and functional impairment, which is not correlated with trauma. The proliferation of hyperplastic synovitis is at first insidious, especially in the nodular forms; this is particularly true in isolated forms where perhaps only one nodule exists. We have fewer differential diagnostic problems in the case of diffuse synovitis, particularly in villonodular forms where there are multiple well-structured and compact nodules with voluminous villous formations.

MRI is particularly useful for differential diagnosis, permitting accurate analysis of the morphologic characteristics, such as the compact aspect of the nodules and their low signal intensity due to the high proportion of iron (3%) in the pathologic tissue (Fig. 9.15). In more aggressive forms, we have observed bone invasion (10% of cases) with the presence of villonodular formations with low signal intensity in the contest of osteolytic areas; at any rate, accurate radiologic study allows recognition of the benign nature because of the presence of sclerotic margins of the destructive bone lesions.

Among the synovial metaplasias of the ankle, the most frequent is chondroid metaplasia, which, because of the calcifications, is readily recognized with conventional X-ray and CT; less easy is diagnosis with MRI, with which it is difficult to recognize the presence of small calcified accumulations inside the hyperplastic synovial alterations and to differentiate

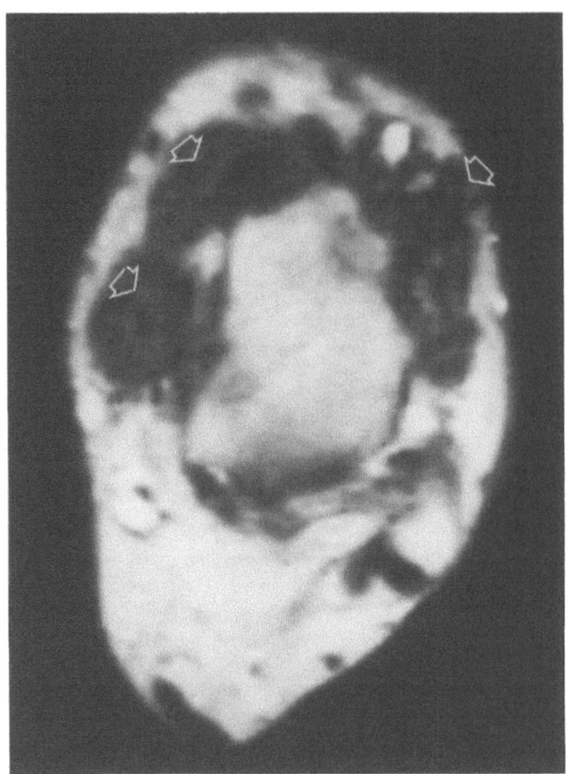

Fig. 9.15. T2-weighted MR image. Nodules appear compact and are of low signal intensity in a diffuse form: giant-cell tumor of the ankle (*open arrows*)

the more voluminous calcifications (which present a low signal intensity in all sequences) from the nodules of PVNS.

It is not very difficult to recognize the aggressive heteroplasias of the synovia; their identification is based on the local aggressivity of the pathologic tissue. Very often, there are calcifications inside the mass, and almost always the pathologic tissue is inhomogeneous. On MRI, differentiation from hemorrhagic synovitis with bone invasion is facilitated by T2-weighted sequences; the inhomogeneous hyperintensity of the heteroplastic tissue cannot be confused with the homogeneous hypointensity of the villonodular formations of PVNS (KONRATH 1994).

References

Bleichrodt RP (1989) Injuries of the lateral ankle ligaments: classification with tenography and arthrography. Radiology 173:347

Cardone BW (1993) MRI of injury to the lateral collateral ligamentous complex of the ankle. J Comput Assist Tomogr 17:102–107

Crim JR (1989) Magnetic resonance imaging of the hindfoot. Foot Ankle Int 10:1–7

Erickson SJ (1990) MR imaging of the tarsal tunnel and related spaces. Normal and abnormal findings with anatomic correlations. AJR Am J Roentgenol 155:323

Faletti C (1995) Magnetic resonance arthrography. Preliminary experience in study technique and main diagnostic applications. Radiol Med 89:211–214

Ferkel RD (1991) Magnetic resonance imaging of the foot and ankle: correlation of normal anatomy with pathologic conditions. Foot Ankle Int 11:289–305

Frost HM (1977) Technique for testing the drawer sign in the ankle. Clin Orthop 123:49

Fussel ME (1973) Ankle arthrography in acute sprains. Clin Orthop 93:278

Geyer M (1993) Stress reactions and stress fractures in the high perfomance athlete. Causes, diagnosis and therapy. Unfallchirurg 96:66–74

Keene JS (1989) Magnetic resonance imaging of Achilles tendon ruptures. Am J Sports Med 17:333–337

Konrath GA (1994) Magnetic resonance imaging in the diagnosis of localized pigmented villonodular synovitis of the ankle: a case report. Foot Ankle Int 15:84–87

Middleton WD (1987) High resolution surface coil magnetic resonance imaging of the joints: anatomic correlation. Radiographics 7:645–683

Munk PL (1992) Current status of magnetic resonance imaging of the ankle and the hindfoot. Can Assoc Radiol J 43:19–30

Resnick D (1974) Radiology of the talocalcaneal articulations. Anatomic considerations and arthrography. Radiology 111:581

Rosemberg ZS (1988a) Computed tomography scan and magnetic resonance imaging of ankle tendons: an overview. Foot Ankle Int 8:297–307

Rosemberg ZS (1988b) Ankle tendons; evaluation with CT. Radiology 166:221

Steinbronn DJ (1994) The use of magnetic resonance imaging in the diagnosis of stress fractures of ankle: four case reports. Foot Ankle Int 15:80–83

Tehranzadeh J (1992) Magnetic resonance imaging of tendon and ligament abnormalities. Part II: pelvis and lower extremities. Skeletal Radiol 2:79–86

Tehranzadeh J (1994) MRI of trauma and sports-related injuries of tendons and ligaments. Part II: pelvis and lower extremities. Crit Rev Diagn Imaging 35:131–200

Vogler HW (1994) Anterior ankle impingement arthropathy. The role of anterolateral arthrotomy and arthroscopy. Clin Podiatr Med Surg 1:425–427

10 Subtalar Instability in Athletes

C. Masciocchi[1] and M.V. Maffey[2]

CONTENTS

10.1
Introduction

The growing popular concern with health and the awareness of the benefits of exercise have led to the participation of more individuals in sports. One of the results of this trend has been an increase in sports-related injuries, a high percentage of which occur in the foot.

In the hindfoot, the subtalar space serves as stabilizer and biomechanical pivot and represents the junction between talar and calcaneal foot. The subtalar joint acts as a hinge between the two biomechanical components, which, having different articular functions, also play different static and dynamic roles.

10.2
The Subtalar Joint

10.2.1
Anatomy

The subtalar joint in the human foot forms a single functional structure consisting of two independent articular zones: the posterior subtalar joint is formed in the calcaneal portion of an ample articular sur-

face, the "talamus". The other joint is the anterior subtalar, which is smaller and situated in front and on the medial aspect of the posterior subtalar joint. This constitutes the "sustentaculum tali," supporting the talus.

In the subtalar joint, a fibrocartilaginous component is found formed by the plantar calcaneo-navicular ligament, or spring ligament, which fills the talar portion between the superomedial articular surface of the calcaneus and the navicular. The spring ligament is a vital stabilizer of the longitudinal arch of the foot; laxity or rupture of this ligament permits plantar flexion of the talus. Medially, the spring ligament is supported by the anterior fibers of the superficial deltoid ligament (tibio-spring fibers) with which it blends.

The posterior tibial tendon runs superficial to the tibio-spring fibers and its plantar expansion provides support to the inferior aspects of the spring ligament. Laterally, the spring ligament is contiguous to the medial band of the bifurcate ligament, also called Chopart ligament, a Y-shaped ligament joining the medial superior aspect of the anterior calcaneus to the neighboring aspects of the navicular bone and the cuboid bone.

The Chopart ligament can be considered the central ligament of the foot since it connects the two systems which depend on talus and calcaneus.

Between the anterior and posterior subtalar joints, the sinus tarsi and the tarsal canal is found. The "sinus tarsi proper" is shaped like a cone with the base on the lateral side, limited at the back by the posterior subtalar and in front by a crest which forms the anterior tuberosity of the calcaneus. The "tarsal canal" is a prolongation in the medial part of the vertex of the sinus; it is found between the anterior and the posterior subtalar joints, and its direction is not exactly perpendicular to the base of the sinus but extends towards the back and the medial side.

Inside the sinus tarsi, ligaments, vessels and nerves surrounded by a variable amount of connective and fatty tissue are found. The sinus tarsi nerve

[1] C. Masciocchi, MD, Department of Radiology, University of L'Aquila, Collemaggio Hospital, 67100 L'Aquila, Italy
[2] M.V. Maffey, MD, Department of Radiology, University of L'Aquila, Collemaggio Hospital, 67100 L'Aquila, Italy

is formed by the lateral terminal branch of the anterior tibial nerve, but also receives fibers from the lateral plantar portion of the posterior tibial nerve. It sends branches to the tarsal canal and the subtalar joints. Vascularization is constant: a vascular arch is formed in the sinus tarsi from a branch of the posterior tibial artery entering medially and a branch of the dorsalis pedis artery entering laterally, although they may not be truly anastomosed.

The ligaments of the ankle not only give stability to the subtalar joint but are important in their intimate biomechanical relationship. The ligamentous structures supporting the lateral aspect of the ankle and the hindfoot can be divided into two main groups: the two anterior components of the lateral collateral ligament (anterior talofibular ligament and calcaneofibular ligament) and the ligamentous structures of the sinus tarsi and tarsal canal which are formed by a few elastic fibers and many collagen fibers, so that they are thick and strong.

The talofibular ligament has a rather horizontal orientation, while the calcaneofibular ligament has a more vertical course, extending from the inferior aspect of the lateral malleolus to the calcaneus.

The tarsal canal contains the ligamentous complex of the sinus tarsi, composed of the interosseous talocalcaneal ligament and the cervical ligament, centrally in the canal and extending medially, and laterally the roof of the inferior extensor retinaculum, which turns downward in the lateral aspect of the neck of the talus and enters the sinus tarsi, where

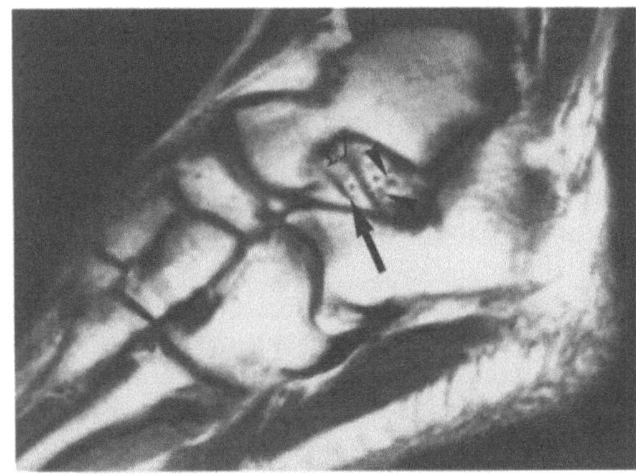

a

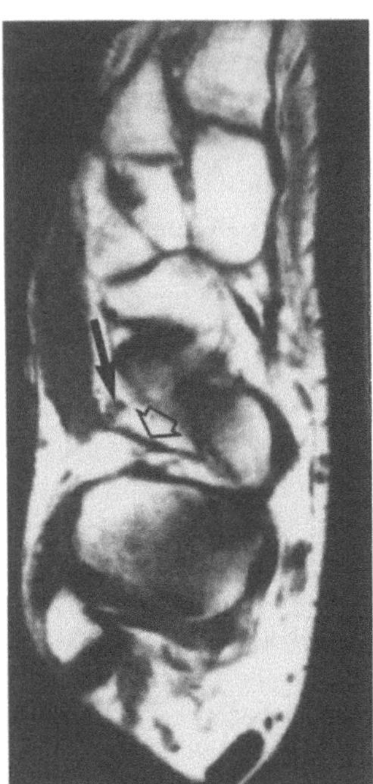

b

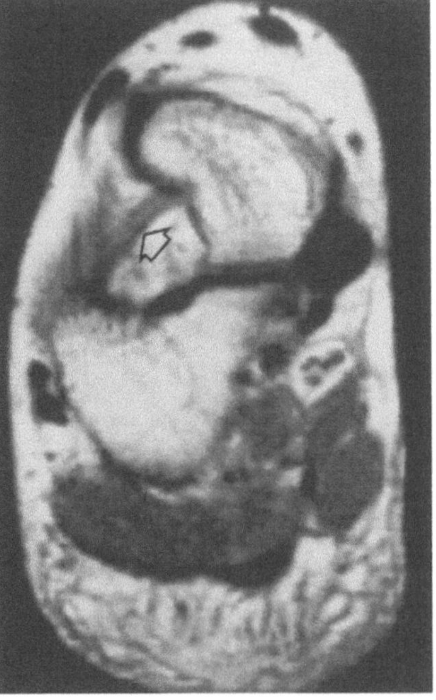

c

Fig. 10.1a–c. MRI anatomy: spin-echo T1-weighted images on sagittal (**a**), axial (**b**), and coronal (**c**) planes showing the ligamentous complex of the sinus tarsi. The cervical (*solid arrow*) and the interosseous (*open arrow*) ligaments appear as dark thin bands; the neurovascular endings are also well evident (*arrowhead*)

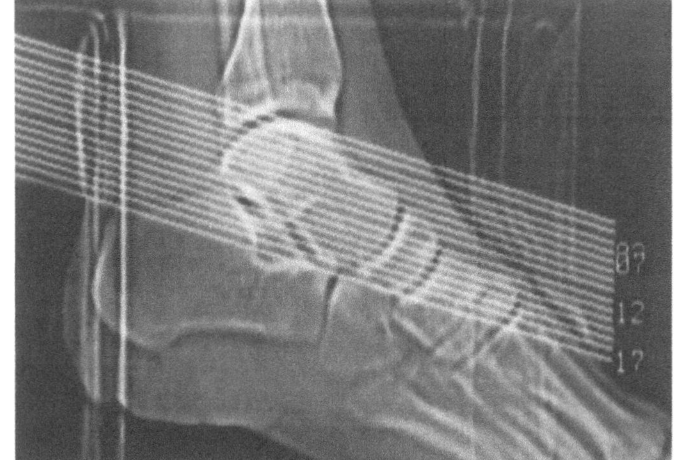

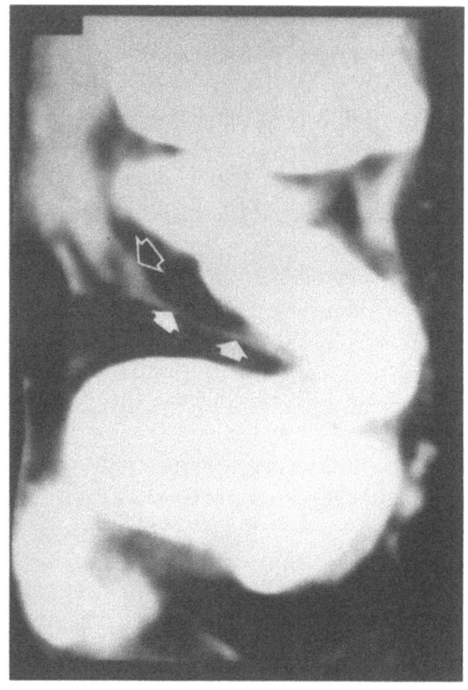

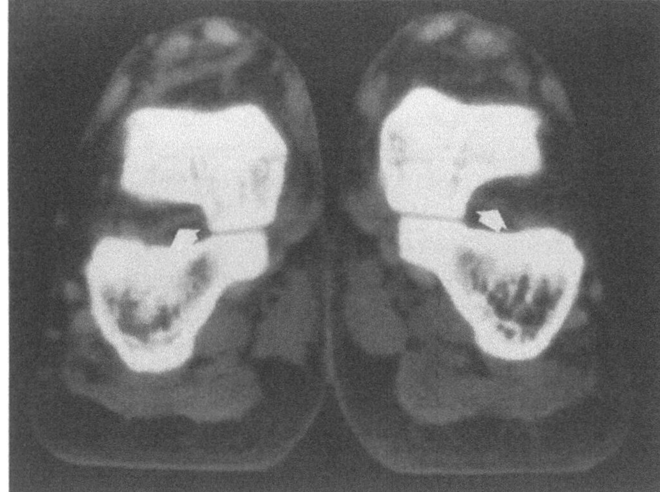

Fig. 10.2a–c. CT: scanogram (**a**); anatomical appearance of interosseous (*solid arrows*) and cervical (*open arrow*) ligament in axial plane (**b**) and coronal plane (**c**)

it divides into three groups: lateral, intermediate, and medial. These retinacula are very lax fibers and easily distensible and do not properly join the talus to the calcaneus, but serve as an insertion to soften formations; they contribute only indirectly to talocalcaneal stability.

The main function of the interosseous talocalcaneal ligament is to limit eversion. By doing so it prevents heel valgus and thus depression of the plantar arch; the multidirectionality of its fibers allows it to control the multiple simple movements that cause eversion of the foot, such as pronation, equinus, abduction, and lysthesis of the talus.

In the sinus tarsi, the cervical ligament extends from the dorsal surface of the calcaneus, medial to the extensor digitorum brevis muscle, to the inferolateral aspect at the neck of the talus: this is the only interosseous ligament that stops inversion, and it continues along the medial portion with the interosseous ligament of the canal.

It must also be considered that, like the cruciate ligament of the knee, the ligamentous complex of the sinus tarsi has terminal vascularization. Thus, once the elastic deformation threshold has been passed, the ligament will be subjected to ischemic processes with subsequent atrophy and structure reabsorption.

Use of magnetic resonance imaging (MRI) has proved reliable in this field, due to its high spatial and contrast resolution and its multiplanar imaging, which is of fundamental value in the study of such different space-oriented structures (Fig. 10.1).

Even though both bony and capsuloligamentous components are well demonstrated by computed tomography (CT), multiplanar and complete imaging of the tarsus is not possible with this technique (Fig. 10.2).

10.2.2
Physiology and Biomechanics

From a biomechanical point of view, the step can be divided into different phases during which the joints are aligned in the distoproximal direction and each skeletal segment moves on the segment next to it.

In the first phase the calcaneus stabilizes to the ground, followed by the calcaneal foot and, in the third phase, by the talar foot. In this phase, subtalar stabilization also starts thanks to the action of the eversion muscles and the ligamentous peritalar complex.

Finally, tibio-fibulo-talar stabilization occurs. When all of these events have ensued, the knee and ankle become involved in the kinetic chain that makes the load-bearing limb become the supporting one during walking. The anterior and posterior subtalar joints function as a double arthrodia. It is geometrically impossible to make two spherical and two cylindrical surfaces glide simultaneously without a loss of contact between the two surfaces. Joint movements of the foot are complex three-plane movements. Hindfoot movement in the sagittal plane is designated dorsiflexion when the anterior part of the calcaneus turns cephalad, and plantar flexion when it turns caudad; in the frontal plane, the movement is designated adduction when the calcaneus turns medially, and abduction when it turns laterally. In the horizontal plane, hindfoot movement is designated internal rotation when the anterior part of the calcaneus rotates medially, and external rotation when it rotates laterally.

The axis along which the movements occur is the result of three elementary movements of the anterior extremity of the calcaneus: pulling down during foot extension, moving inwards during abduction, and leaning on the external portion during supination.

Geometrically, the resulting movement is represented by a double frustum, and the resulting axis along which the movement occurs penetrates the superointernal aspect of the talar neck, passes through the sinus tarsi, and issues from the posteroexternal tuberosity of the calcaneus. This is the so-called Henke's axis.

The movements that occur at the subtalar joint are those of eversion and inversion. Eversion is not under the control of any specific muscle group, while inversion is controlled by the tibialis posterior muscle, one of the main stabilizers of the hindfoot and the gastrocnemius-soleus muscles. However, the

mechanism of the plantar aponeurosis, the external rotation of the lower extremity, and metatarsal break also contribute to the inversion of the subtalar joint.

The talus is the joint that transmits forces from the leg to the foot. It lacks muscular attachments and is kept in place and partially stabilized by the peritalar ligamentous complex. Moreover, more than 70% of its surface is covered by articular cartilage.

In contrast, the calcaneus has eight muscular attachments constituting agonist and antagonist groups that coordinate the movements: triceps versus extensors, and peroneus versus medial flexors of the leg.

The interosseous ligament is the central pivot of the system, not the geometrical centre. In fact, it lies closer to the calcaneocuboidal joint and more distant from the tibiotarsal ligament. The interosseous ligament is stimulated during both torsion and elongation. For this reason, the ligament is not only a rotatory stabilizer, but also a torsional stabilizer, at the level of Henke's axis, during the complex movements of calcaneal inversion/eversion. Moreover, the interosseous ligament has proprioceptive fibers from which the proprioceptive action of the peroneal muscles originates, in the case of blunt foot inversion.

The two peroneal muscles are controlled by proprioceptive endings constituted by the ligamentous complex of the sinus tarsi: the peroneus longus is controlled by the posterior aspect of the ligament, and the peroneus brevis by the anterior one. The subtalar joint is the pivot between talar and calcaneal foot whose balance is determined by the supporting action of the glenoid fossa, formed by navicular, spring ligament and articular surface of the sustentaculum tali, and talar head.

All skeletal, ligamentous, and muscular components of this structure play a fundamental dynamic role. Subluxations or protrusions occurring at this level lead to the main alterations of the foot.

10.2.3
Pathological Findings

Pathological alterations caused by trauma or generative processes of the different anatomical components of the subtalar region can lead to clinical syndromes. In particular, due to the skeletal structures of the hindfoot and to traumatic diseases, it is possible that inversion disorders of the tibiotarsal or subtalar joints, or of both, are more frequently observed. In contrast, degenerative capsuloligamentous processes or inflammatory osteoarticular processes can more frequently lead to eversion instability of the coxa pedis (talo-calcaneo-navicular joint), tibiotarsal joint, or subtalar joint.

The most frequent traumatic event during sports activity (basketball, soccer, volleyball, rugby, tennis, etc.) is inversion sprain, which leads to tearing of the lateral ligamentous components. The resulting condition can be a diastasis between talus and calcaneus with subsequent traumatic involvement of the stretched capsuloligamentous structures of the subtalar joints and in particular of the ligamentous complex of the sinus tarsi. The subtalar capsuloligamentous diseases mainly concern the ligamentous complex of the sinus tarsi (cervical and interosseous) which is stretched by the talocalcaneal diastasis brought about by the trauma.

Clinical joint instability may be correlated to lesions of these ligaments, and several statistics suggest not only a high degree of association between the ligaments of the sinus tarsi and tarsal canal and the lateral collateral ligament, but also a high frequency of sinus tarsi and tarsal canal ligament tears with inversion injury.

Diffuse lateral foot pain, perceived hindfoot instability, usually with lack of clinical or radiographic evidence of subtalar joint instability, focal pain on palpation, and alleviation of the pain by local anesthetic injection into the sinus tarsi are common criteria for sinus tarsi syndrome, which is usually reported as a post-traumatic event in middle-aged sportsmen and sports women, even though about 30% of cases are not related to trauma.

Inversion trauma will first cause an elastic deformation with subsequent tearing of the anterolateral bundle of the ligamentous complex of the sinus tarsi (cervical ligament). Subsequently, if trauma is severe, tearing of the posterolateral component (interosseous ligament) will follow. Therefore, there may be acute trauma with involvement of a single bundle or severe acute trauma with lesion of both ligamentous components. Chronic outcomes of lesions concerning one or both bundles can also be found.

Ligamentous tears and laxity can be followed by articular instability, which in turn leads to biomechanical functional overload, particularly at the level of subtalar joint cartilages and neurovascular structures of the tarsal canal, with long-term consequences including weakness, pain, osteochondral fracture, and loose body formation.

At the sinus tarsi level, the traumatic event causing the ligamentous lesion may induce zonal bleeding, leading to reactive celluloadipositis and formation of granulation and scar tissue.

Stretching of the ligamentous, capsular, and vascular structures may cause "truncation" of the nerve endings with subsequent pain. The latter event is clinically indistinguishable from post-traumatic sinus tarsi syndrome, even though pain is dull and resistant to analgesics and anti-inflammatory therapy. At subtalar level, the anterior and posterior articulations may be affected by different pathological alterations leading to pain and/or articular instability. Even though trauma seems to be the main cause of pain and instability, primitive anatomopathological alterations cannot be ruled out.

As already stated, ligamentous laxity may induce functional overload of articular cartilages, in particular at the level of the posterior subtalar joint, which plays a fundamental biomechanical role and is at risk from degenerative processes.

Functional overload therefore causes alterations of cartilaginous components as well as subchondral bone.

10.2.4
Imaging

Currently, diagnosis of the specific ankle ligament injured and the severity of the injury is based on: (a) the history of the injury and the findings on physical examination and (b) stress radiography (whose diagnostic parameters are not fully agreed on), or more invasive procedures such as arthrography and tenography.

The degree of talar tilt can be measured accurately on anteroposterior radiographs obtained with inversion stress. However, there is no general agreement on correlation of the degree of tilt with the specific ligament injury, because sometimes it is impossible to differentiate between isolated injuries to one ligament and injuries to combined ligaments (Fig. 10.3).

Complicating furthermore the interpretaton of radiographic stress tests of acute injuries is the accompanying pain and muscle spasm, which tend to restrict motion. Some investigators claim that stress radiography is of little use unless performed after administration of local nerve block or general anesthesia. Ankle arthrography has been useful in diagnosing some acute ankle-ligament injuries, but some

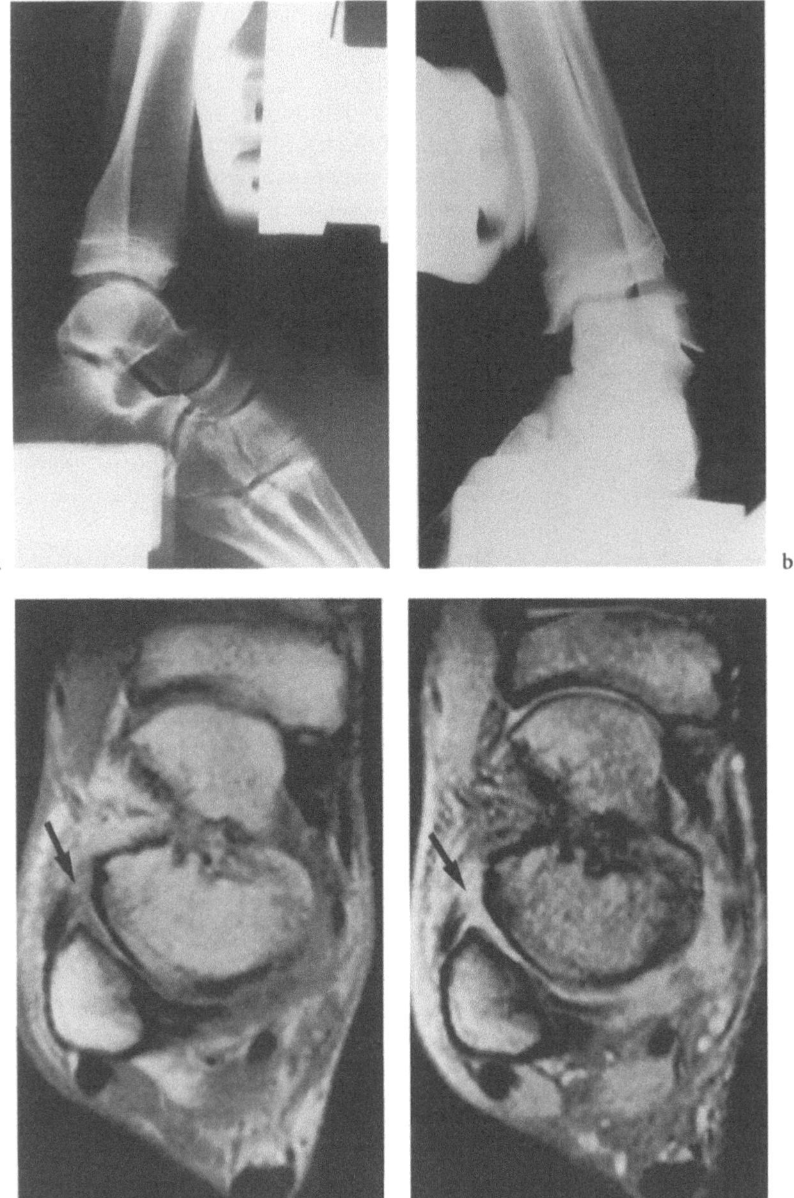

Fig. 10.3a–d. Varus stress lateral (a) and AP (b) views of an injured ankle demonstrating increased talar tilt. The lesion of the anterior talofibular ligament (*black arrows*) is well evident on MRI SE T1-weighted (c) and GE T2-weighted (d) images on axial plane. *AP*, anteroposterior; *SE*, spin echo; *GE*, gradient echo

authors contend that if it is not performed within the first few days after injury the arthrogram is likely to be negative since either organized clots or the repair process will have sealed the capsular rent.

The introduction of new diagnostic techniques such as CT and MRI has been of great help in the study of the subtalar joint and the sinus tarsi, which represents its biomechanical pivot.

Both techniques, particularly MRI, are fundamental for definition of the damage entity and for correct therapeutic planning. However, detection of gross alterations of the components of the subtalar joint,

in particular of the ligamentous complex of the sinus tarsi, is possible with CT in transverse and coronal planes (Fig. 10.4).

With MRI, acute traumatic involvement of the ligamentous complex of the sinus tarsi must always be evaluated in axial planes, using both T1- and T2-weighted sequences (Fig. 10.5). Generally, spin-echo T1-weighted sequences in the sagittal plane aid in demonstrating the type and degree of the ligamentous lesion, due to the natural contrast between the fatty tissue of the sinus tarsi and the ligamentous structure (Fig. 10.6).

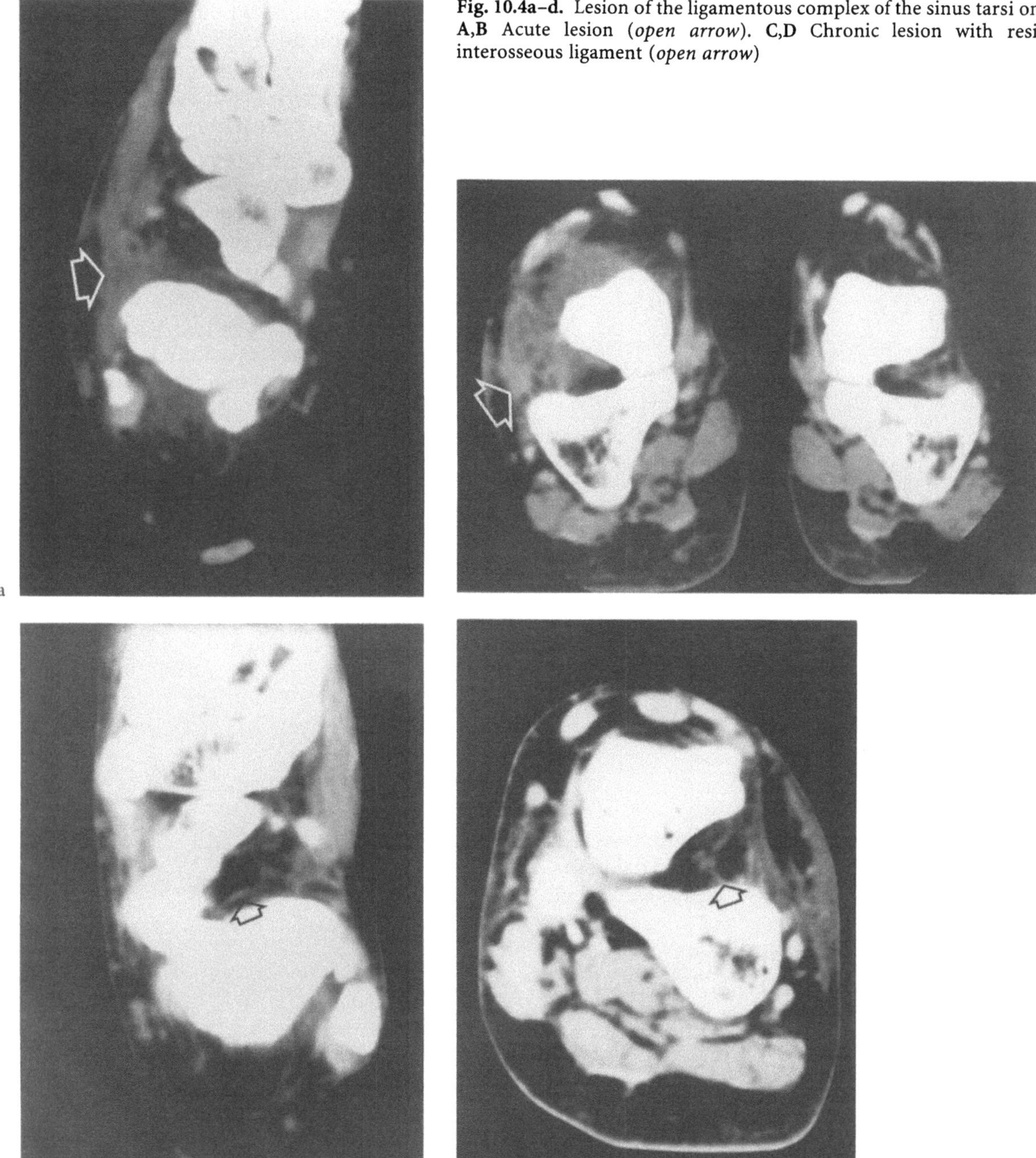

Fig. 10.4a–d. Lesion of the ligamentous complex of the sinus tarsi on CT. **A,B** Acute lesion (*open arrow*). **C,D** Chronic lesion with residual interosseous ligament (*open arrow*)

On the other hand, T2-weighted sequences will be employed when a more accurate evaluation is needed, as in cases where several structures of the sinus tarsi are involved by fibrotic or reactive processes. In such cases, the ligament can be readily recognized by its low signal intensity (SI) on these sequences compared to the surrounding reactive hyperplastic and fibrotic tissue, which is characterized by high SI (Fig. 10.7).

Although T2-weighted sequences allow, in these cases, visualization of the ligament, it is not always possible to distinguish its principal components be-

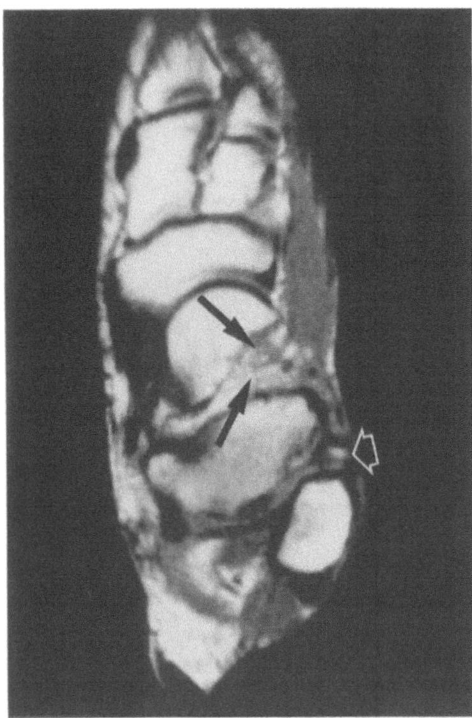

Fig. 10.5. MRI SE T1-weighted image on oblique axial plane shows the complete lesion of the ligamentous complex of the sinus tarsi (*black arrows*). Fibrotic scar is present on the lateral aspect due to chronic lesion of the lateral collateral ligamentous complex (*open white arrow*)

cause inflammatory and/or reparative processes may compress both bands and conceal the partial lesion. Diagnostic difficulties are encountered as the fibrous tissue reaches an advanced stage and presents low SI similar to that of the ligament on both T1- and T2-weighted sequences (Fig. 10.8).

For a better assessment of the MR image, it is advisable to distinguish among different events and to consider trauma and severity or chronic nature of the pathological condition: acute trauma with involvement of a single band; acute trauma with involvement of both ligamentous components; chronic outcomes of lesions involving one or both bands. A partial lesion in the acute phase always concerns the cervical ligament, which will not appear tense on MR images, but is documented by higher SI and a dishomogeneous and stretched appearance due to phenomena of serohemorrhagic filling. The interosseous talocalcaneal ligament will be easily recognizable and characterized by low and homogeneous SI.

It is important that the lesion of the subtalar ligamentous complex always be evaluated on both transverse and sagittal images in order to avoid possible

misinterpretation and allow more accurate evaluation of the ligamentous structures.

When acute traumas induce a complete tear of the subtalar ligamentous complex, there are two possible findings: (a) visualization of the size of the lesion and of the residual stumps, or (b) no evidence of the ligamentous structures, but only of small multiple fringes (Fig. 10.9). Depending on the type of trauma, a demarcated lesion or complete destruction and fibrillation of the whole ligament can be induced.

In late phases, when atrophic processes of ischemic nature are predominantly found, there will be no evidence of the ligament inside the tarsal canal, but residual fringes will be observed.

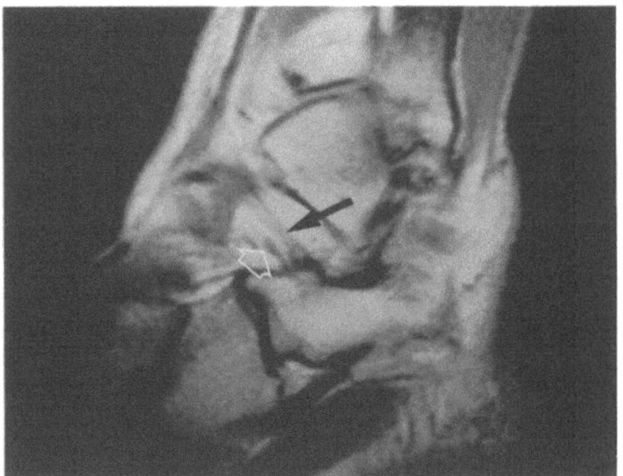

a

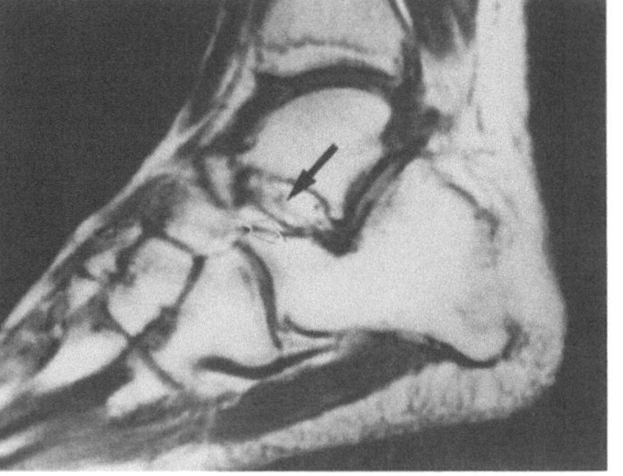

b

Fig. 10.6a,b. MRI SE T1-weighted images on sagittal planes. **a** Acute traumatic involvement of the cervical ligament which appears frayed with a distal residual portion (*open white arrow*). Interosseous talocalcaneal ligament is normal (*black arrow*). **b** Partial lesion of the ligamentous complex of the sinus tarsi: in the sinus tarsi only the cervical ligament is present (*open white arrow*), while the interosseous talocalcaneal ligament is reabsorbed (*black arrow*)

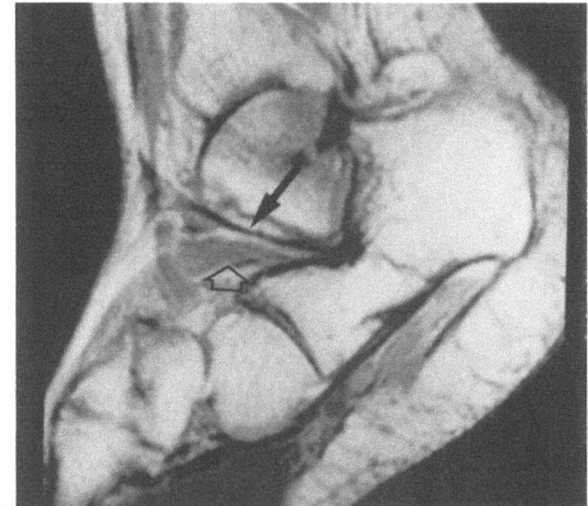

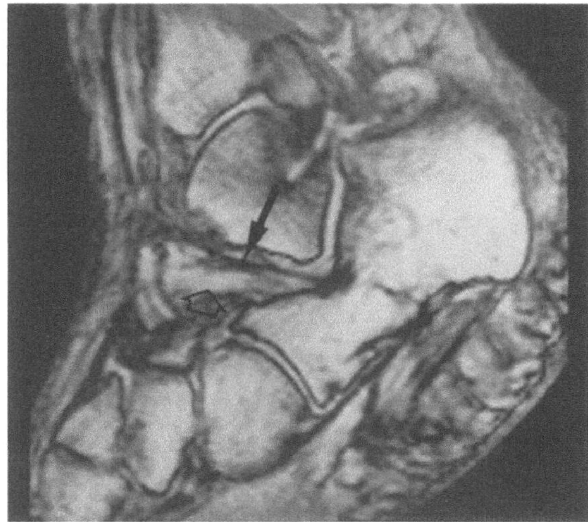

Fig. 10.7a,b. MRI sagittal planes showing the traumatic involvement of the cervical ligament on SE T1-weighted image (**a**) with reactive processes in the sinus tarsi recognized by high SI on GE T2-weighted image (**b**; *open arrow*). The interosseous ligament is not involved (*solid arrow*). *SI*, Signal intensity

Besides involving the ligamentous complex of the sinus tarsi, the traumatic event may induce reactive processes concerning the fatty components of the sinus; as already mentioned, the sinus contains fatty tissue supporting multiple vascular structures and nerve endings.

In the case of trauma, subtalar ligamentous tear can be associated with reactive processes involving the fatty tissue. Trauma responsible for a damaged ligament can lead to serohemorrhagic effusion, inducing a reactive fatty tissue process which produces fibrotic degeneration (Fig. 10.10).

Both parts of the inflammatory process, the stromal component involving the fatty tissue and the fibrous component, occupy the sinus tarsi, causing compression and stretching of the ligamentous, vascular, and nervous structures and narrowing of the nerve endings.

The painful syndrome is therefore due to inflammatory and reactive processes concerning the fatty tissue and the "chopping" effect exerted by the fibrous and granulation tissue on the nerve endings.

For better assessment of the MR image, two different conditions must be distinguished: acute findings and the outcome of chronic fibrosis. In the acute phase, the MR image is predominantly characterized by an adipose reactive process which appears with low SI on T1-weighted sequences. The process completely occupies the sinus tarsi and involves its components. On T2-weighted sequences the inflammatory change of the fatty tissue shows a high SI, when edematous phenomena outweigh the fibrotic ones.

In the chronic phase it is possible to identify, on both T1- and T2-weighted sequences, a tissue with inhomogeneous low SI covering all the structures contained in the sinus tarsi. In these cases it is not possible to say whether subtalar ligament lesions are present because the ligaments are completely

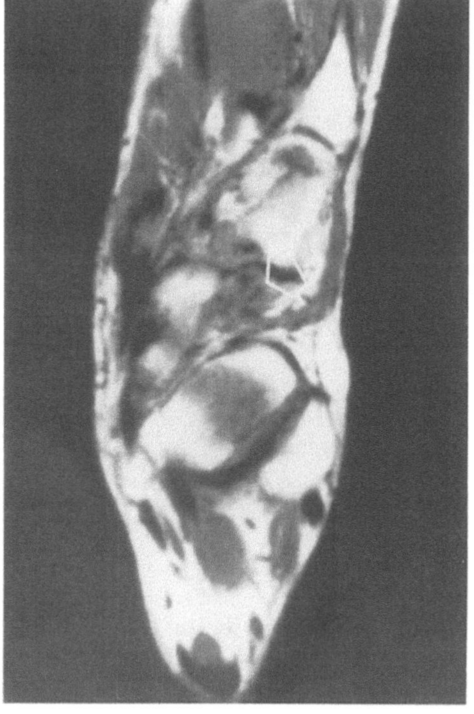

Fig. 10.8. Chronic lesion. MRI SE T1-weighted image on axial plane: low-SI area in the sinus tarsi representing fibrotic tissue (*arrow*)

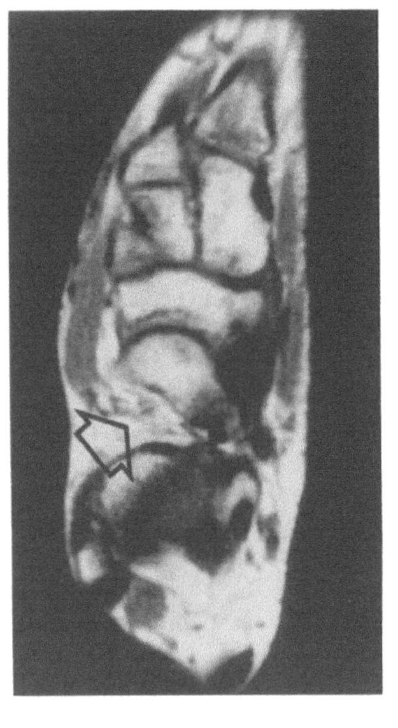
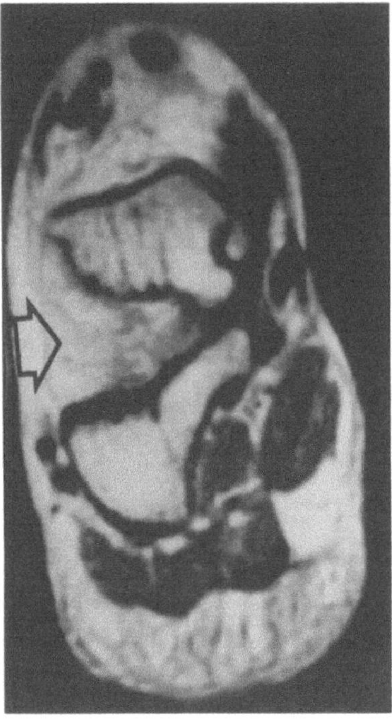

Fig. 10.9a,b. Complete ligamentous tear. SE T1-weighted images in axial (a) and coronal (b) planes show ischemic and atrophic degeneration of the cervical and the interosseous ligaments (*arrow*)

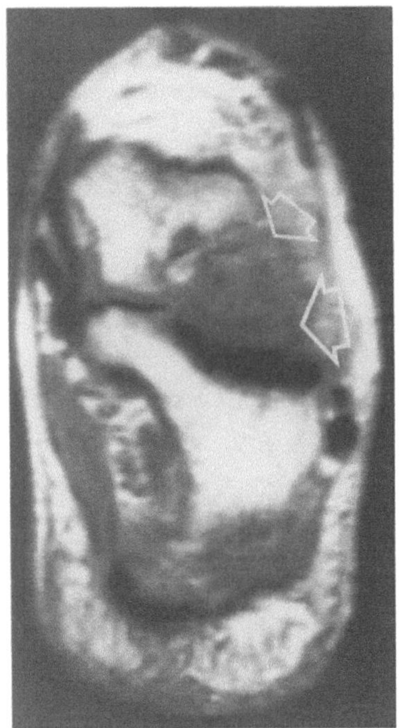
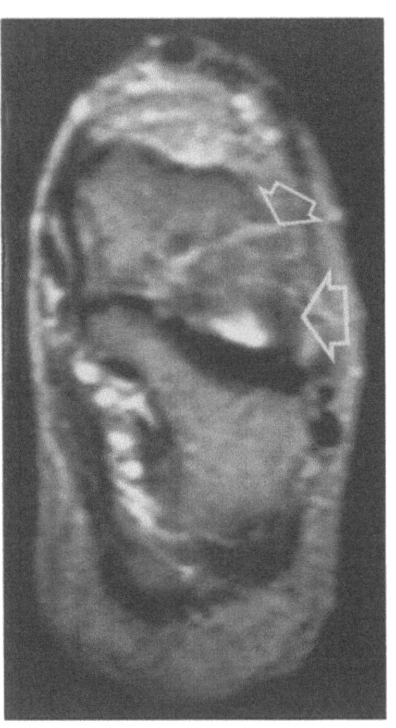

Fig. 10.10a,b. MRI coronal planes demonstrate reactive fatty tissue processes with low SI both on SE T1-weighted (a) and T2-weighted (b) images (*arrows*)

masked by the fibrotic process. It is advisable, however, to perform T2-weighted sequences in both transverse and sagittal planes to distinguish between the ligamentous component and the surrounding reactive process. Sometimes, mostly under edematous circumstances, this process can be documented by slightly higher SI, allowing differentiation of the diverse structures.

CT still plays an important role in the diagnosis of the diseases which bring about a sinus tarsi syndrome not necessarily associated with lesions of the ligamentous complex of the sinus tarsi.

In this case, in fact, MRI does not help in the diagnosis, since it is not always possible to characterize dystrophicodysplasic tumor-like lesions on the basis of SI and morphology alone (synovial cysts, neuromas, etc.).

Although a rare occurrence, the possibility of neuromas occupying the sinus tarsi must be taken into account. Clinically, they induce a painful syndrome that is indistinguishable from post-traumatic sinus tarsi syndrome, although a possible factor of differentiation could be represented by the type of pain, which is dull, slowly exacerbating, and does not respond to anti-inflammatory therapy.

The assessment of SI and morphological appearance alone does not contribute to characterizing the lesion on MR images. For differential diagnosis, therefore, two further pathological conditions must be considered: (a) a post-traumatic adipose inflammatory process in the acute or subacute phase, and (b) synovial cysts originating from the subtalar joints with extension into the sinus tarsi. Considering that on MR images neuromas present high SI on T2-weighted sequences and homogeneous low SI on T1-weighted sequences with regular morphological appearance, sometimes multilobar or clearly divided, differentiation from a post-traumatic inflammatory and reactive process in the acute phase is readily accomplished (Fig. 10.11).

The distinction between neuroma and synovial cyst may be very difficult. Clinically, both lesions may lead to the same symptoms, and in both cases there can be an absence of trauma. Moreover, as in neuromas, synovial cysts can appear roundish or lobated. They are always regular, with homogeneous low SI on T1-weighted sequences and homogeneous high SI on T2-weighted sequences. Differential diagnosis may be achieved on the basis of their location and morphology. Synovial cysts are directly connected to the articular surfaces, whereas neuromas present a cleavage plane with the surrounding articular structures.

As to the painful subtalar syndromes and in particular the overload and instability conditions secondary to trauma in athletes, MRI has proved more sensitive than CT in recognizing pathological patterns. Even though CT can demonstrate severe alterations, early evaluation of ischemic subchondral areas that cause severe pain is impossible (Fig. 10.12).

Arthrography and arthro-CT of the subtalar joint clearly show the cartilaginous component, but they do not allow evaluation of the subchondral bone. Functional overload of the posterior subtalar joint causes alterations of both cartilage and subchondral bone. These findings have the same MR characteristics as chondropathies and subchondral ischemic areas already observed in other anatomical territories. The articular cartilage therefore tapers.

Tapering associated with large areas of degeneration with low SI is identified at subchondral level secondary to ischemic process. As the process advances, it is possible to identify subchondral cystic lesions with regular morphology and low SI on T1-weighted sequences and high SI on T2-weighted se-

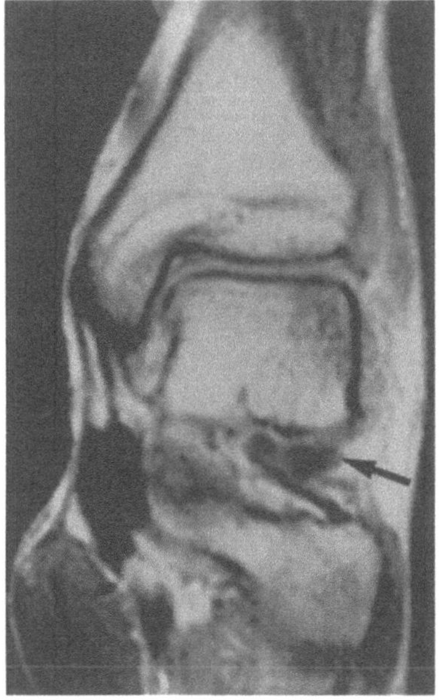
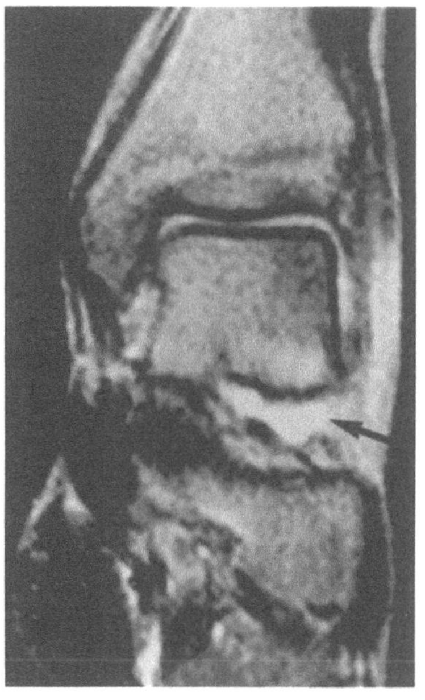

Fig. 10.11a,b. Synovial cyst: MRI coronal planes on SE T1-weighted (**a**) and T2-weighted (**b**) images (*arrow*)

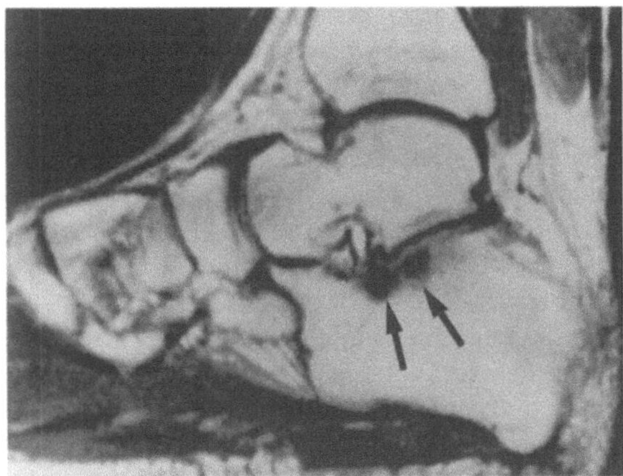

Fig. 10.12. MRI SE T1-weighted image well demonstrates the ischemic subchondral lesion at the level of subtalar joint in a patient with chronic hindfoot instability (*arrows*)

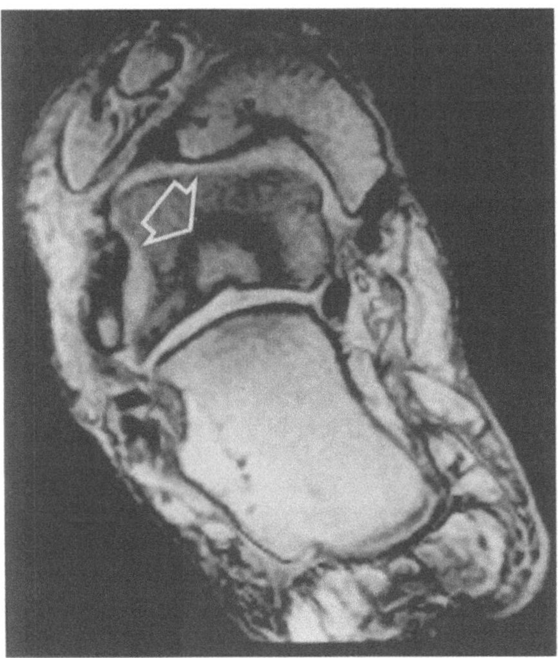

Fig. 10.13. Subchondral cystic lesion of the talus at the level of the posterior subtalar joint (*arrow*)

quences (Fig. 10.13). From a technical point of view, the T1-weighted sequences are particularly helpful in visualizing alterations in the subchondral bone.

T2-weighted gradient-echo sequences provide more detailed information on the cartilaginous component. Osteochondral changes are better visualized on sagittal and coronal oblique planes with slices perpendicular to the posterior subtalar rim.

MRI has higher sensitivity in identifying such pathological conditions than the other imaging techniques, including CT, which, although able to visualize severe alterations, does not allow evaluation of early subchondral lesions.

On the basis of certain clinical findings of frank subtalar instability, reparative treatment may be suggested, including replacement of the talocalcaneal ligament with a prosthesis or tendinous components. In such cases, it is wise to examine the prosthesis at regular intervals by means of MRI.

Although a wide spectrum of surgical procedures is available, the ligamentous prosthesis is usually positioned through two bony tunnels whose inlet and outlet holes are located on the calcaneal-floor base and on the talar vault of the sinus. In such cases, it is necessary that levels of data acquisition are defined for proper evaluation of surgical procedure, status, and trophism of the ligamentous prosthesis.

The osseous tunnels and the prosthesis status must be evaluated. Transverse planes oriented at different angles seem to be best suited for providing good visualization of the new ligament along its interosseous course. On the basis of the information acquired using oblique transverse planes, it is sometimes possible to employ longitudinal planes (sagittal and coronal) to visualize the entire osseous tunnel.

Moreover, MRI allows evaluation of the presence or absence of compression or rubbing along the new ligament tunnel.

10.3
Conclusions

In conclusion, MRI offers promise as an objective, noninvasive means of identifying the site and degree of ligament injury in both acute trauma and chronic instability of the ankle. MRI may be useful in patients in whom significant instability is detected, in the evaluation of injured ligaments and of the severity of injury, and in the evaluation of apparently stable acute ankle injuries in professional and amateur athletes.

A correct diagnostic approach to subtalar region diseases includes the employment of MRI for diagnostic certainty and proper therapeutic planning.

Suggested Reading

Andersen P, Wethelund J, Helmig P, Soballe K (1988) The stabilizing effect of the ligamentous structures in the sinus and tarsal canal on movements in the hindfoot. Am J Sports Med 16:5

Beltran J, Munchow AM, Khabiri H, Magee DG, McGhee RB, Grossman SB (1990) Ligaments of the lateral aspect of the ankle and sinus tarsi: an MR imaging study. Radiology 177:455–458

Burks RT, Morgan J (1994) Anatomy of the lateral ankle ligaments. Am J Sports Med 22:72–77

Clanton TO (1989) Instability of the subtalar joint. Orthop Clin North Am 20:583–592

Deutsch AL, Mink JK, Kerr R (1992) MRI of foot and ankle. Raven, New York

Erickson SJ, Smith JW, Ruiz ME, et al. (1991) MR imaging of the lateral collateral ligament of the ankle. AJR Am J Roentgenol 156:131–136

Forrester DM, Kerr R (1990) Trauma to the foot. Radiol Clin North Am 28:423–433

Forrester DM, Kricun ME, Kerr R (1988) Imaging of the foot and ankle. Aspen, Gaithersburg

Goossens M, De Stoop N, Claessens H, Van der Straeten C (1989) Posterior subtalar joint arthrography. A useful tool in the diagnosis of hindfoot disorders. Clin Orthop 249:48–55

Harper MC (1992) Stress radiographs in the diagnosis of lateral instability of the ankle and hindfoot. Foot Ankle Int 13:435–438

Kato T (1995) The diagnosis and treatment of instability of the subtalar joint. J Bone Joint Surg [Br] 77:400–406

Kjaersgaard-Andersen P, Wethelund JO, Helmig P, Soballe K (1988) The stabilizing effect of the ligamentous structures in the sinus and canalis tarsi on movements in the hindfoot. An experimental study. Am J Sports Med 16:512–516

Klein MA, Spreitzer AM (1993) MR imaging of the tarsal sinus and canal: normal anatomy, pathologic findings, and features of the sinus tarsi syndrome. Radiology 186:233–240

Louwerens JW, Ginai AZ, van Linge B, Snijders CJ (1995) Stress radiography of the talocrural and subtalar joints. Foot Ankle Int 16:148–155

Lowy A, Schilero J, Kanat IO (1985) Sinus tarsi syndrome: a post-operative analysis. J Foot Surg 24:108–112

Pisani G (1990) Trattato di chirurgia del piede. Minerva Med

Rule J, Yao L, Seeger LL (1993) Spring ligament of the ankle: normal MR anatomy. AJR Am J Roentgenol 161:1241–1244

Sarrafian SK (1993) Biomechanics of the subtalar joint complex. Clin Orthop 290:17–26

Schneck CD, Mesgarzadeh M, Bonakdarpour A (1992) MR imaging of the most commonly injured ankle ligaments. Radiology 184:507–512

Terk MR, Kwong PK (1994) Magnetic resonance imaging of the foot and ankle. Clin Sports Med 13:883–908

Viladot A, Lorenzo JC, Salazar J, Rodriguez A (1984) The subtalar joint: embryology and morphology. Foot Ankle 5:••

Volpe A (1984) Anatomia e fisiologia della articolazione sottoastragalica. Chir Piede 8:••

11 Impingement Syndrome of the Upper Limb

S. SINTZOFF

CONTENTS

11.1
Shoulder Impingement

11.1.1
Introduction

Rotator cuff disorders in athletes have been documented only in recent years. The history of rotator cuff disorders dates back to 1931, when E.A. CODMAN published his comprehensive work "*The Shoulder*", in which he suggests traumatic origin of shoulder impingement.

MEYER in 1934 argued against CODMAN's theory and proposed for the first time the idea that repeated minor trauma caused the pathologic findings. He also described the concept of impingement as narrowing the interval between the acromion and the humeral head and damaging the intervening tissue. No references to rotator cuff involvement as a result of sporting endeavors were made in these early years. The first such report by GILCREST was of biceps tendon rupture associated with significant trauma in pitchers and lifters (1925).

NEER, in his classic paper in 1972, suggested that pitching and overhead sports may be related to the etiology of the first two stages of impingement syndrome.

11.1.2
Epidemiology

It is difficult to obtain accurate data on the incidence of rotator cuff problems (HAWKINS and MOHTADI 1994). Cuff tears have been documented in up to 39% of cadaver specimens; however, this figure may not reflect cuff problems in the general population. Shoulder pain has been reported in up to 80% of competitive swimmers. Football injuries to the shoulder are usually dislocations, with a lesser incidence of rotator cuff or bicipital tendinosis (HILL 1983). In a series of world-class tennis players, more than 50% suffered shoulder problems, mainly involving the rotator cuff and biceps tendon (NIRSCHL 1988). The shoulder is involved primarily in many other overhead sporting activities such as volleyball, javelin throwing, golf, and baseball. Although rotator cuff problems were originally described in manual workers, they are of considerable concern in athletes, especially those involved in overhead sports.

Concepts relating to the causes of rotator cuff disorders in athletes are evolving at a rapid rate. Since the 1970s it has been taught that impingement is the primary pathology underlying rotator cuff disorders. This primary impingement results from narrowing of subacromial and coracohumeral spaces due to repeated chronic compression of the cuff or encroachment from the overlying coracoacromial arch.

S. SINTZOFF, MD, PhD Professor, Brussels Free University, Department of Radiology and Medical Imaging, Erasmus Hospital, avenue Prince de Ligne 116, 1180 Brussels, Belgium

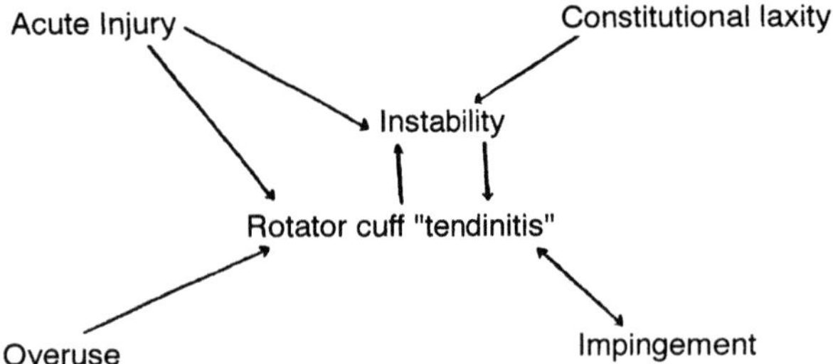

Fig. 11.1. Causes of tendinopathies

Frequently, and perhaps more commonly, impingement is a secondary phenomenon in athletes. In secondary impingement there is a relative narrowing of the available space that is usually related to eccentric overload of the cuff or glenohumeral instability (Fig. 11.1).

Overuse and fatigue related to eccentric overload resulting in intrinsic fiber failure of the rotator cuff and biceps tendon constitute a common etiology in the young athletic population (FOWLER 1988). This initial failure of the fibers due to repetitive overuse of the extremity in sports may lead to secondary impingement as forces pull the cuff superiorly. Shoulder instability may also be related to both rotator cuff and bicipital disorders (HAWKINS and KUNKEL 1990). Patients with anterior subluxation (GARTH et al. 1986) are at risk of developing secondary im-

pingement because of the architectural setup of the subacromial region. Those with loose shoulders or classic multidirectional instability may develop cuff tendinopathy due to overwork and overstretching (Fig. 11.1).

11.1.3
Anatomy

The shoulder is a ball-and-socket joint that provides the link between the trunk and the upper extremity. It is the most mobile joint of the body and as such allows precise positioning of the hand in space for an unlimited number of functions. As a result, the shoulder absorbs the majority of the forces in sports that require propulsive action of the upper extremity. The rotator cuff is vitally linked to these motions in terms of both precision and propulsion.

11.1.3.1
The Subacromial or Subperihumeral Space

The humeral head and its tuberosities, surrounded by the musculotendinous cuff, move by rotation and gliding in the coracoacromial space, which is inextensible and especially narrow in its medial part.

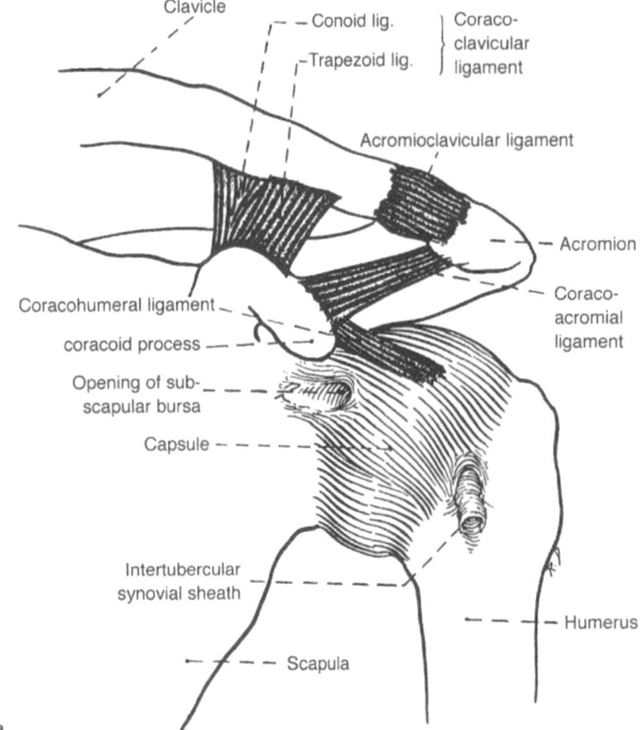

Fig. 11.2. a Ligaments of the shoulder joint and distal end of the clavicle. **b** Superior axial view of the coracoacromial ligament

Fig. 11.2. *Continued*

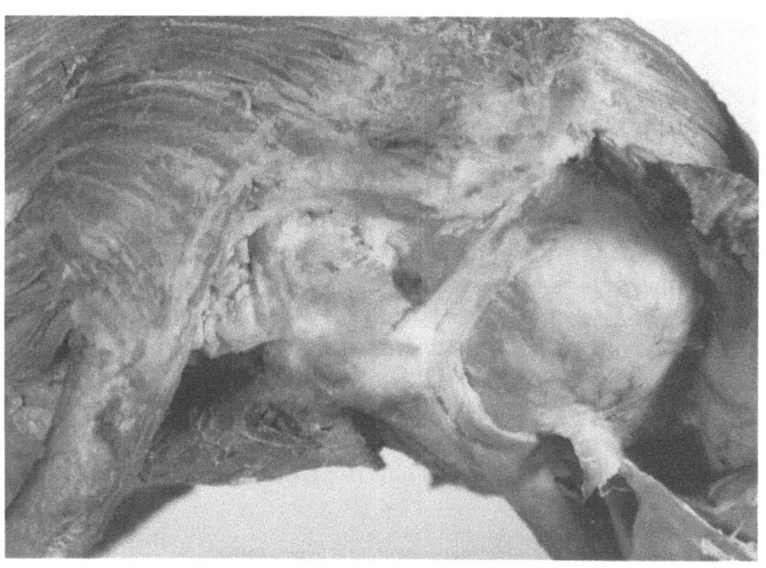

Fig. 11.3a,b. Anatomy of the glenohumeral ligaments and inferior glenohumeral ligament complex. **a** Open anatomic specimen in axial view of the glenoid cavity: *1*, glenoid cavity; *2*, glenoid groove; *3*, inferior glenoid labrum; *4a*, axillary pouch of the inferior glenohumeral ligament (IGHL); *4b*, anterior band of IGHL; *4c*, posterior band of IGHL; *5*, superior glenohumeral ligament; *6*, tendon of the long head of the biceps brachii muscle; *7*, coracoacromial ligament. **b** Anatomical depiction of the glenohumeral ligaments and inferior glenohumeral ligament complex (*IGHLC*). *P*, posterior; *A*, anterior; *SGHL*, superior glenohumeral ligament; *MGHL*, medial glenohumeral ligament; *AB*, anterior band of IGHLC; *PB*, posterior band; *AP*, axillary pouch; *B*, biceps tendon; *PC*, posterior capsule

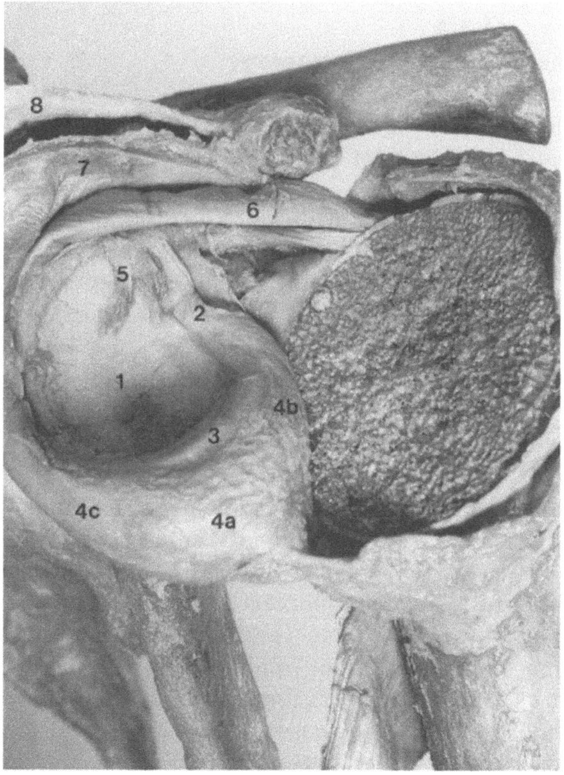

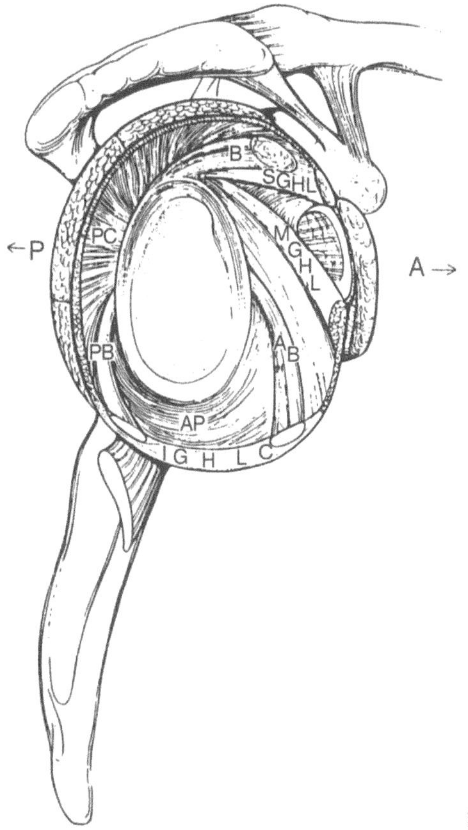

The roof consists of the acromiocoracoid arch formed by bone and ligaments, the clavicle, the acromioclavicular joint, ligaments at the back of the acromion, and the scapular spine (Fig. 11.2). In the latter are inserted the trapezoid and the deltoid muscles. This space is divided into two compartments by the coracohumeral ligament which, owing to its coracoid insertion and the cuff, constitutes part of the dome with its humeral end. The subacromial compartment proprio sensu lies between the acromioclavicular dome and the humeral pivot. It is filled with the interposed subacromiosubdeltoid bursa, which is the widest of the whole body and plays the role of a synovial joint. The bursa separates two muscle layers whose efficiency is provided by this gliding space:

- The external layer concerns mainly the deltoid and the teres major muscle.
- The internal layer, forming the cuff of the short rotator muscles, consists of the subscapularis, supraspinatus, infraspinatus, and teres minor.

In the middle of its base, the bursa adheres to the greater tuberosity of the humerus and to the insertion area of the cuff with part of its roof along the inferior side of the acromion and the coracoacromial ligament.

The bursa is independent and moves with the humeral head, which is surrounded by its cuff, towards the narrow anterior part with internal rotation.

11.1.3.2
The Anteromedial Compartment

The anteromedial compartment consists of the coracohumeral space between the coracoid process and the lesser tuberosity. It lies before the anterior outline of the coracohumeral ligament.

The distance between the lesser tuberosity and the coracoid ligament is reduced by 2 mm by flexion or internal rotation (GERBER et al. 1985).

This impinged position of the soft tissues increases the anatomic narrowness, especially in the superior part lying under the coracoid process. This situation corresponds with the thicker part of the subscapularis tendon, following the superior glenohumeral ligament and the central region of the medial glenohumeral ligament close to the insertion of the long head of the biceps tendon (Fig. 11.3).

The subscapularis recess communicates with the glenohumeral joint in line with the superior edge of the subscapularis tendon (the Weitbrecht foramen)

and the subcoracoid web enveloping the subscapularis tendon. Owing to its superficial and deep synovial cover, it acts as an intra-articular structure.

The coracohumeral ligament lying between the supraspinatus and the subscapularis makes up the roof of this narrow, deep area called by PATTE (1990a,b) "the crossroad area," where two synovial systems may be contiguous without being continuous (Figs. 11.2, 11.3).

This space is filled with vascularized and innervated fatty tissue.

Lesser tuberosity hypertrophy (Fig. 11.4), false orientation, and length of the coracoid process may reduce the coracohumeral space. The ideal method of measurement is not clear. CT anatomical evaluations made in supine position are not available. They do not take into account morphology, functional position, volume, and situation of the humeral head.

11.1.4
Rotator Cuff Pathology

11.1.4.1
Impingement Syndrome

Impingement syndrome is a common condition in which the soft tissues filling the subacromial space (i.e., supraspinatus tendon, biceps tendon, and subacromial bursa) and coracohumeral space (i.e., subscapularis tendon, coracoid and subscapularis recess, and biceps tendon) are chronically entrapped between the humeral head and the acromion, and between the coracoid process and the lesser tuberosity.

The two anatomic compartments explain the two clinical situations: first, an anterosuperior or proper subacromial impingement and second, an anteromedial, subcoracoid, or coracohumeral impingement. NEER (1972) has identified three progressive stages of impingement and has stated that 95% of cuff tears result directly from compression and not from osseous, vascular, or degenerative changes. He suggests that pitching and overhead sports may be related to the etiology of the first two stages. Each stage has its proper demographic, clinical, and pathologic signs (Fig. 11.5).

Stage I consists of edema and hemorrhage in the tendon and is usually found in patients under 25 who strain their shoulder in swimming competitions and throwing sports. The clinical differential diagnosis concerns acromioclavicular arthropathy and shoul-

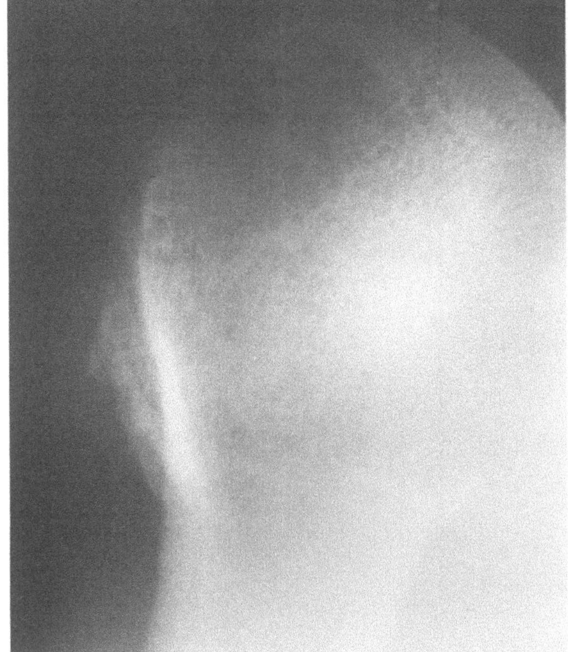

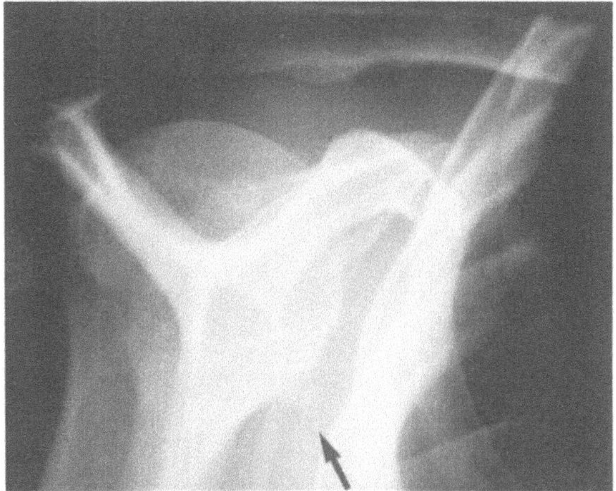

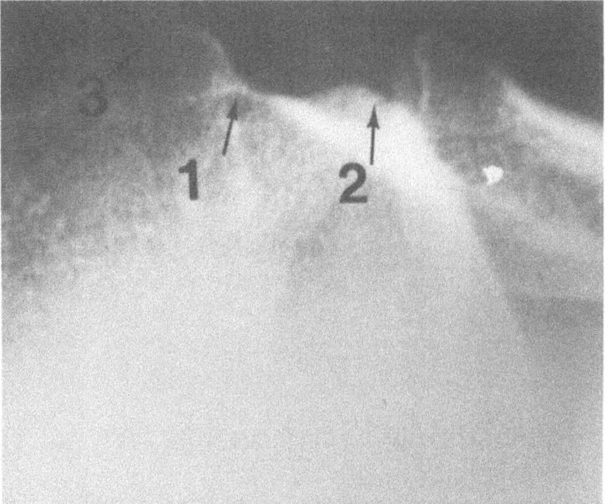

Fig. 11.4a–c. Hypertrophy of the lesser tuberosity on the insertion of the subscapularis tendon. **a** In external (lateral) rotation. **b** Y view (*black arrow*). **c** Bicipital groove view: *1*, groove; *2*, lesser tuberosity; *3*, greater tuberosity

der instability. This stage is potentially reversible with conservative therapy.

Stage II is the result of repetitive strain. It consists of thickening and fibrosis of the subacromial soft tissues with widening of the subacromiodeltoid bursa. The patients are older (25–40 years). The differential diagnosis includes calcifying tendinosis and capsulosis. A conservative therapy is usually applied; in cases that are refractory to treatment, surgeons perform the resection of the acromion or the acromiocoracoid ligament. Surgical management that includes acromioplasty and bursectomy is controversial.

Stage III represents complete rotator cuff tear, biceps tendon rupture with bone alterations, hypertrophy of the greater tuberosity at the insertion of the supraspinatus tendon, and traction osteophytes along the anterior surface of the acromion and the acromioclavicular joint. These injuries cause depression of the supraspinatus tendon, a certain degree of sclerosis, and roughness of the greater tuberosity due to compression with the dome by abduction-

elevation of the humerus. The process develops in a rotatory fashion: first subacromial osteoarthritis called "rotator cuff arthropathy" develops, followed by glenohumeral osteoarthritis.

11.1.4.1.1
ANTEROSUPERIOR IMPINGEMENT

Anterosuperior impingement concerns tendinosis or tears of supraspinatus muscles and tendons as well as the tendons of the long head of the biceps brachii muscle, a subacromial bursitis.

11.1.4.1.2
ANTEROMEDIAL OR CORACOHUMERAL IMPINGEMENT

Anteromedial or coracohumeral impingement results via anatomic internal rotation from compression of the subscapularis muscles and tendons and the anterior and posterior recesses with variation in the length and orientation of the coracoid process.

Anatomic variations may cause a narrowing of the coracohumeral space, making it vulnerable to any

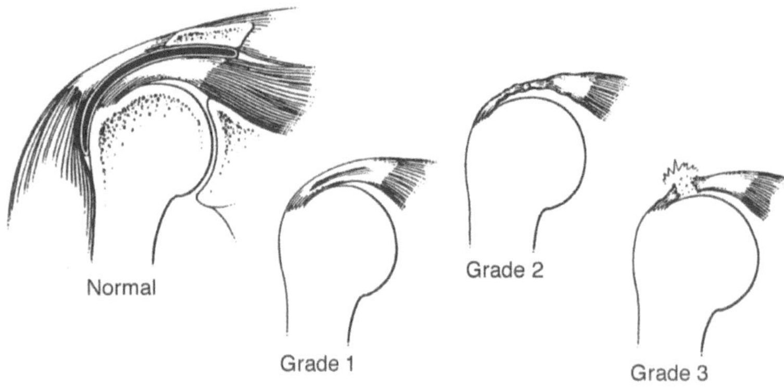

Fig. 11.5. Illustration of *normal, grade 1* (edema/hemorrhage), *grade 2* (thinning and fibrosis), and *grade 3* (cuff tear) rotator cuff injuries

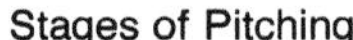

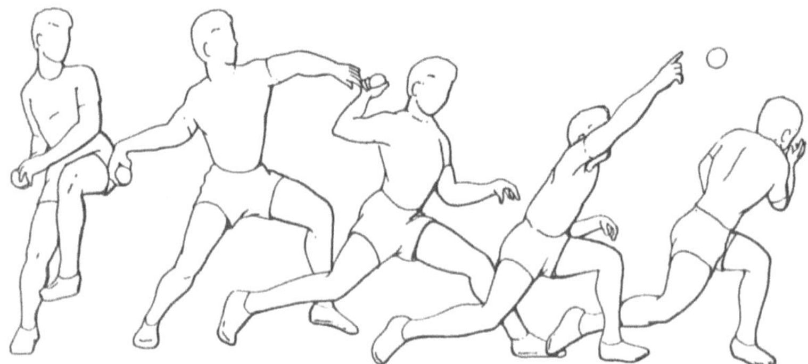

Fig. 11.6. Stages of pitching. The five phases of throwing: wind-up, early cocking, late cocking, acceleration, and follow-through

repetitive strain of the arm in the course of flexion or medial rotation.

The most frequent factors are the decentering of the humeral pin as well as incompetent, perforated, or broken cuffs and constitutional or acquired hyperlaxities.

The contents of the coracohumeral space might be the cause of impingement, originating a traumatic, inflammatory, crystal-induced or rheumatoid bursitis.

11.1.4.2
Acute Rotator Cuff Tear

Acute rupture results from a major sport-related trauma, without impingement syndrome. It results also from overuse in sports. Overhead motion, as in throwing, is the most common motion affecting the shoulder in sports (Nicholas et al. 1977). This action, such as in pitching, passing (football), or serving (tennis), can be divided into five phases (Fig. 11.6). The actions comprising the overhead throw, the tennis serve (Fig. 11.7a), the javelin throw, and the various swimming strokes (Fig. 11.7b,c) are all made up of relatively similar mechanisms. Differ-

ences exist in the equipment involved, the associated body motions, and the position of the shoulder in each action. Important are the degree, repetitiveness, and nature of the forces involved and whether any impact occurs, such as in spiking a volleyball. Because of the biomechanical action of the rotator cuff, dysfunction due to injury or disease can easily lead to significant problems, particularly in the athlete's shoulder, in which stress is very great (Hawkins and Mohtadi 1994).

Acute tears occur by repetitive professional strain (repair of motors in vehicles, in supine position with stretched arms; movements of painters and carpet layers).

Other lesions are the result of trauma of various origins:

– A fall on the shoulder stump or a forward fall with the arm in strained anterior elevation, or a side fall with a laterally elevated arm; such falls may cause a tendon rupture in the cuff of a "healthy" or "nearly healthy" young athlete. These ruptures may be partial or complete (Fig. 11.8). Partial tears may lie deep in the inferior cuff surface; they may be intratendinous or superficial in the superior cuff face. Complete ruptures may

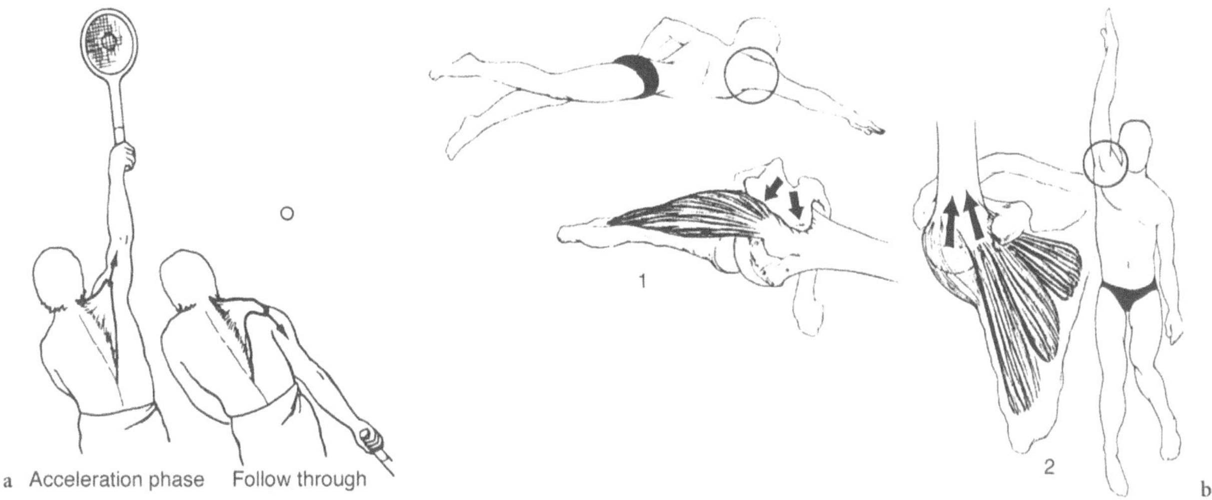

Fig. 11.7. a Tennis shoulder results from stretching of the shoulder elevator muscles during both the acceleration and follow-through phases of overhead serve. **b** Swimmer's shoulder: *1*, during the beginning of the pull-through phase, the humeral head forces the rotator cuff against the acromion (*arrows*), creating impingement in this area; *2*, in the backstroke, with initiation of the pull-through phase there is a tendency to place tension on the anterior portion of the glenohumeral capsule (*arrows*)

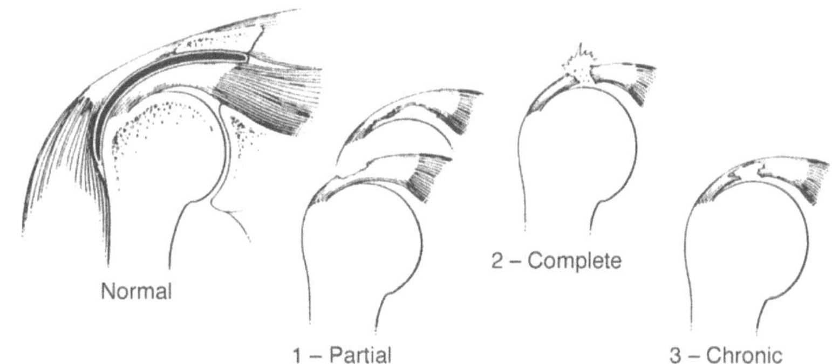

Fig. 11.8. Illustration of normal, partial-thickness (inferior and superior), full-thickness, and chronic rotator cuff tears

concern a single tendon, usually the supraspinatus, occasionally the subscapularis or even several tendons.

- An ascensional trauma (upwards) due to a fall on the elbow or the hand; it involves impaction of the humeral head into the acromial dome, which might result in subacromial impingement.
- A minor trauma or a single, sport-related "forceful" movement that may cause a cuff tear in athletes with a long history of chronic impingement and is often treated by local corticoid injections.

The acute tear has a characteristic clinical presentation without any X-ray findings; the diagnosis is usually confirmed by ultrasonography owing to its localization in the critical area.

The traumatic lesion of the long head of the biceps tendon usually concerns an internal luxation of the latter, associated, or not, with a partial or complete tear of the subscapularis tendon.

11.1.4.3
Clinical Evaluation

An athlete initially diagnosed as having a chronic rotator cuff or tendon problem of the shoulder may present with one or a variety of chief complaints. It is usually possible to place these complaints into two main categories: (1) acute or macrotraumatic presentation that makes it necessary to identify as clearly as possible the mechanism of injury, and (2) overuse or microtraumatic presentation, where it is helpful to analyze the pattern of training and competition (JOBE 1983). It is also important to realize that an acute episode may be superimposed upon a chronic situation. The most common complaint is that of pain.

Establishing history in the athletic population does not lead to a clear-cut diagnosis as easily as it does in more sedentary people. This is a direct result of the fact that rotator cuff and biceps tendon pathology can be attributed to a number of different causes (Fig. 11.1). Stress placed upon the shoulder joint by the athlete can lead to problems such as eccentric overload of the surrounding musculature, either primary or secondary impingement, acute traumatic injury, or uni- or multidirectional instability (JOBE and BRADLEY 1988). This understanding, when combined with constitutional factors, the severity of the complaint, and the specific sporting activity involved, constitutes the diagnostic process during history taking.

The main concern with respect to differential diagnosis is ruling out glenohumeral instability of one form or another (JOBE and BRADLEY 1988). This can be particularly difficult, and indeed instability may be combined with rotator cuff or biceps tendon pathology (Fig. 11.1). Referred pain from the surrounding joints should always be considered. Radicular pain, numbness, or paresthesias may point to cervical pathology, thoracic outlet syndrome, or a primary neurologic problem such as suprascapular neuropathy (BROWN 1983).

Finally, it should be stated that a diagnosis of rotator cuff impingement based on the history alone is not as specific or sensitive as is a diagnosis of other athletic injuries made in this way. Confirmation by physical examination and further investigation and imaging is usually required.

11.1.4.4
Routine X-Rays

11.1.4.4.1
TECHNIQUES

"Static" Views
Anteroposterior View with Double Obliqueness. The first obliqueness concerns a rotation of the patient by 45° towards the side studied, thereby exposing the glenohumeral joint line (i.e., posterior oblique position); the second obliqueness includes a downward beam of 25°, exposing the subacromial space by aligning the acromion and the lateral end of the clavicle (Fig. 11.9).

The view is performed in three positions of the humerus. The first position involves a neutral rotation of the arm alongside the body; the hand runs parallel with the thigh, the thumb pointing forwards; this position reveals the upper face of the greater tuberosity, the cortical layer of which is slightly thickened and also the insertion area of the supraspinatus tendon. The quality criterion of the view is an external paracentral position of the bicipital groove.

The incomplete edge of the lesser tuberosity superposes itself on the external, paracentral region of the humeral head. The subacromial space is filled with the anterior part of the supraspinatus tendon and the long head of the biceps tendon. The subacromial space is normally 7–15 mm wide. The anteroposterior view of the opposite side is performed in a neutral rotation.

The second position in external rotation discloses the anterior surface of the humeral head, the protrusion of the lesser tuberosity, and the anterior part of the cuff within the subacromial space.

The third internal (medial) rotation analyzes the posterior surface of the greater tuberosity with the insertion of the infraspinatus and teres minor tendons. The lesser tuberosity, seen in profile, stands out on the inferomedial outline of the humeral head. Here the subacromial space is filled with the infraspinatus tendon.

"True Lateral Scapular View". In this view (synonyms: Y view, true lateral view of rotator cuff, tangential view, lateral view of NEER or LAMY), the horizontal beam, tangential to the subcutaneous subscapularis region, superposes the scapular shell on the humeral diaphysis when we remove the contralateral shoulder from the imaging plane (Fig. 11.10). This view is acquired at a 60° anterior oblique patient position. The humeral head is centered over a Y shape made up of the wing of scapula, the scapular spine, and the coracoid process. This view is used to analyze the morphology of the acromion and the lesser tuberosity (Fig. 11.4), and it localizes the calcifications on the anterior (subscapularis) and posterior surface [infraspinatus (Fig. 11.11) and teres minor] of the humeral head.

Likewise, the projection shows the localization of inferior partial or complete cuff tears on the arthrogram.

Axillary View. The axillary view provides profile information on the glenohumeral joint and transverse axial information of the acromioclavicular joint. The

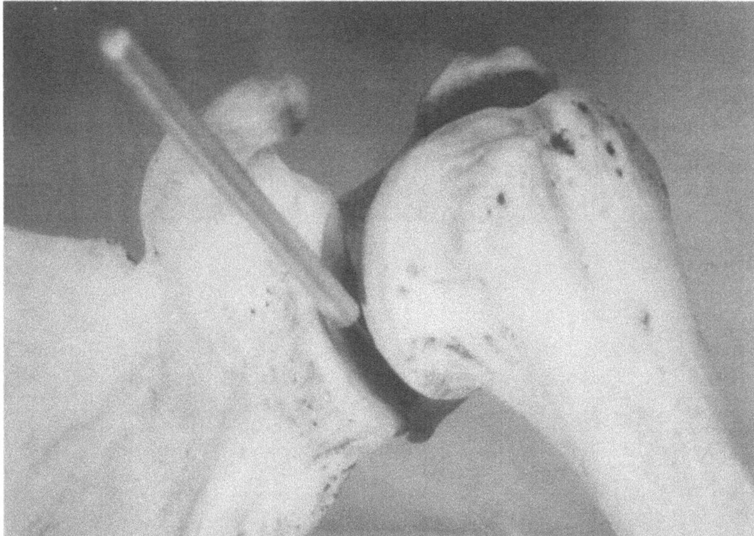

Fig. 11.9a–c. Anteroposterior (AP) view with double obliqueness. a Gleno-humeral and subacromial spaces on anatomic specimen. b Technique. c Image: *1*, glenohumeral space; *2*, subacromial space; *3*, acromion; *4*, lesser tuberosity; *5*, greater tuberosity

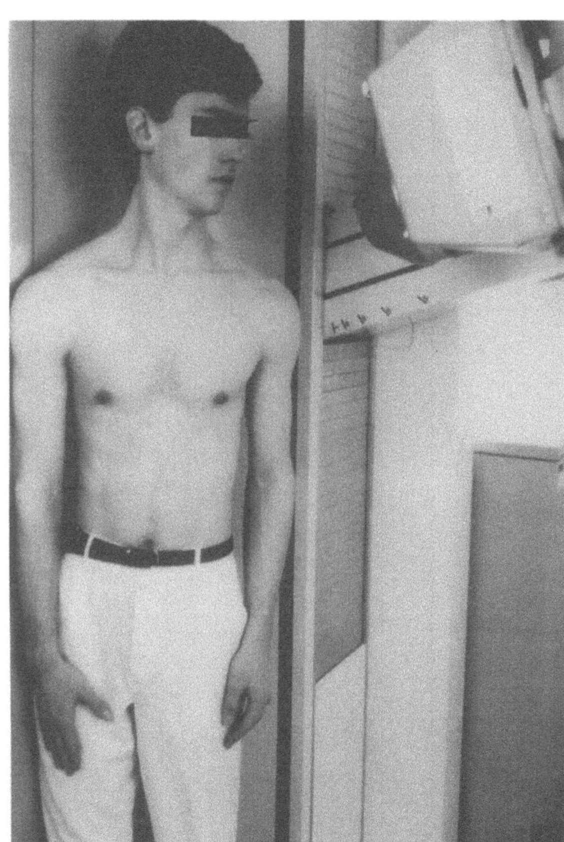

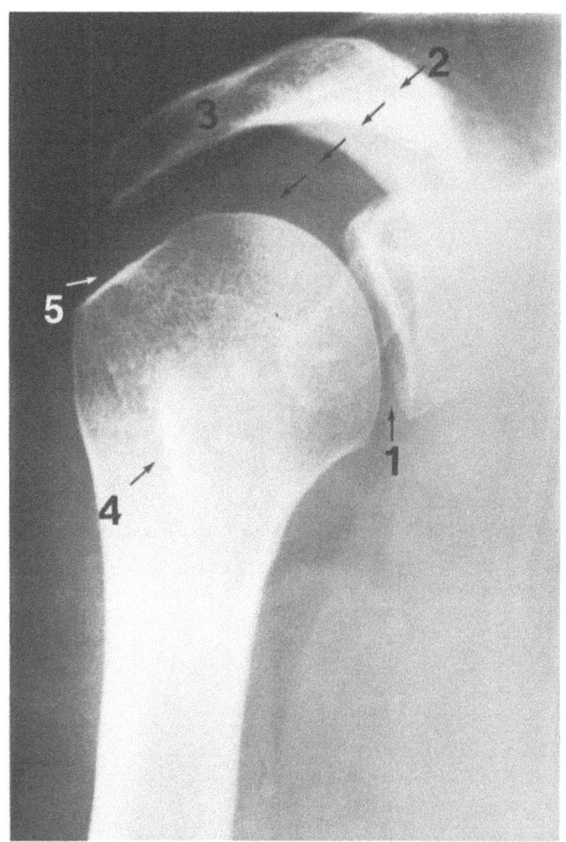

view controls the congruence of the head in the socket and makes us understand the morphology of the lesser tuberosity by unrolling it.

What makes Bernageau's view or "glenoid rim profile view" interesting is not that it replaces the axillary view, but that it provides a better definition of the anterior glenoid rim morphology. The axillary view is the gold standard for the "os acromiale."

Acromioclavicular Joint. This joint, one of the upper parts of the rotator cuff, is disclosed by a cranial beam of 25° without any displacement of the body

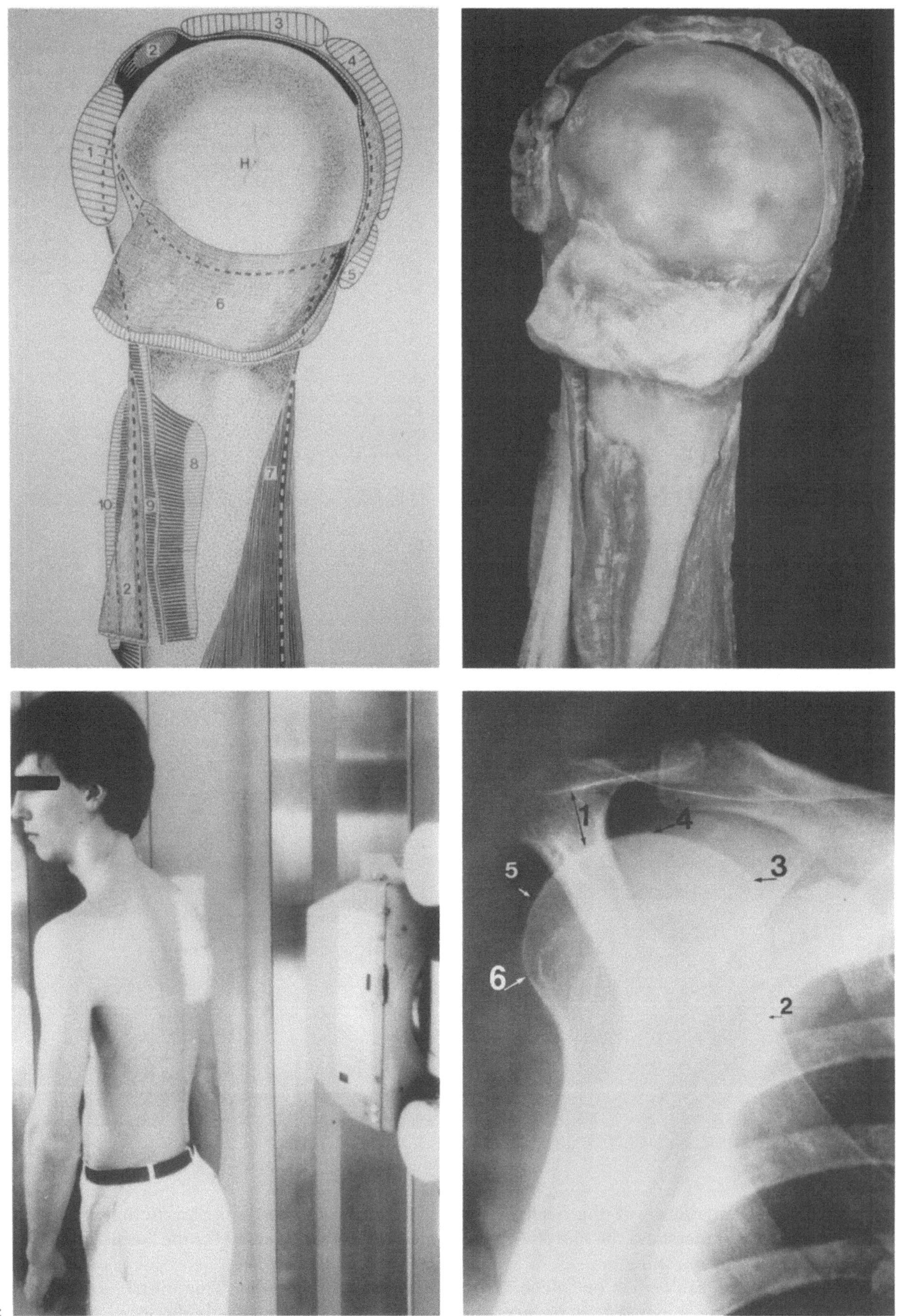

Fig. 11.10a–d. True lateral scapular view (synonyms: Y view, true lateral view of the rotator cuff, tangential view, lateral view of Neer or Lamy). **a** Anatomic drawing: *1*, subscapularis tendon; *2*, tendon of the long head of the biceps brachii muscle; *3*, supraspinatus tendon; *4*, infraspinatus tendon; *5*, teres minor tendon. **b** Photography of the anatomic specimen. **c** Technique. **d** Image: *1*, subacromial space; *2*, lesser tuberosity and subscapularis tendon; *3*, anterior part of supraspinatus tendon; *4*, posterior part of supraspinatus tendon; *5*, infraspinatus tendon; *6*, teres minor tendon

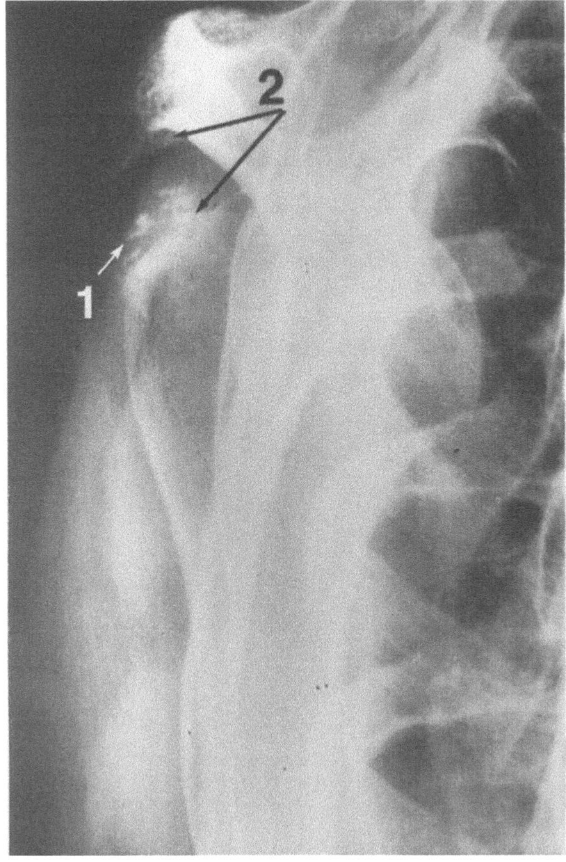

Fig. 11.11. Calcifications in the infraspinatus tendon: *1*, calcifications; *2*, subacromial space

(without turning the patient). It is strained by a traction of both upper limbs carrying a weight of 10 lb (4.5 kg). The acromioclavicular joint is also analyzed in one view by the Railhac technique.

Dynamic Techniques

Leclercq Maneuver. The Leclercq maneuver involves on AP view in double obliqueness. In his original paper in 1950 about the diagnosis of the supraspinatus tendon, LECLERCQ performed, in external rotation, a humeral abduction of 30°–45°, resulting in a physiological subacromial narrowing owing to the external rotation, so that the greater tuberosity crossing under the acromion did not allow evaluation of the thickness of the cuff.

This maneuver of "impeded abduction" was redescribed in 1965 by WELFLING, who also performed a humeral abduction of 40°–45° that made any measure between the head and the acromion in accurate

because of the gliding of the greater tuberosity into the subacromial space.

As a matter of fact, the humeral head is fixed in the glenoid cavity in the abduction sector from 0° to 20°. The modified test includes, by neutral rotation against a resistance or owing to a downward traction of the upper limb, an opposed abduction of less than 20°, keeping the superior surface of the greater tuberosity and the cuff in a vertical position above the acromiocoracoid vault. The arm and the chest are enclosed in a strap, which prevents abduction. The strap may be replaced by a lateral buttress or by having the patient carry a weight of 4 lb (1.8 kg). The patient then makes an abduction in the coronal (frontal) plane, limited by the strap, the lateral buttress, or the weight in the first 20° (Fig. 11.12). A subacromial thickness equal or inferior to 7 mm would signal a cuff tear and would obviate any further diagnostic imaging.

True AP View in Supine Position. This technique, proposed by RAILHAC and RIGAL, includes a vertical beam perpendicular to the table (RIGAL 1994). This view with the patient in supine position exposes the recentering action on the glenohumeral joint of the arm's weight and reveals the pull of the humeral head superiorly only when there is a complete supraspinatus tendon tear (Fig. 11.13).

11.1.4.4.2
CRITICAL REMARKS

Static Views. The AP view, with double obliqueness and neutral, internal, and external rotations, exposes the subacromial space and the glenohumeral joint space, providing a comparative evaluation of rotator cuff thickness. It visualizes the insertion areas of the cuff tendons and allows the localization of calcifications and tears on arthrography. As far as anterosuperior impingement is concerned, the useful and essential views are the neutral and external rotations. The internal rotation indeed releases the posterior cuff segment, which is free from impingement. Its usefulness is limited to the morphological assessment of the lesser tuberosity and calcifications.

The true lateral view of the cuff (also called Y view, subacromial view, or lateral view of NEER or LAMY) shows the acromiohumeral connections (Fig. 11.14) and allows localization of calcifications and, on arthrography, the extent of partial or total cuff tears. The classification of acromion morphology into three groups proposed by BIGLIANI et al.

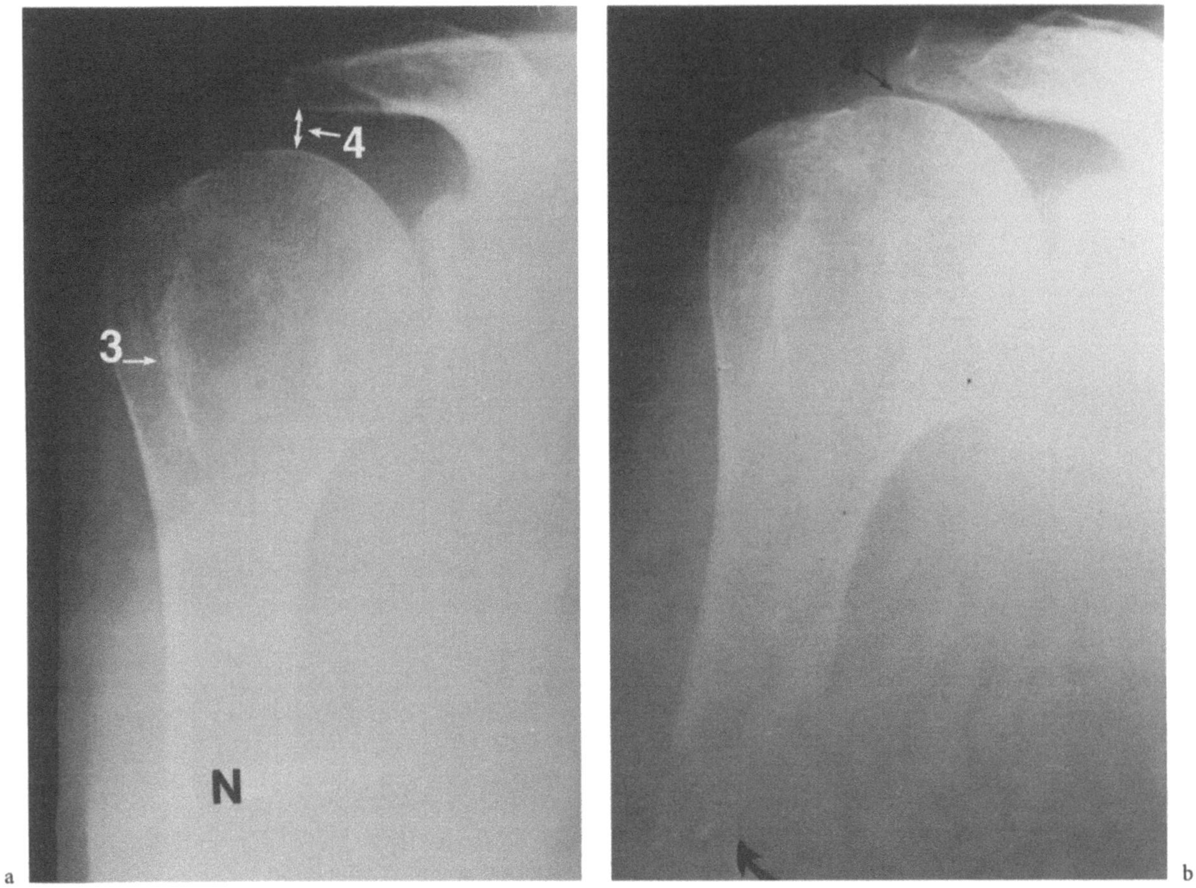

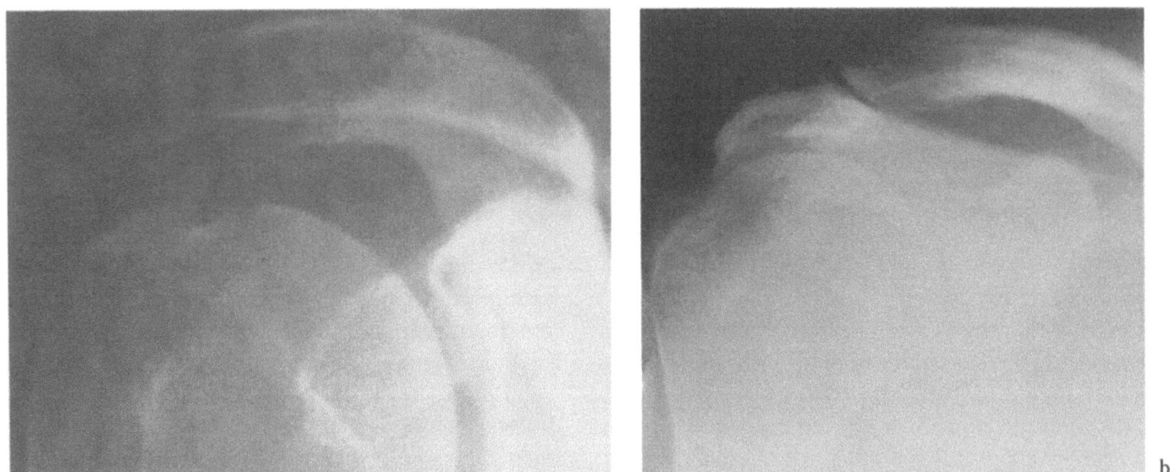

Fig. 11.12a,b. Leclercq maneuver. a Neutral position. b Impeded abduction

Fig. 11.13a,b. Railhac and Rigal maneuver. a AP view with double obliqueness in erect position. b Perpendicular vertical beam in supine position

(1986) remains artificial. The authors are not able to demonstrate a significant difference in the distribution of the anatomic variants between the normal reference population and the patients with an impingement syndrome without cuff tear. This classification is discussed in the literature by HAYGOOD et al. (1994) and EDELSON (1995) and is nonexistent.

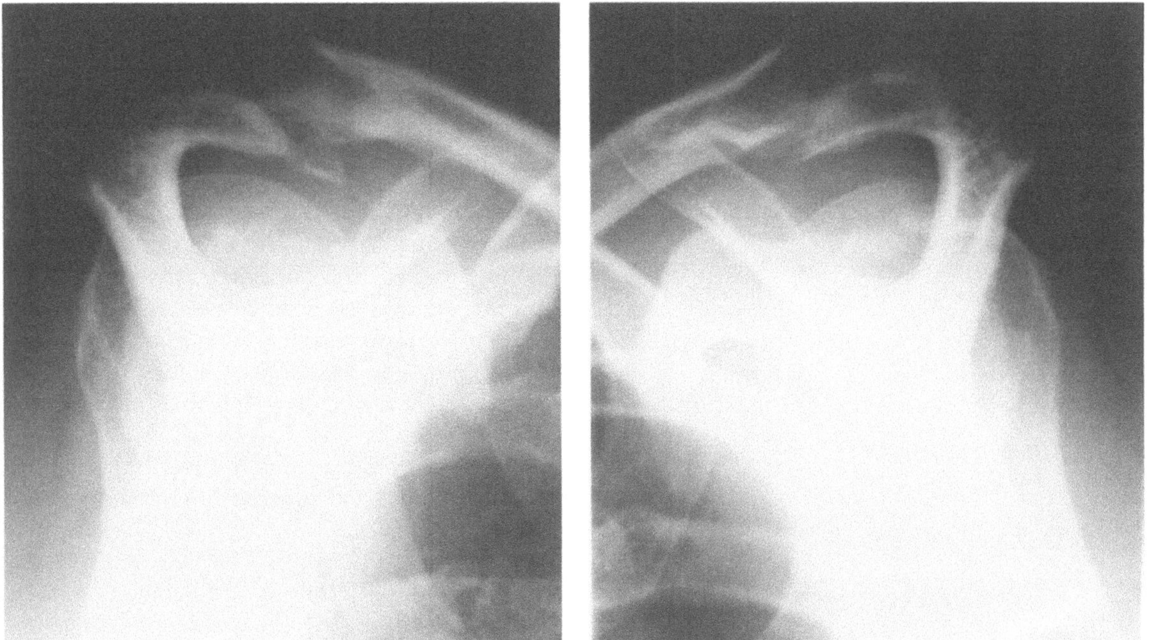

Fig. 11.14a,b. True lateral scapular view or Y view. **a** Right subacromial impingement. **b** Left normal subacromial space

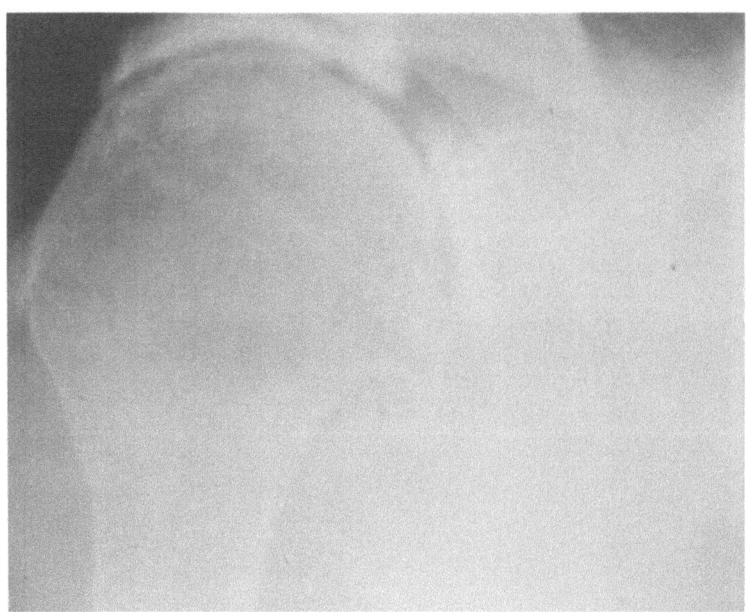

Fig. 11.15. Loss of the subacromial space, complete chronic rotator cuff tear, and secondary "rotatory" glenohumeral joint osteoarthritis

The true lateral view of the rotator cuff, or Y view, or lateral view of NEER or LAMY, also shows the width of the coracohumeral space compared to the other side (Fig. 11.9). The normal values are being discussed in the literature and are not fixed yet. The only practical use is the observation of space asymmetry between both sides.

These "static" views sometimes disclose the sign of a cuff tear, i.e., collapse (Fig. 11.15) or reduction of the subacromial space (Fig. 11.16). In a normal stage, this space is filled with the tendons of the higher part of the cuff, especially the supraspinatus tendon, topped by the thin subacromiosubdeltoid bursa. Its thickness varies according to the authors from 7 mm to 15 mm with a mean value of 10.5 mm. In a retrospective study of the shoulders of 93 patients investigated by arthrography, GOUPILLE (GOUPILLE et al. 1993) establishes that, if the threshold value indicat-

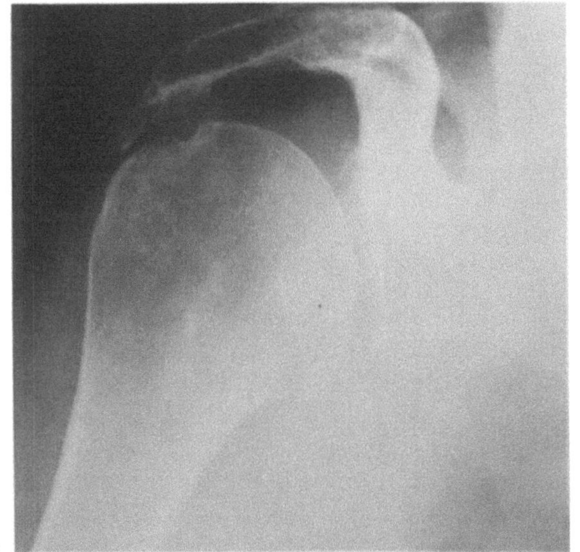

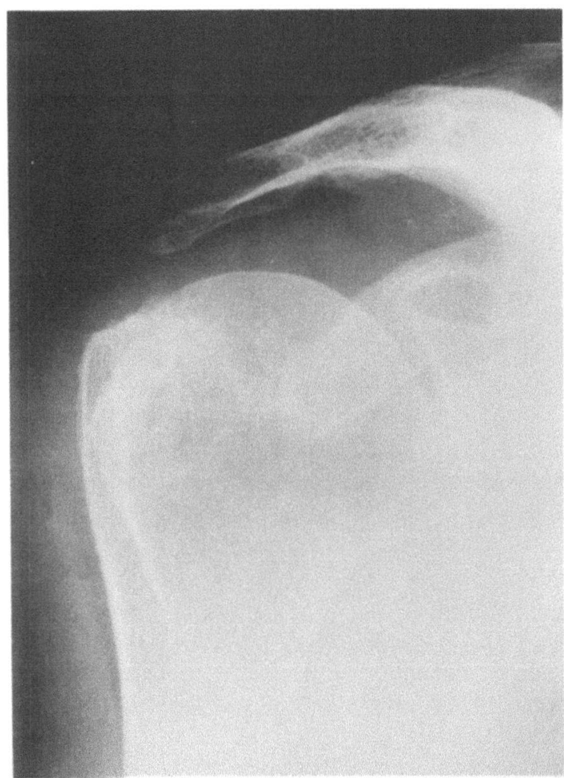

Fig. 11.16. Subacromial or anterosuperior impingement. a Loss of the subacromial space, osteophytes, and "geodes" of the greater tuberosity. b Sclerosis and hypertrophy of the greater tuberosity in external (lateral) rotation

ing a cuff tear is fixed at an acromiohumeral width equal or inferior to 7 mm, sensitivity reaches 24% and specificity 75%. RESNICK (1995) emphasizes that there is no routine X-ray sign of acute cuff tear if there is no glenohumeral dislocation. The fat layer

may be filled in acute tears just as well as in inflammatory processes extending into adjacent tissues, including rheumatoid arthritis and calcifying tendinopathy. RESNICK strictly limits the diagnostic value of indirect signs of chronic cuff tears.

Severe degenerative evolution, i.e., atrophy of the rotator cuff without tear, may create changes similar to those seen in chronic tears. RESNICK reminds us of the fact that such X-ray alterations may be present in other entities especially when they include capsulosis. The signs considered as indirect and predictive should not be used as a diagnostic tool for chronic rotator cuff tear, whether in clinical or in forensic matters. These signs follow a degenerative senescent involution, i.e., a chronic tendinopathy, whether there is decompensation by complete tear or not.

Nevertheless, in spite of cuff tear, static views may be normal or not reveal a diagnostic collapse of subacromial space. The dynamic views allow superior migration of the humeral head.

Dynamic Techniques

Modified Leclercq Maneuver. The modified Leclercq maneuver reveals the reduction of the subacromial space, visualizing as such an indirect sign of rupture of the higher part of the cuff, especially the supraspinatus tendon. The maneuver allows assessment of the extension of the rupture. It abolishes the necessity of arthrography or diagnostic MRI; however, the latter proof remains justified in the preoperative setup with regard to the site and extension of the rupture. Recent studies (COTTY and FOUQUET 1994; RIGAL 1994) evaluate the modified "Leclercq maneuver." According to RIGAL (1994), the mean value ($\pm$2.0 SD) of the subacromial space on films of opposed abduction in healthy subjects is 9.5 mm ($\pm$1.5 mm), as opposed to 8.8 mm ($\pm$1.4 mm) when there is a localized rupture of the supraspinatus tendon and 4.6 mm ($\pm$2.4 mm; $p = 0.0001$) with associated tear of the supraspinatus and the infraspinatus tendons. According to COTTY and FOUQUET (1994), the thickness of the acromiohumeral space without any rupture is evaluated as 10.5 $\pm$ 1.8 mm, and as 8.0 $\pm$ 2.5 mm with rupture. If a threshold value of the acromiohumeral space is fixed at 7 mm, its sensitivity varies, in different studies, from 62% to 81%, and the specificity varies from 82% to 100%. The reduction in thickness of the acromiohumeral space is considered as diagnostic if greater than or equal to 4 mm compared to the static findings and 2 mm compared to the contralateral shoulder. Reduction in thickness should be associated with cranial migration of the humeral head of more than 3 mm in relation to the neutral position and the opposite shoulder.

The drawbacks of the maneuver are operator dependence, incomplete understanding of the maneuver by the patient so that correct application is not possible, and major shoulder pain, eliciting false-negative results. For these reasons the true AP view in supine position (Fig. 11.13) is the best choice.

True AP View in Supine Position (Railhac-Rigal). The vertical beam examines only the supraspinatus muscle and tendon. The AP view improves detection of complete supraspinatus tendon tear by the spontaneous cephalad migration of the humeral head, free from muscular and tendinous restraints and from the arm's weight. It is also used to analyze the morphology of the acromioclavicular joint, avoiding another specific view.

A prospective study has been carried out by FOURCADE et al. (1996) in 57 patients with a suspected, nonoperated cuff tear. The results are compared with the data of routine arthrography: 19 patients did not show any cuff lesion on arthrography; 23 patients showed a partial or isolated tear of the supraspinatus tendon; seven patients showed associated lesions of the supraspinatus and the infraspinatus tendons. Regarding associated lesions of the supraspinatus tendon and the infraspinatus tendon, the optimal discriminatory threshold of the subacromial space is fixed by the ROC curve, which is 6 mm wide with a sensitivity of 90% and a specificity of 90%. As for the isolated lesions of the supraspinatus tendon, there is a relatively significant difference ($p < 0.02$) between the group without any cuff lesion and the group with a rupture, but overlapping of the measurements makes analysis difficult in routine practice. Regarding isolated lesions of the supraspinatus tendon, the modified Leclercq maneuver does not reveal any diagnostic difference in the thickness of the subacromial space when compared to thickness in the normal population.

11.1.4.4.3
CONCLUSIONS

In routine X-ray imaging of the rotator cuff, static views sometimes detect the direct tear sign, a collapse (Fig. 11.15) or a reduction of the subacromial space (Fig. 11.16). They may, however, be normal and not reveal any diagnostic narrowing. The technique in supine position improves detection of the

tear. The method is at least equivalent to, if not better than, the modified Leclercq maneuver, the acromiohumeral collapse indicating a complete tear of the supraspinatus tendon (FOURCADE and RAILHAC 1996). A normal X-ray appearance of the acromiohumeral space does not exclude a partial or complete cuff tear, the diagnosis of which is possible with noninvasive techniques such as ultrasonography in the extra-acromial part of the cuff, or MRI.

11.1.4.5
Arthrography and Arthro-CT

Single- or double-contrast arthrography (Figs. 11.17–11.20) is currently considered the gold standard for determining the presence of a full-thickness rotator cuff tear (Fig. 11.21). However, in high-level athletes this technique is replaced by ultrasonography and MRI. Arthrography is used to diagnose other pathologic conditions such as capsulosis or "frozen shoulder" (Fig. 11.21). The combination with CT is helpful in diagnosing intraarticular pathology such as labral changes indicating instability.

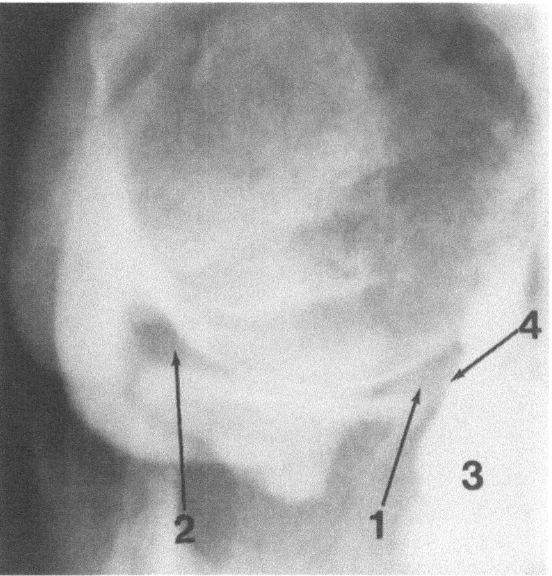

Fig. 11.17. Normal single contrast arthrography on Bernageau view or glenoid profile view: *1*, anterior glenoid rim; *2*, posterior glenoid rim; *3*, subscapularis recess; *4*, inferior glenohumeral ligament complex

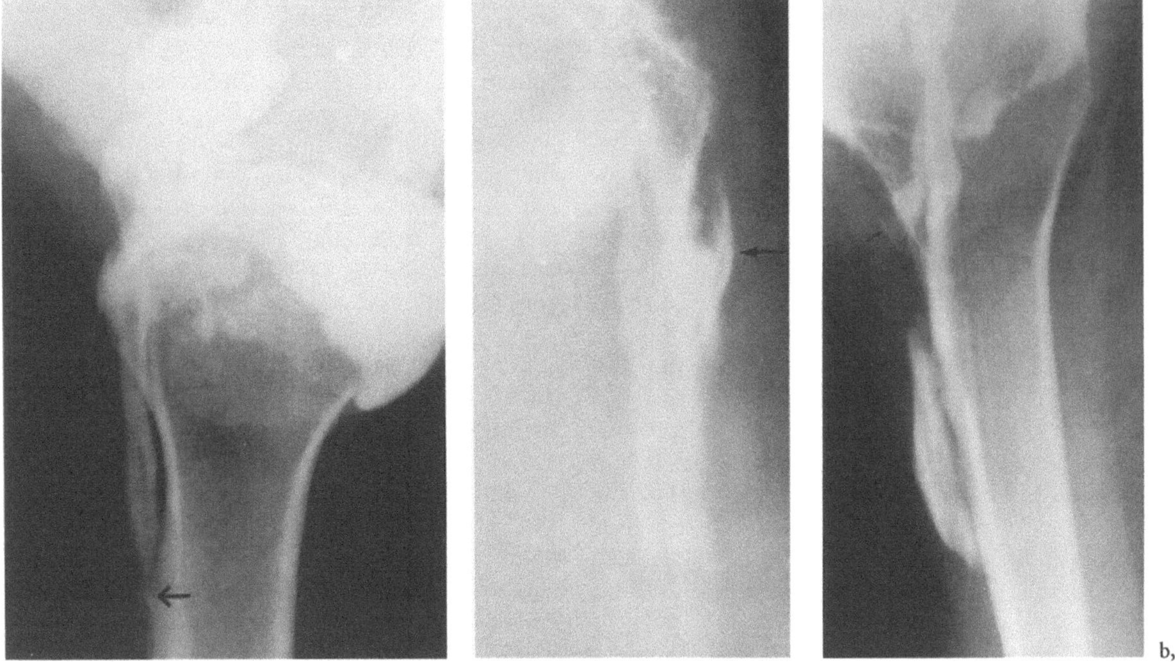

Fig. 11.18a–c. Partial tear in the tendon of the long head of the biceps brachii muscle (*black arrow*)

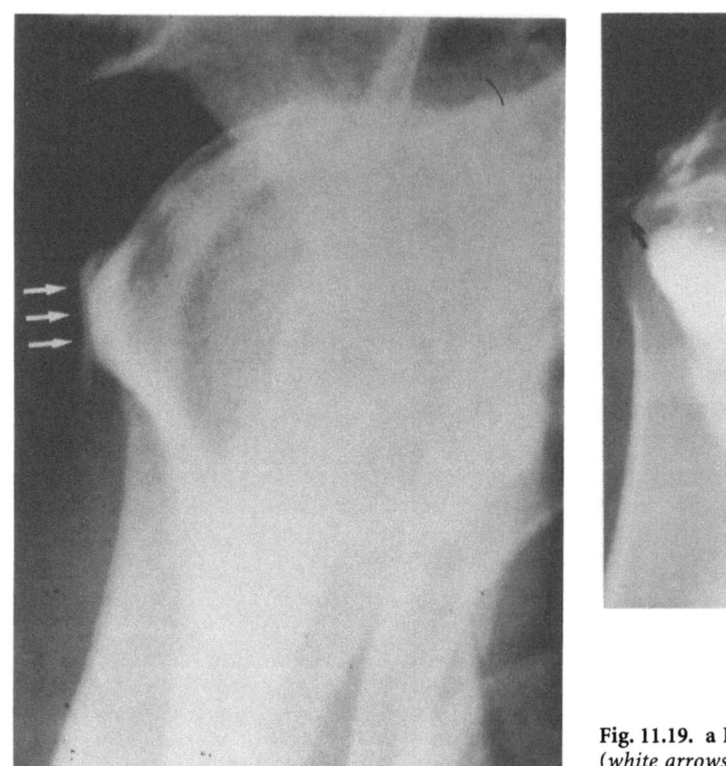

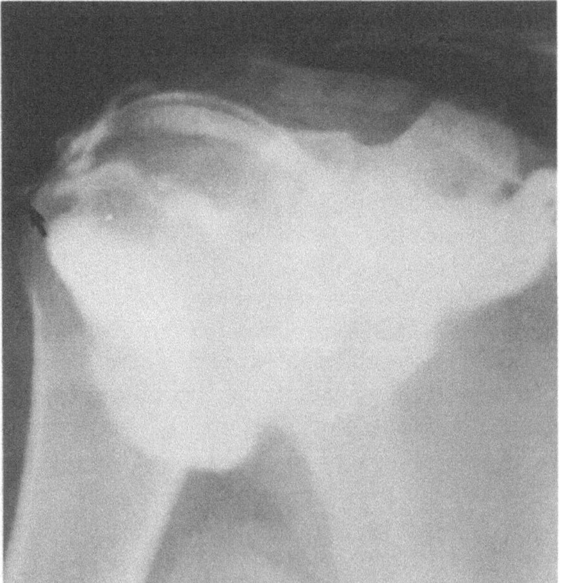

Fig. 11.19. a Partial tear of the teres minor tendon on Y view (*white arrows*); **b** Partial tear of the supraspinatus tendon on the greater tuberosity (*black arrow*)

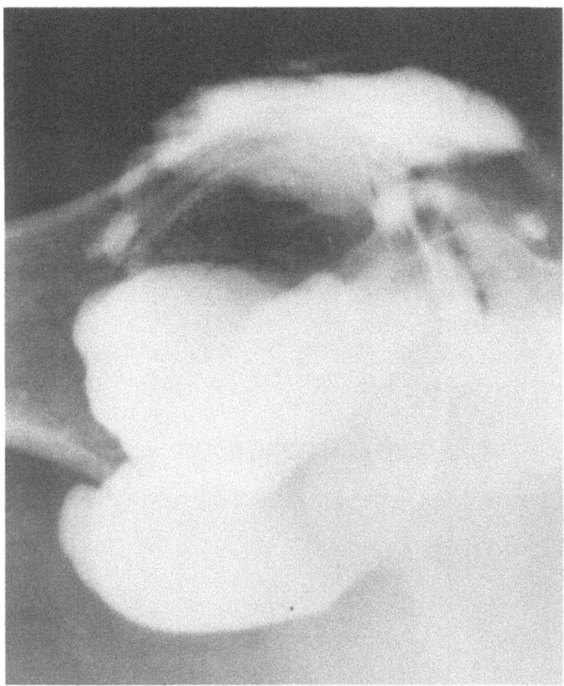

Fig. 11.20. Complete tear of the supraspinatus tendon on the greater tuberosity insertion; humeral abduction producing compression of the opacified subacromial subdeltoid bursa

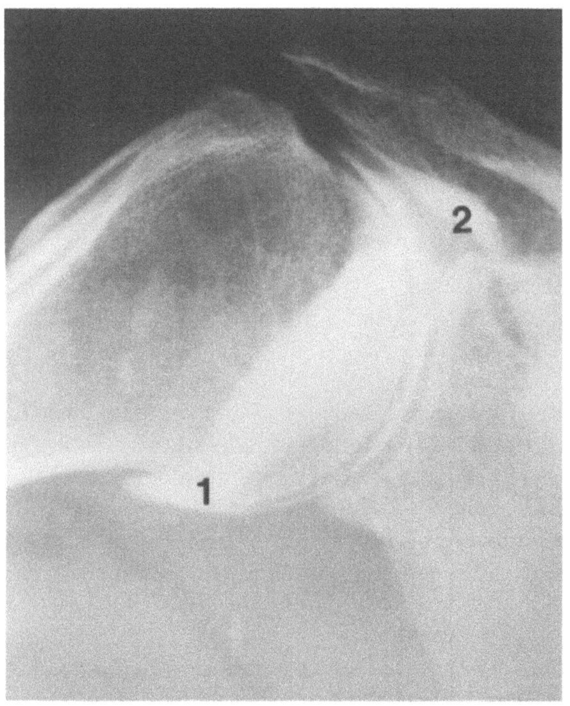

Fig. 11.21. Adhesive capsulosis or frozen shoulder: *1*, inferior recess; *2*, subcoracoid recess. Retraction of the joint cavity

11.1.4.6
Ultrasonography

Diagnostic ultrasound (US) (Fig. 11.22) is a non-invasive method for screening the rotator cuff.

In experienced hands, sonography can be a useful technique for the evaluation of shoulder tendons lesions. It is important to note that rotator cuff sonography is characterized by a significant "learning curve," and novices are encouraged to begin performing the technique immediately after single-contrast arthrography. As a screening tool for rotator cuff disorders US has advantages, including its noninvasive nature, relatively low cost, and potential availability at the time of clinical consultation.

US of the rotator cuff has been shown to be of value in diagnostic full thickness rotator full thickness cuff tears in a series of 500 patients. All subjects were examined with the hyperextended internal rotation view using commercially available high-resolution real-time US equipment. Rotator cuff tear was diagnosed if a focal echogenic lesion or a defect in the rotator cuff was identified (Fig. 11.22). Accuracy, sensitivity, and specificity all exceeded 90%, and results correlated with surgical findings. The results were superior to those of arthrography in the same patient population.

US allows comparison with the contralateral side and compared with arthrography, can evaluate a greater amount of anatomic detail. It has a reported 91% sensitivity and specificity (BURK 1989) with a 100% positive predictive value when it shows nonvisualization or focal thinning (MACK 1988). It has also been reported to be very useful in diagnosing bicipital pathology (MIDDLETON 1986) and is helpful in patients who have previously undergone rotator cuff repair. The results are related to the operator's experience, and the technique has inherent limitations because of the surrounding bony anatomy.

11.1.4.7
Magnetic Resonance Imaging

11.1.4.7.1
INTRODUCTION

Magnetic resonance imaging (MRI), the most sophisticated imaging modality, has revolutionized diagnostic imaging. It has an impact on musculoskeletal imaging unparalleled by any other imaging modality, owing to its exquisite resolution of soft tissue structures and its multiplanar capability – all

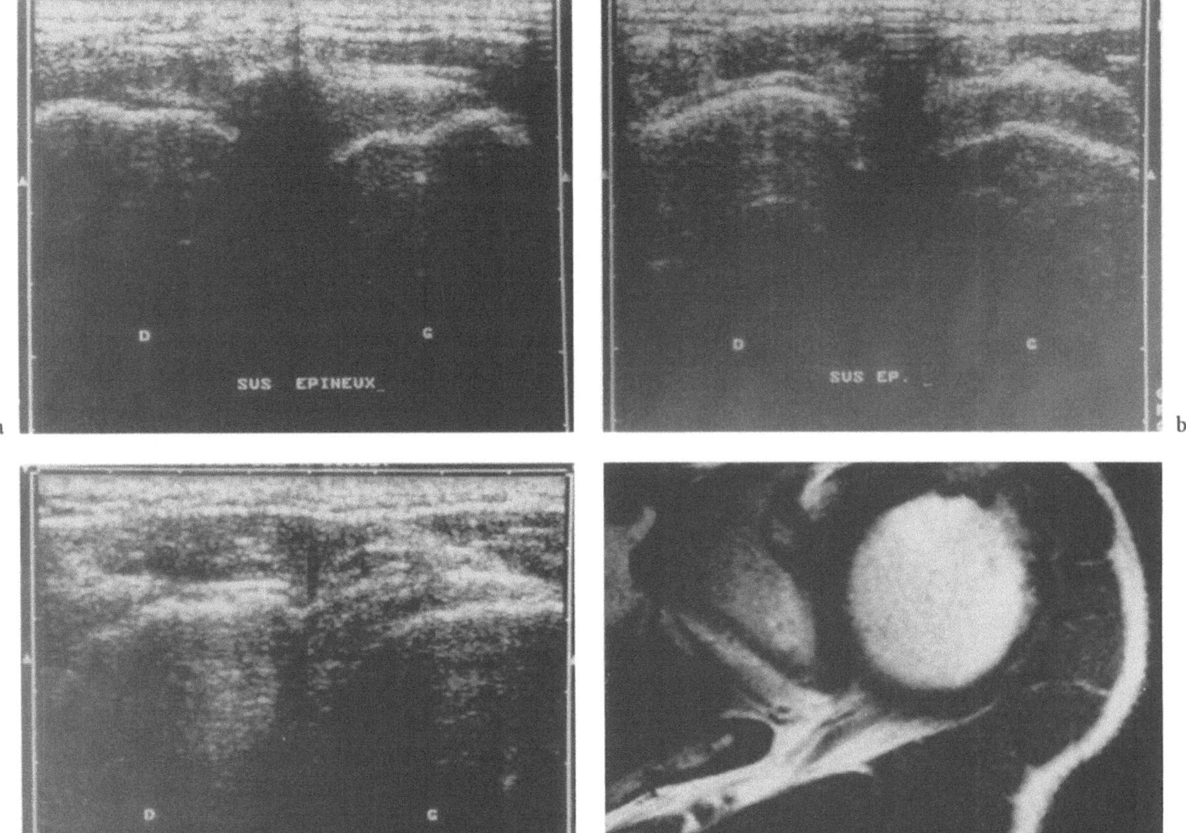

Fig. 11.22a–d. Ultrasonography. a Complete tear of the right supraspinatus tendon on coronal view, normal left supra spinatus tendon. b The same tear on axial view, right and left. c Complete tear of the right infraspinatus tendon. d The same tear of the infraspinatus tendon on axial MRI in T1-weighted images

this noninvasively. Perhaps the most significant improvement provided by MRI is the imaging of articular disorders. For many diagnostic applications MRI has replaced arthrography, proving more accurate. Furthermore, MRI has expanded the horizon of diagnosis to a variety of other articular and intrinsic soft tissue disorders that cannot be visualized by other imaging modalities.

MRI has recently been used in the investigation of rotator cuff pathology with promising results. Sensitivity has ranged from 80% to 91%, with specificity of 88%–94%. These studies are operator-dependent, and the newer technology has improved diagnostic capabilities. MRI can detect size, location, and characteristics of pathology of the cuff. The drawbacks of MRI are that it is time-consuming and costly, and there is an occasional patient intolerance because

of the required lack of movement and because of claustrophobia.

11.1.4.7.2
SEMIOLOGY

When the subacromial bursa and supraspinatus and subscapularis tendons and muscles are chronically entrapped, changes occur in these structures. The alterations are manifested on MRI as thickening of the subacromial bursa, thinning of the supraspinatus (Fig. 11.23) and subscapularis tendons and muscles, and an abnormally increased signal within the tendon that is indicative of tendinosis (Fig. 11.24). Further lesions to the supraspinatus and subscapularis tendons are partial or small full-thickness tears (Fig. 11.25). Findings characteristic of full-thickness rotator cuff tears (Figs. 11.26, 11.27) include fluid within

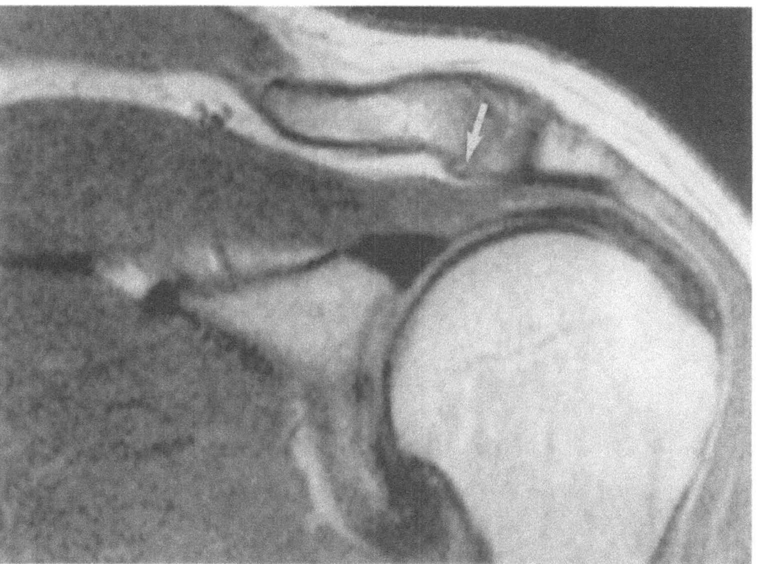

Fig. 11.23a,b. Anterosuperior or subacromial impingement on MR imaging. a Acromioclavicular impingement on supraspinatus muscle (*white arrow*). b Acromioclavicular impingement on supraspinatus muscle (*arrow*) and partial tear of supraspinatus (*arrow*)

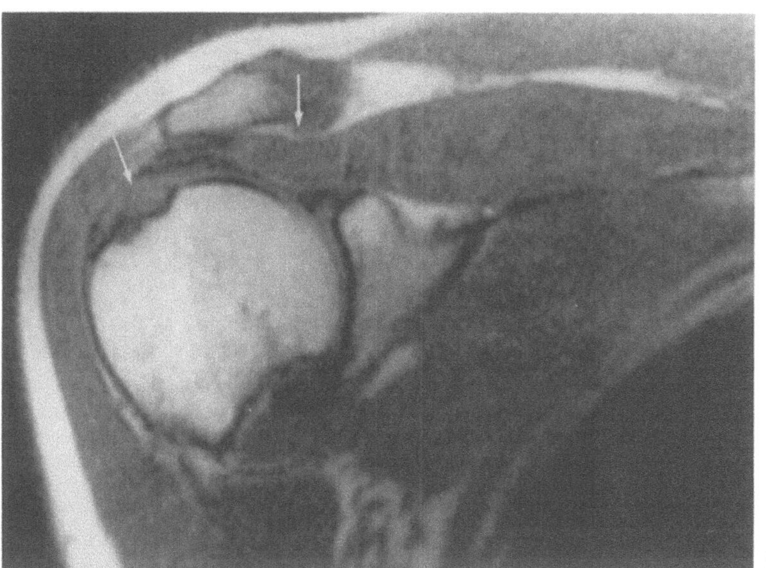

the subacromial bursa (bright on T2-weighted images), increased signal within the supraspinatus tendon on T2-weighted images (consistent with fluid within a tear; Fig. 11.24), and loss of the normal signal of the fat plane that surrounds the subacromial-subdeltoid bursa. Musculotendinous retraction at the margins of the tear may also be demonstrated, and effusion may be detected within the glenohumeral joint (Figs. 11.25–11.28).

Partial-thickness tears involve only the upper or lower surface of the rotator cuff tendons (Figs. 11.18, 11.24). MRI allows detection of these tears, although sometimes they may be mistaken for full-thickness tears. Distinguishing between upper and lower partial tears is difficult; secondary signs (fluid within the subacromial bursa and loss of the peribursal fat plane) as well as primary signs (abnormal signal within the tendon and disruption of the tendon) demonstrate the accuracy of MRI in identifying the full spectrum of rotator cuff disease. ZLATKIN and colleagues (1989) found MRI to be more sensitive and specific than arthrography in diagnosing rotator cuff tears.

11.1.4.7.3
ANATOMIC VARIANTS AND PITFALLS

Another variation of signal intensity in the supraspinatus tendon involves the anterior aspect of the tendon approximately 1 cm from the greater tuberosity. In this region, constituting the critical zone of

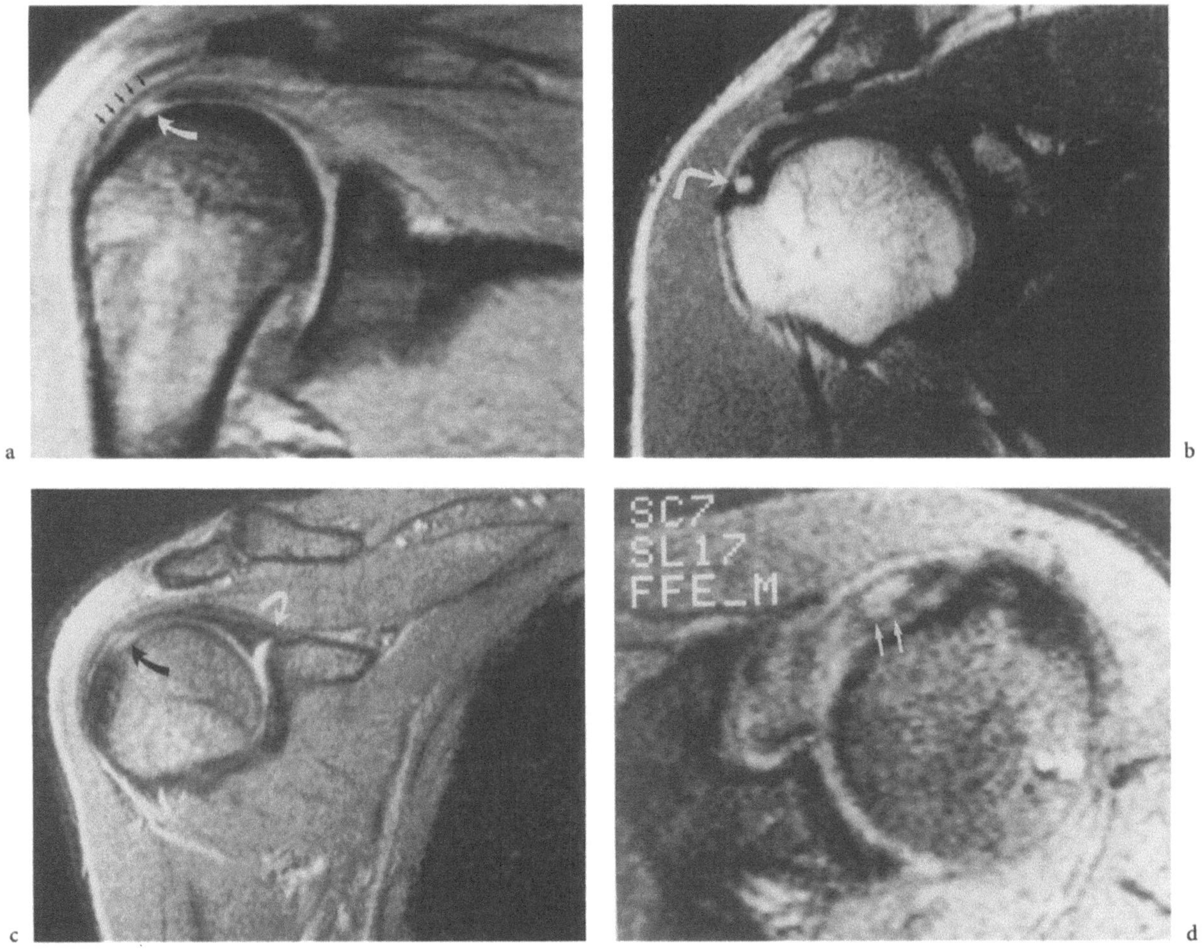

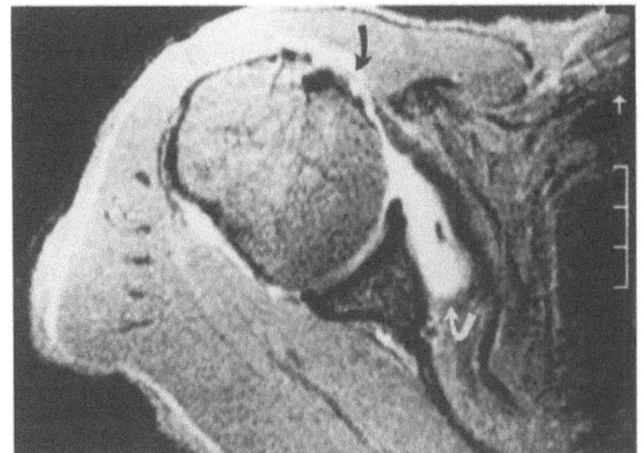

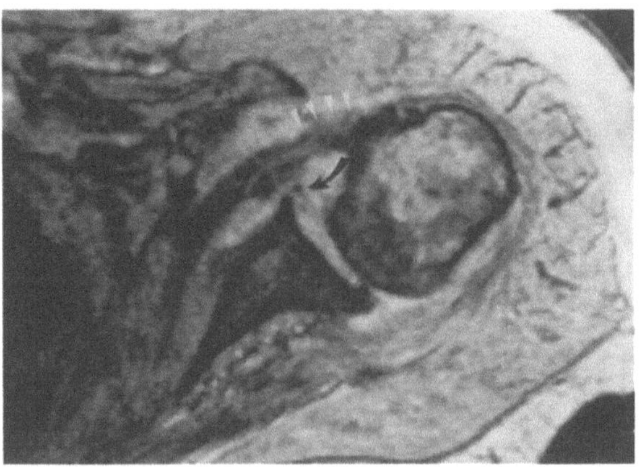

Fig. 11.24. a Partial tear of the inferior surface of the supraspinatus tendon (*curved white arrow*); superior surface of the supraspinatus tendon (*short black arrows*). **b** High signal intensity into the supraspinatus tendon in accordance with partial tear or tendinosis (*curved white arrow*). **c** Partial tear or tendinosis of the supraspinatus tendon (*black arrow*); tear of the superior glenoid rim (*curved white arrow*) **d** Partial tear or tendinosis of the subscapularis tendon (*white arrows*)

Fig. 11.25. a Axial plane in T2, complete tear of the subscapularis tendon on the lesser tuberosity insertion (*curved black arrow*); tear of the medial capsular insertion (*curved white arrow*). **b** Axial plane in T2, tear of the subscapularis tendon (*white arrowheads*); tear of the anterior glenoid rim (*curved black arrow*)

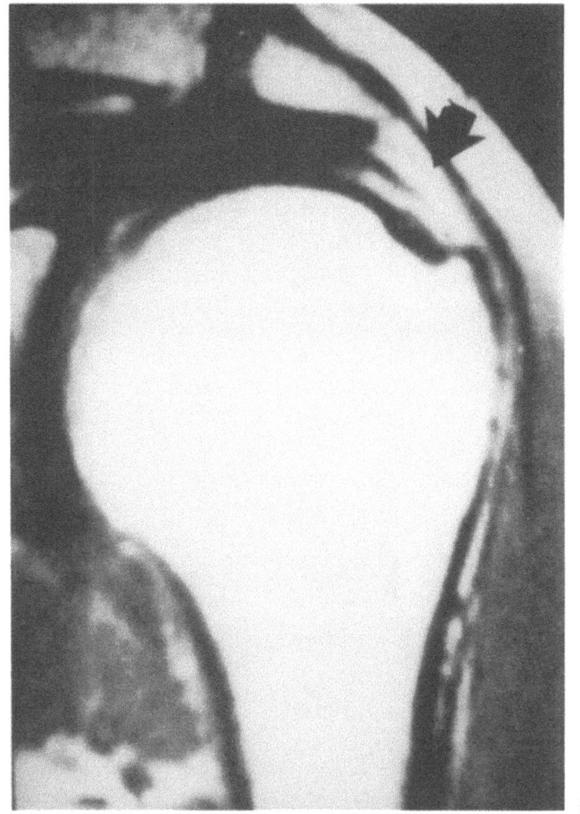

Fig. 11.26. a Complete acute tear of the supraspinatus tendon in a coronal oblique plane in T1 (*black arrowhead*). **b** Complete tear of the supraspinatus tendon in a coronal oblique plane in T1 (*curved white arrow; black arrowheads*). **c** The same tear in T2 (*curved white arrow*). **d** The same tear in coronal oblique plane in T2 muscle retraction (*curved black arrows*). **e** Sagittal oblique plane in T2, tear of the supraspinatus tendon and supraspinatus muscle retraction (*black arrow*)

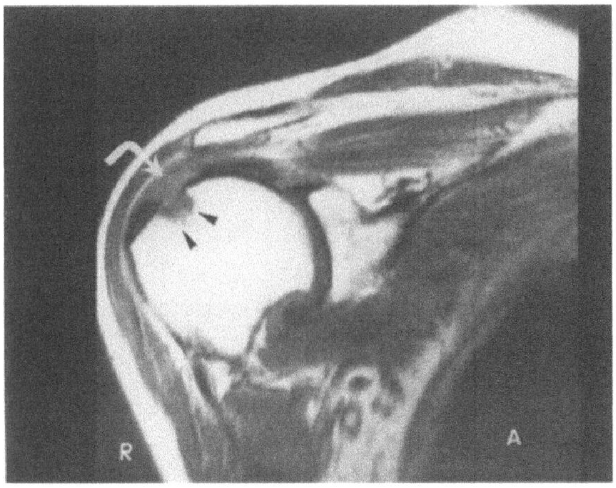

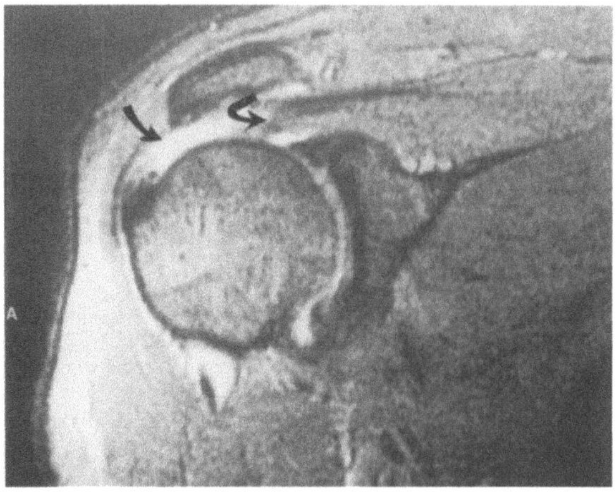

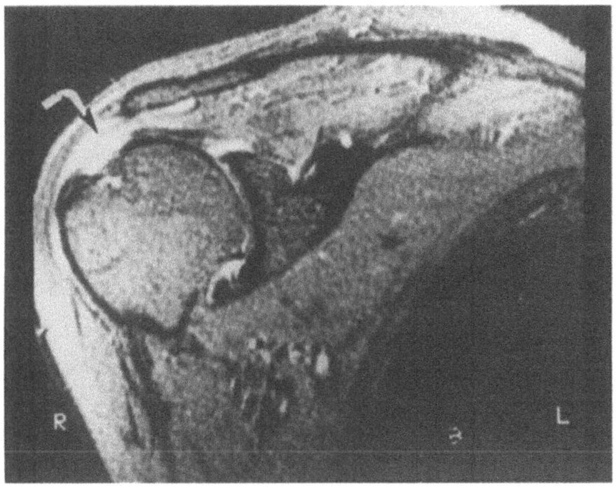

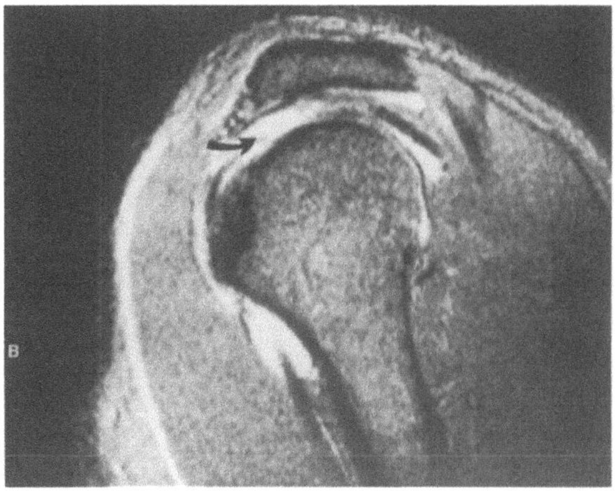

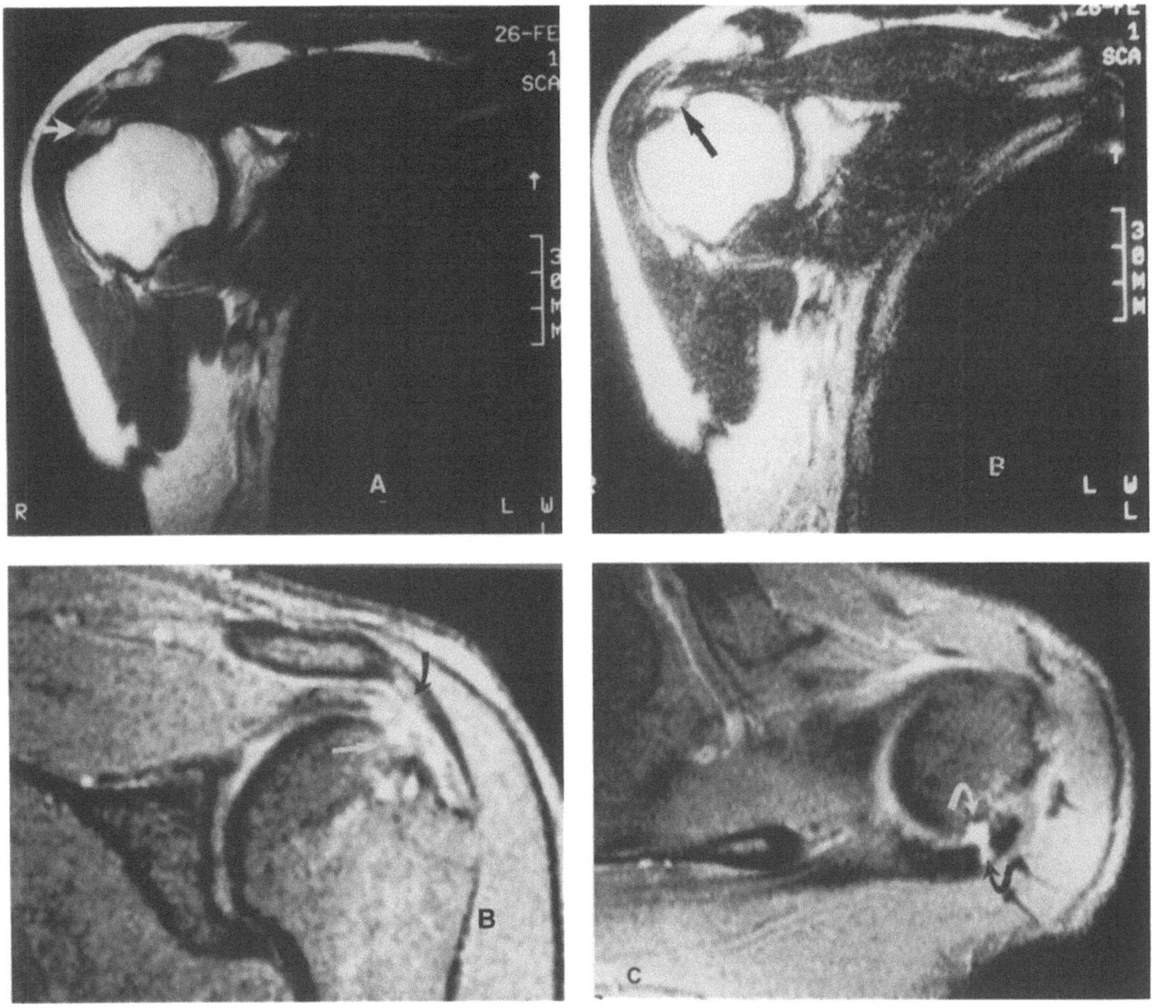

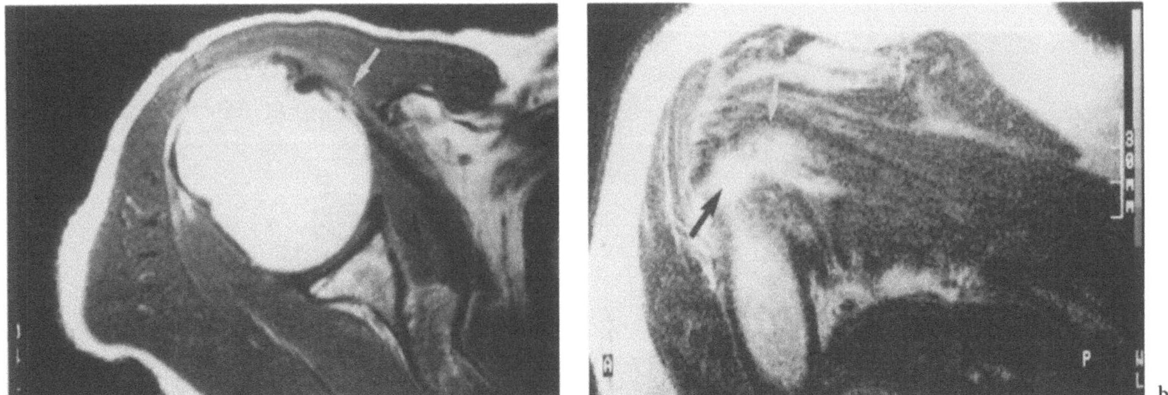

Fig. 11.27a–d. Complete tear of the supraspinatus tendon. **a** Coronal oblique plane in T1 (*white arrowhead*). **b** The same tear in T2 (*black arrow*). **c** Coronal oblique plane in T2, complete tear of the supraspinatus tendon (*black arrow*), and greater tuberosity avulsion (*white arrow*). **d** The same shoulder in axial plane in T2; tear of the infraspinatus tendon insertion (*curved white* and *black arrows*)

Fig. 11.28a,b. Complete tear of the subscapularis tendon insertion on the lesser tuberosity in T1-weighted images. **a** Axial plane (*white arrow*). **b** Coronal oblique plane (*black* and *white arrows*)

the supraspinatus, a round or oval area of high signal intensity is occasionally observed on T1-weighted and proton density images. This focal area of increased signal intensity is more prominent on images acquired with fat suppression or gradient-echo sequences. No increase in signal intensity, however, is observed on T2-weighted images, and the focus appears isointense with skeletal muscle on all sequences. Two explanations have been offered for this finding. One is aberrant vascularity of the critical zone or the presence of subclinical tendon degeneration. This hypothesis is supported by the fact that the hypovascular critical zone of the supraspinatus is the predominant site for development of pathologic changes in impingement syndrome. Another explanation is based on the "magic angle" theory. Based on this theory, artifactual increased signal intensity of tendons may be observed when the tendon fibers are oriented at 55° to the main magnetic field (ERICKSON et al. 1991). This phenomenon may contribute to increased signal intensity of the anterior supraspinatus tendon because the tendon deviates anteriorly at or near this position.

11.1.4.7.4
CONCLUSIONS

MRI is fully accurate in diagnosing complete rotator cuff tear (Figs. 11.25–11.28). The intraarticular injection of paramagnetic contrast solution in order to improve visualization of tendon injury is a matter of discussion in the athletic population. MRI arthrography may be selectively utilized when routine MRI has failed to clearly identify or exclude an expected lesion, i.e., labral lesion or inferior glenohumeral unit lesion.

11.2
Elbow Impingement

11.2.1
Introduction

Chronic overuse injuries of the medial and lateral tendons (tendinosis or peritendinitis) are common around the elbow. Partial (second-degree strain) and complete (third-degree strain) ruptures of muscle or muscle-tendon units are uncommon. Tendon injury at the elbow can be classified in a manner similar to that for rotator cuff injuries. The initial stage is inflammation, followed by fibroblastic degeneration and finally partial or complete disruption. The last is unusual.

Tendinosis or peritendinitis may involve the medial or lateral origins at the epicondyles or, less frequently, the triceps tendon posteriorly. Patients present with local pain and tenderness that can be triggered by contraction of the involved muscle groups. Flexion contractures of the elbow are present in 50% of professional athletes. Patients with tendinosis are usually 30–55 years old and frequently play racquet sports or golf (tennis elbow). We suggest a classification similar to that for the rotator cuff, into lateral, medial, anterior, and posterior impingement.

11.2.2
Lateral Impingement

Injuries to the lateral side of the elbow, collectively known as "tennis elbow," are manifested as pain over the radiohumeral joint owing to repetitive flexion, extension or pronation, supination activity, compression, and shearing forces.

A macroscopic tear of the extensor carpi radialis brevis tendon, possibly with a contribution from the extensor digitorum communis, either superficial or deep, can be singled out as the pathologic anatomy most commonly producing the pain. Fifteen microscopic pathologic features reported as characterstic of lateral epicondylitis were identified from the literature (MORREY and REGAN 1994).

In athletes over 40 years old, edematous changes or thickening of the common extensor tendon result from tearing, and traction enthesophytes are common. Occasionally (approximately 1% of cases), the radial nerve is involved.

Routine AP and lateral radiographs are usually of little help in diagnosis; however, the gun-sight oblique view of the medial or lateral epicondyle often shows irregularity or punctate calcification (Fig. 11.29; COONRAD 1986). NIRSCHL (1985) has reported calcification of some degree in 22% of cases in a single series; however, gross calcification is very uncommon in this disorder (Fig. 11.29).

Lateral impingement is also involved in the lateral presentation of "little league elbow," i.e., a complex of injuries due to recurrent microtrauma. Pitchers may present with medial tendinosis, lateral impingement, posterior impingement, or ulnar nerve compression.

The entity termed little league (or little leaguer's) elbow was initially used in 1960 by BRODGON and CROW (1960) to describe the clinical and radio-

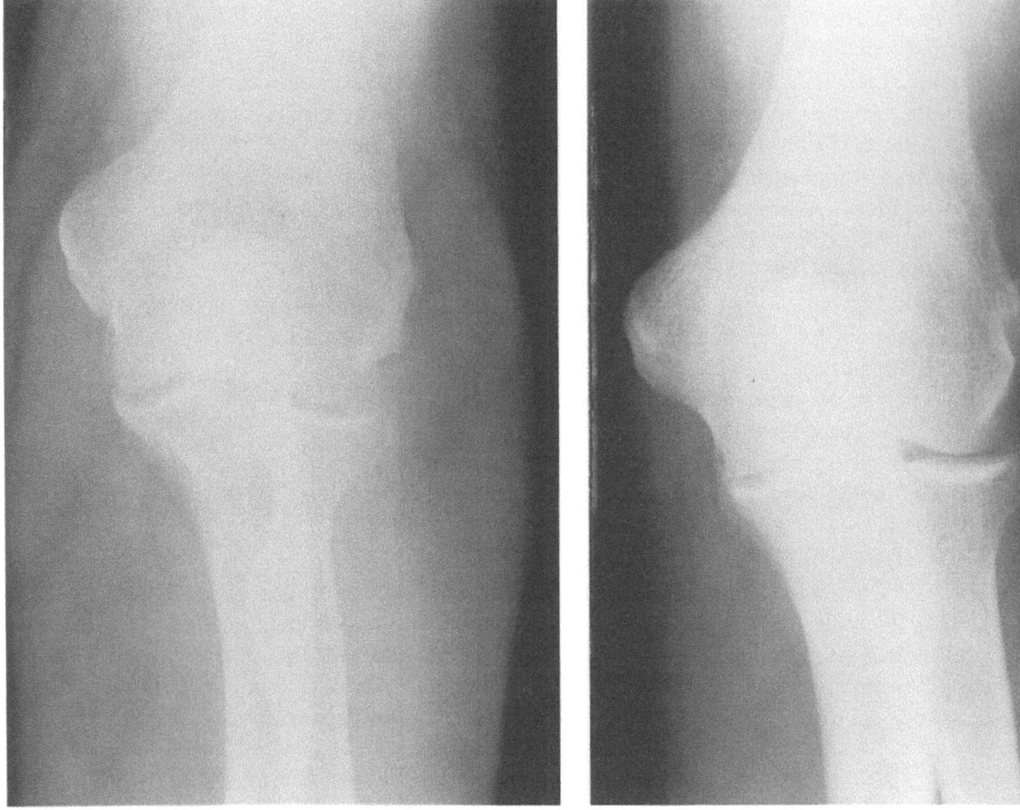

Fig. 11.29. a Lateral epicondyle calcifications. **b** Ossification above the lateral epicondyle

graphic changes on the medial side of the elbow in young baseball pitchers. ADAMS (1965) expanded the entity to include all of the problems that he associated with pitching, including lateral injuries, and correctly focused attention on the damage occurring to the immature elbow. The sports medicine community rightly became concerned with what appeared to be an epidemic of potentially harmful injuries occurring as a result of an activity that was intended to be fun and safe for children.

Pitching is divided into five phases (Fig. 11.6). Phase 1 is the wind-up or preparation phase, ending

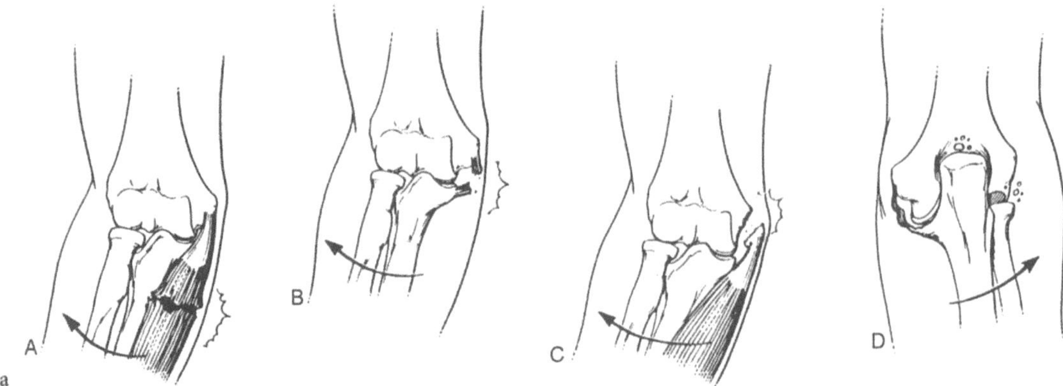

Fig. 11.30. a Throwing injuries of the elbow. *Arrows* indicate the direction of force application. *A*, flexor muscle injury; *B*, medial ligament tear; *C*, medial epicondyle avulsion fracture; *D*, ulnar spur formation with loose bodies. **b** During early and late cocking, the forces that usually cause injury during throwing are compression of the capitellum against the radial head and tension on the medial collateral ligament, flexor muscles, and ulnar nerve medially. **c** The sites of injury during the acceleration phase of throwing (*arrowheads*). **d** Osteophyte from the coronoid process after avulsion injuries

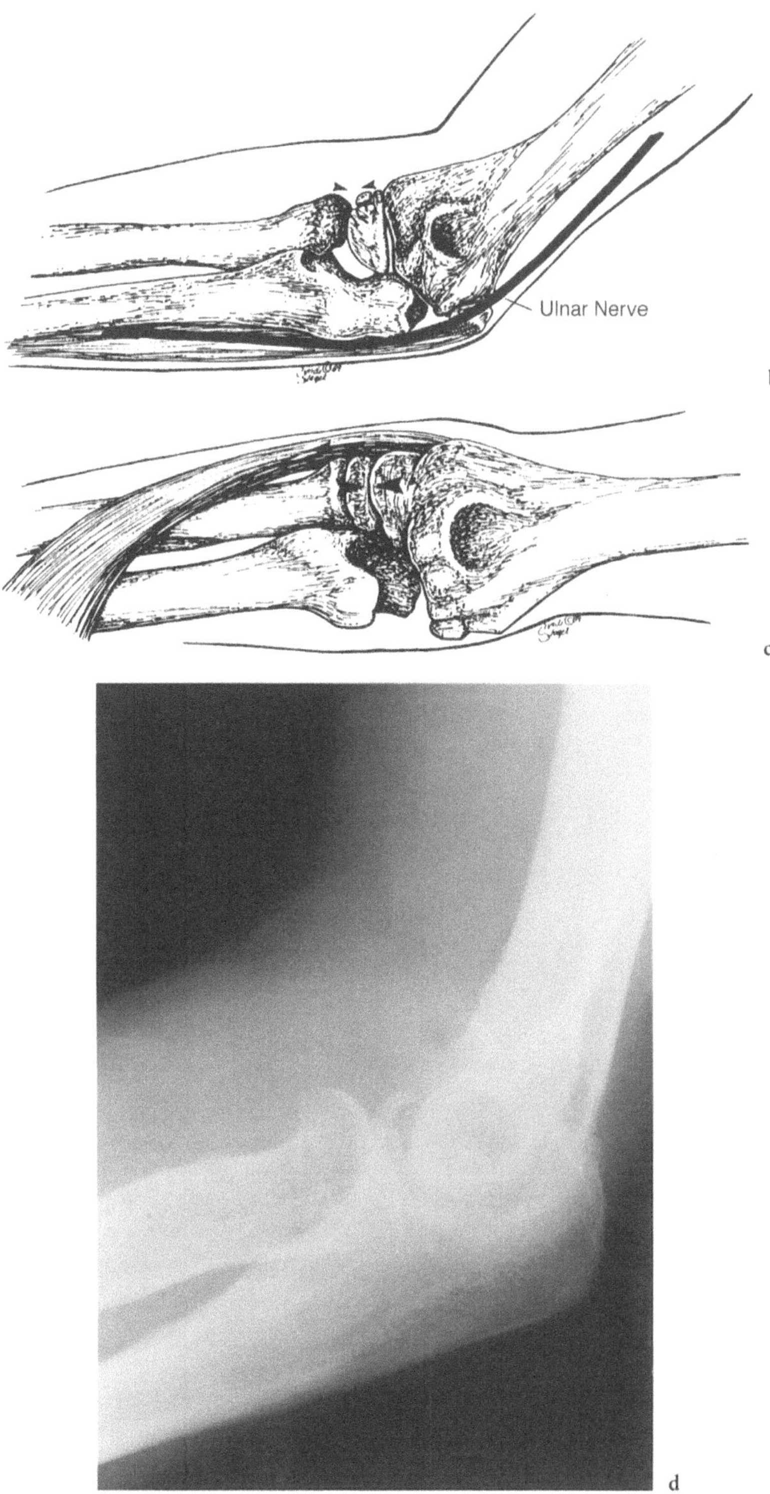

Fig. 11.30. *Continued*

when the ball leaves the glove hand; phase 2, termed "early cocking," is a period of shoulder abduction and external rotation that begins as the ball is released from the nondominant hand and terminates with contact of the forward foot to the ground; phase 3, the late cocking phase, continues until maximum external rotation at the shoulder is obtained; phase 4 is the short propulsive phase of acceleration that starts with internal rotation of the humerus and ends with ball release; and phase 5 is the follow-through phase, which starts with ball release and ends when motion has ceased.

The injuries that occur from throwing may be divided into medial tension injuries, lateral compression injuries, and posterior injuries (Fig. 11.30).

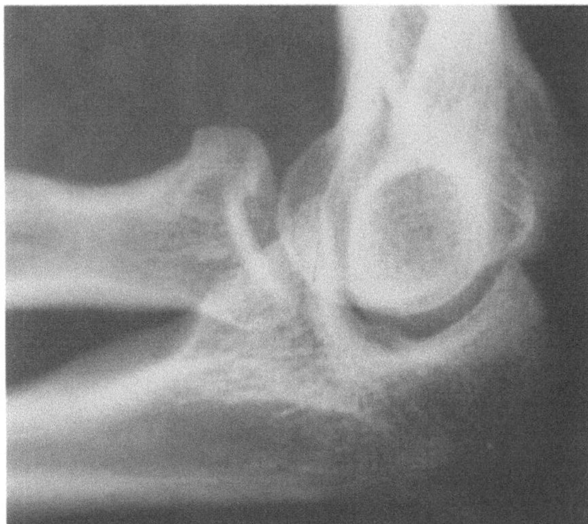

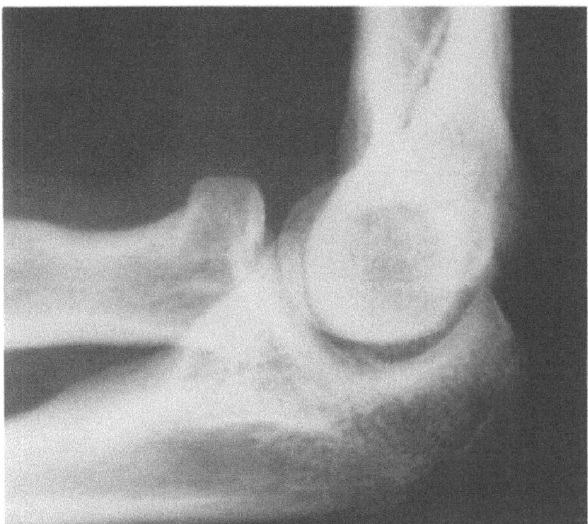

Fig. 11.31a,b. Radial head fracture better seen on **a** the oblique cranial (25°) profile view than on **b** the true profile view

As the arm is forced into valgus at the elbow, high compression and shear stresses are created between the radial head and the capitellum. The capitellar side is more susceptible to injury, and osteochondral fractures of the capitellum and, rarely, the radial head occur (Figs. 11.31, 11.32). Little league elbow also occurs in golfers and in tennis players who use exaggerated top spin requiring excessive pronation of the forearm.

11.2.3
Medial Impingement or Medial Tennis Elbow

Medial epicondylitis is an example of medial tension overload of the elbow. This results from direct (dislocation; Figs. 11.34–11.40) or indirect trauma as in young throwing athletes, in whom repetitive valgus stress and flexor forearm muscle pull can produce an overuse syndrome in the common flexor origin, secondary to forceful flexion and distraction. Medial tendinosis predominantly involves the flexor carpi radialis, but in 10% of cases the flexor carpal ulnaris is involved. Partial rupture may occur in 3% of cases. Calcification of the pericondyle may be evident on radiographs in up to 25% of patients with chronic medial epicondylitis (Fig. 11.41).

Sporting activities producing medial impingement include squash, racquets, and particularly tennis. The activities of tennis or any racquet sport most likely to initiate difficulty are the serve and forearm strokes.

Medial elbow impingement, also occurs in golfers and in tennis players who use exaggerated top spin requiring excessive pronation of the forearm.

During the acceleration phase, the medial aspect of the elbow is placed under tension and the lateral side is subjected to high compression forces (Figs. 11.31, 11.32). On the medial side, the resulting valgus stress causes tension on the ligament, which also attaches to the medial epicondyle, and thus strong static forces are also transmitted to the medial epicondyle (Fig. 11.42). Traumatic avulsion of the medial epicondyle through the epiphyseal plate can occur with a single throw, or damage can be caused more gradually by repetitive throwing maneuvers, as in the classic little league elbow.

Just before and during the release of the ball, the wrist flexors contract forcefully, adding to the stresses on the medial ligament, the forearm flexor muscles, and the medial epicondyle.

The common flexor-pronator group is the first line of defense against the valgus strain of throwing

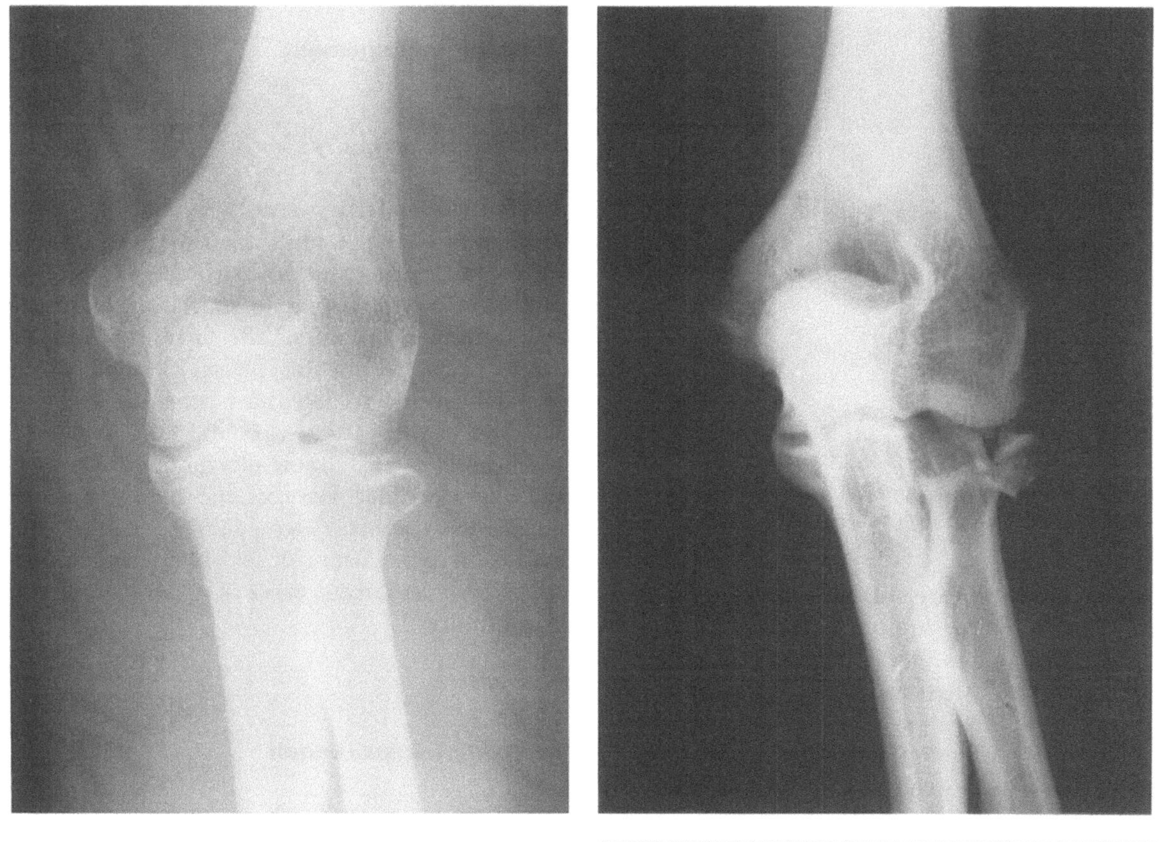

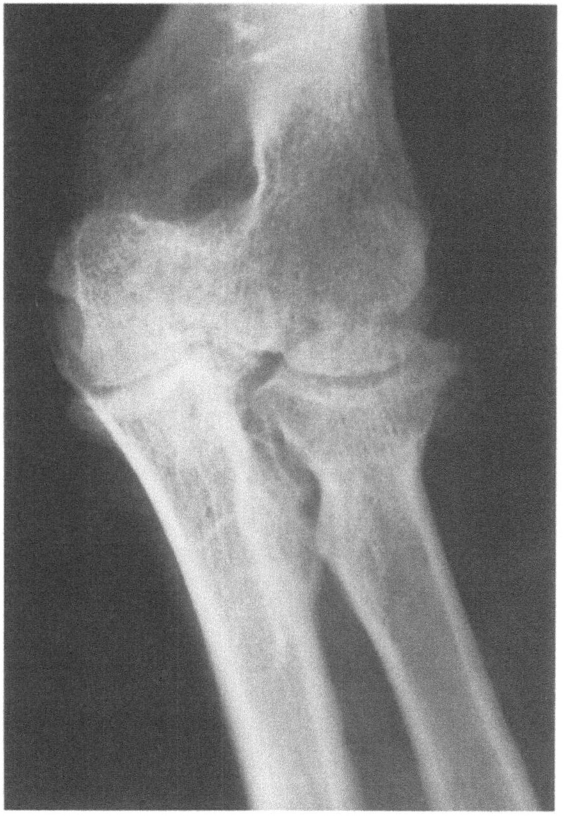

Fig. 11.32. a Osteochondral fracture of the radial head. b Complex fracture of the radial head. c Post-traumatic ulnohumeral and radiohumeral osteoarthritis and impinge-ment 2 years later

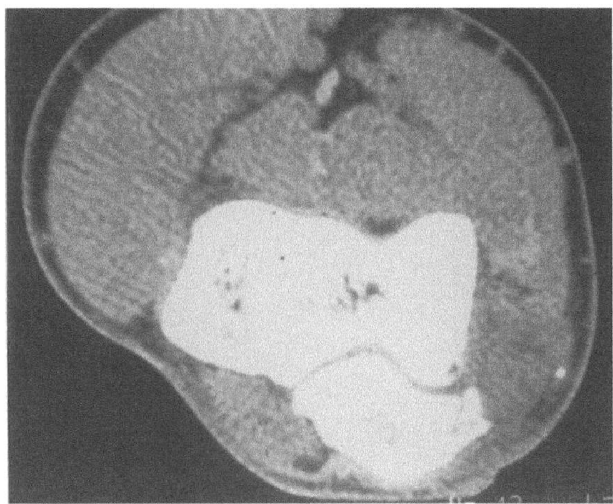

Fig. 11.33. Axial CT: partial medial fracture of the olecranon not depicted by routine ulnar nerve impingement

while the ligaments are still lax and can become inflamed (myositis) or ruptured. Occasionally, severe displacement of the medial epicondyle associated with elbow dislocation can result in entrapment of the fracture fragment in the joint after reduction. This entrapment is often difficult to diagnose on the lateral view but is suggested by medial joint widening or visualization of the loose body on the radiograph. When this occurs, closed reduction is unsuccessful; open reduction with anatomic pinning must be undertaken.

11.2.4
Anterior Impingement

Anterior impingement is the result of brachialis anterior tendon impingement directly on the elbow joint and the bicipitalis tuberosity of radius after acute complete tear or chronic complete tear, whether following heteropic ossification or not (Fig. 11.40).

11.2.5
Posterior Impingement

11.2.5.1
Triceps Tendon Injury

Triceps tendon injury usually results from a fall or forceful throwing in adults. During the acceleration phase, the triceps contracts strongly to forcibly extend the elbow, exposing the muscle, its tendon, and its olecranon attachment site to injury. Very large forces occur during this phase; angular velocities averaging over 4000 deg/s have been reported in professional pitchers (PAPPAS et al. 1985). As the elbow reaches full extension, the olecranon strikes against the supracondylar fossa of the humerus, causing additional trauma (Figs. 11.32, 11.42). Triceps rupture is rare. ANZEL et al. (1989) reported eight triceps ruptures in 856 cases of upper extremity tendon ruptures.

11.2.5.2
Snapping Triceps Tendon

Snapping triceps tendon is an uncommon disorder. The condition occurs most commonly in young athletes. Snapping typically occurs medially and posteriorly. The sensation of snapping may be due to anomalous triceps insertions or subluxation of the ulnar nerve. Most frequently, snapping is due to subluxation of the medial head of the triceps over the medial epicondyle (DREYFUS 1978).

11.3
Wrist and Hand Impingement

There are numerous soft-tissue and osseous overuse syndromes that may affect the hand and wrist.

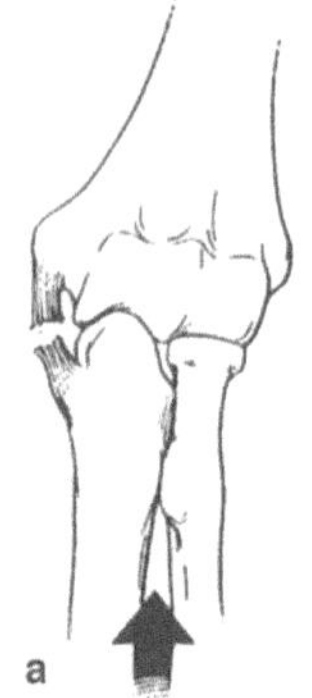
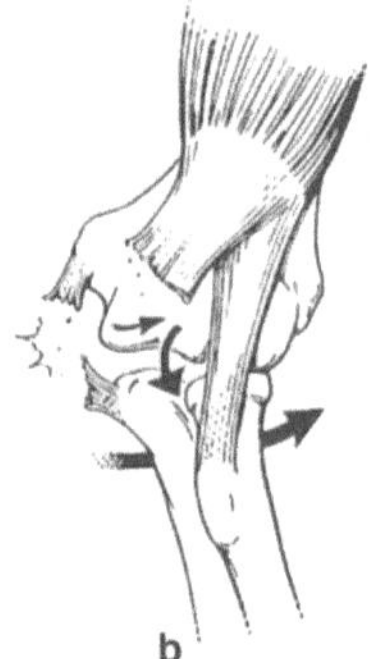
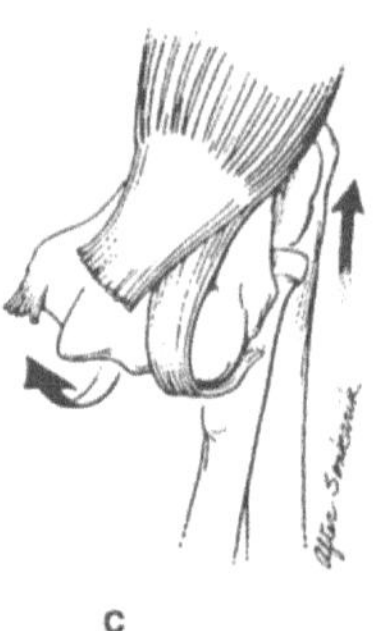

Fig. 11.34. Elbow dislocations. *Arrows* indicate the direction of force application. *A*, hyperextension with medial ligament disruption; *B*, posterolateral ulnar displacement; *C*, posterior dislocation with biceps tendon trapped over the trochlea

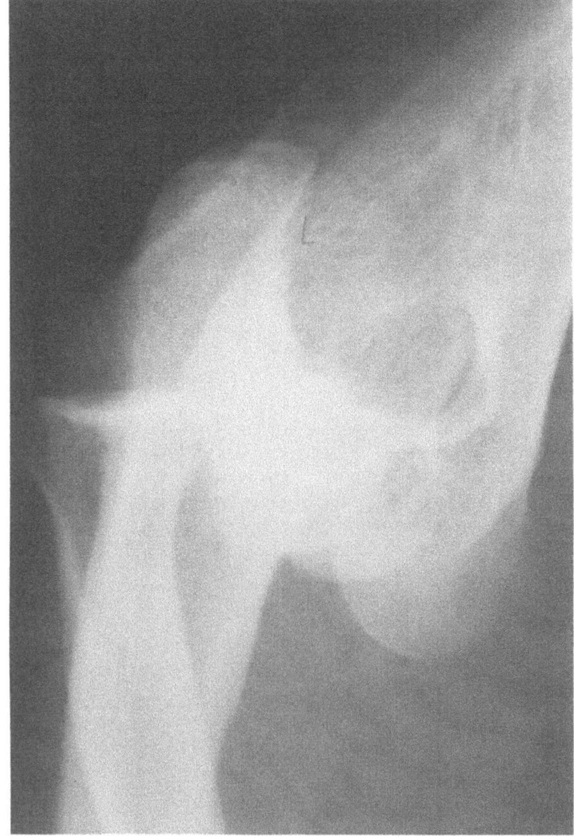

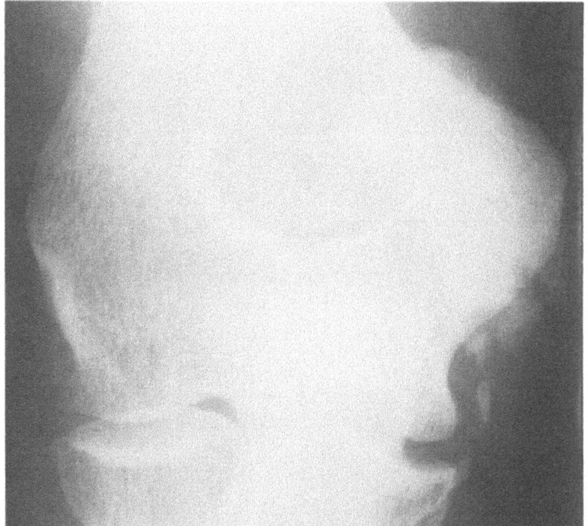

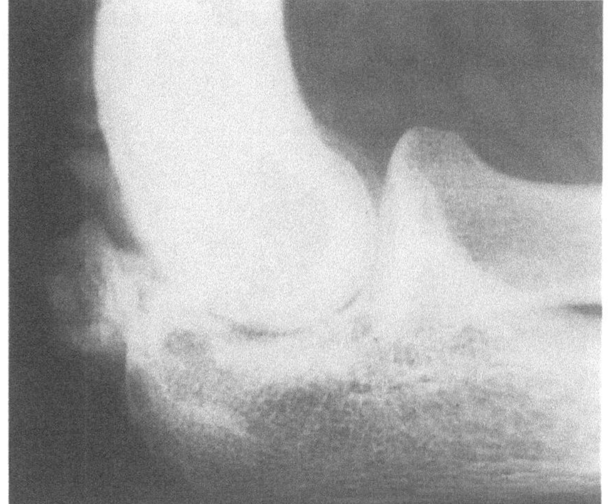

Fig. 11.35. a Elbow dislocation, Eight months later, periarticular ossifications on the **b** medial and **c** posterior site; nerve and tendon impingement

11.3.1
Introduction

Tendinosis or peritendinitis of the wrist is the most frequent sports injury to require medical attention. Symptoms often begin some time after an inciting event, which is usually overuse of some kind. Tendinosis is common in athletes participating in racquet sports, rowing, and weight lifting.

11.3.2
Thumb Injuries

Thumb injuries are particularly common in skiers.

Bowler's thumb – traumatic neuroma of the ulnar digital nerve to the thumb – occurs almost exclusively in bowlers. The cause appears to be repeated friction between the thumb and the edge of the thumb; the ulnar digital nerve lies superficial to the sesamoid bone and can be trapped during repeated insertion and withdrawal of the thumb during bowling. This condition may also result from repetitive pressure on the ulnar digital nerve during racquet sports. Presenting complaints usually include sensitivity over the ulnar digital nerve and hypesthesia in the area of irritation. Atrophy of the overlying skin or callus formation is usually present, and the indurated area of the nerve can almost always be palpated. "Rolling" of the nerve over the metacarpophalangeal joint prominence reproduces the

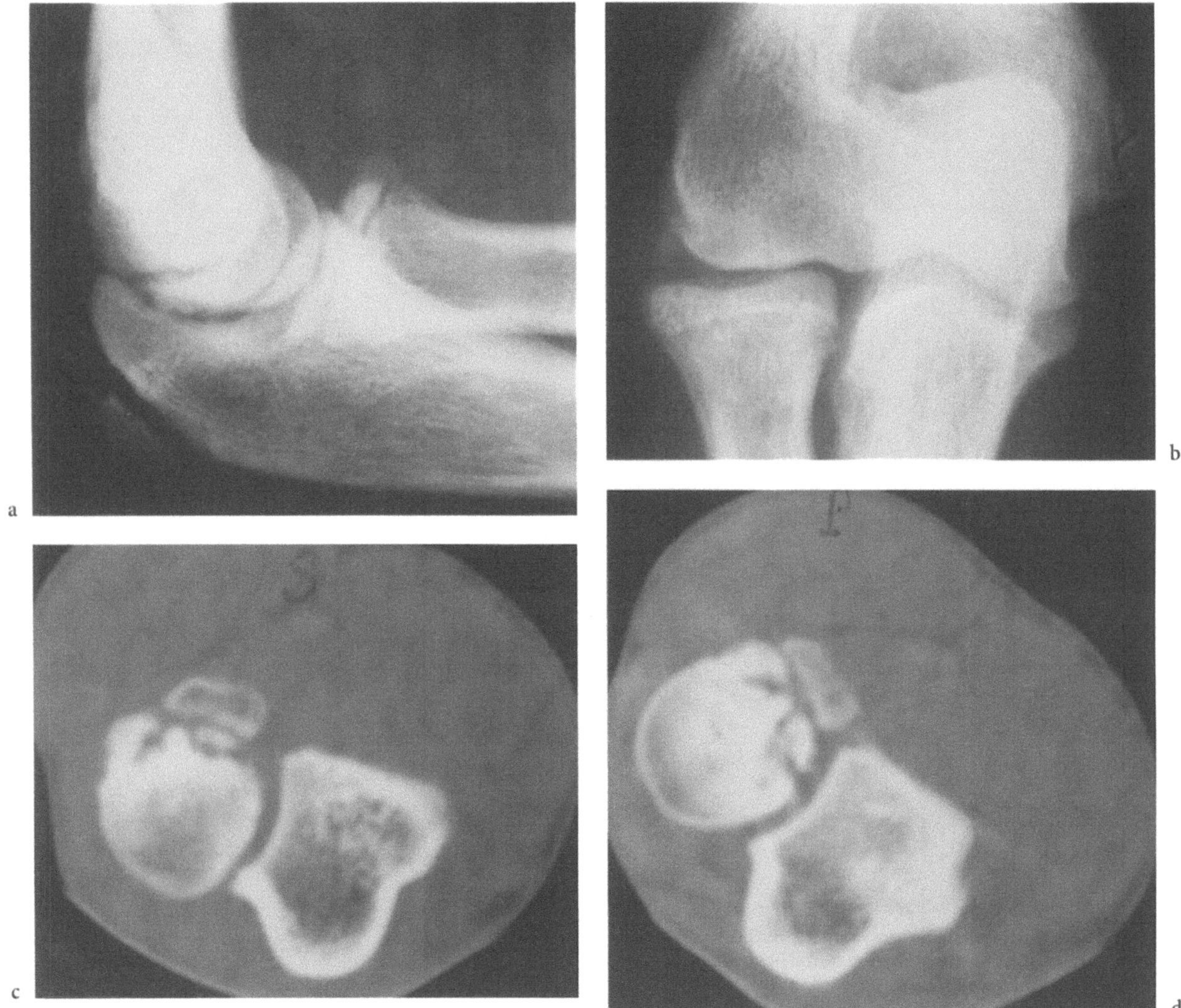

Fig. 11.36. a Medial condyle and radial head fractures in a 13-year-old boy. Loss of **b** pronation and **c** impingement. **d** Axial CT

patient's complaints (GREEN and STRICKLAND 1994).

Diagnosis of these disorders is often based on the history and physical findings. Imaging and diagnostic or therapeutic injections are frequently required, however. X-rays are usually negative except in chronic cases, in which calcification may occasionally be present in the soft tissues. Calcification is much more common in the supraspinatus tendon of the shoulder.

11.3.3
Flexor Carpi Ulnaris and Flexor Carpi Radialis

Tendinosis of the two wrist flexors is relatively common. It is caused by chronic repetitive trauma. Lo-

calized tenderness and swelling are present over the tendon, and pain is increased with passive dorsiflexion or resisted palmar flexion. Crepitus may be noted with movement.

11.3.4
Extensor Carpi Ulnaris and Extensor Carpi Radialis

Tendinosis may also involve extensor carpi radialis longus and brevis. This condition is frequently associated with carpal boss. The carpal boss, an unmovable bony protuberance, is located on the dorsum of the wrist at the base of the second and third metacarpals adjacent to the capitate and trapezoid bones. This bony prominence may represent degenerative

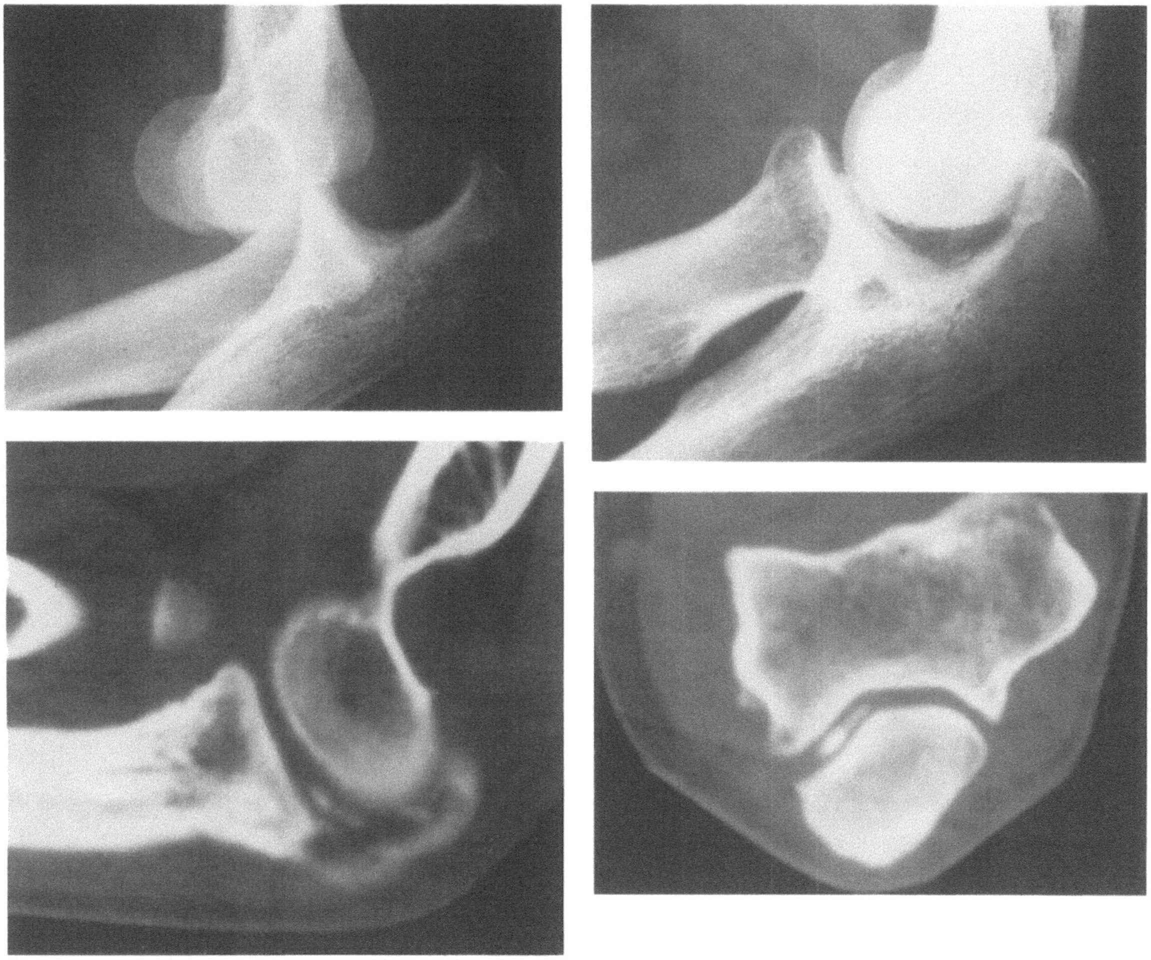

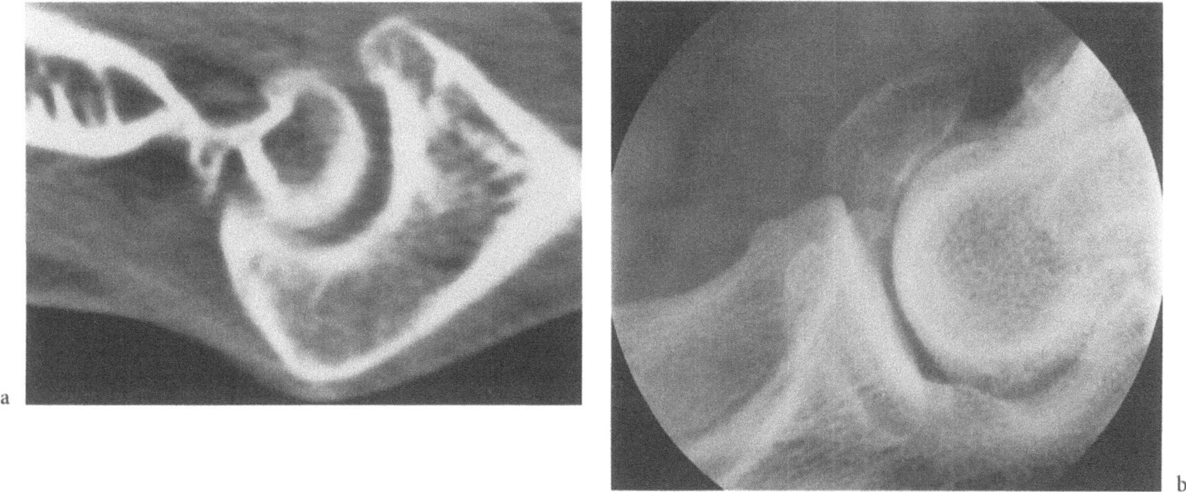

Fig. 11.37. a Elbow dislocation. b Articular incongruity, intra-articular loose bodies. c Sagittal CT. d Axial CT

Fig. 11.38. a Cristae ossea humeralis reduces extension after elbow dislocation, sagittal CT. b Osteochondral loose body in the anterior part of the joint space, lateral X-ray view

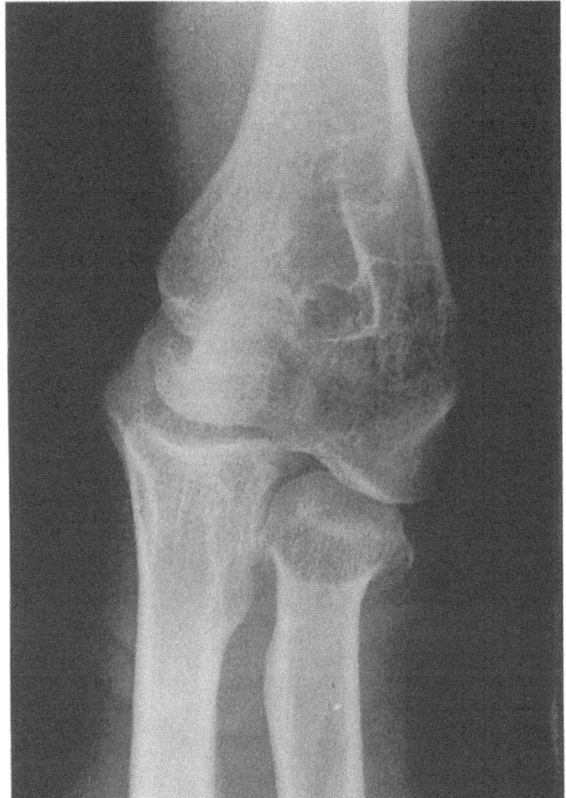

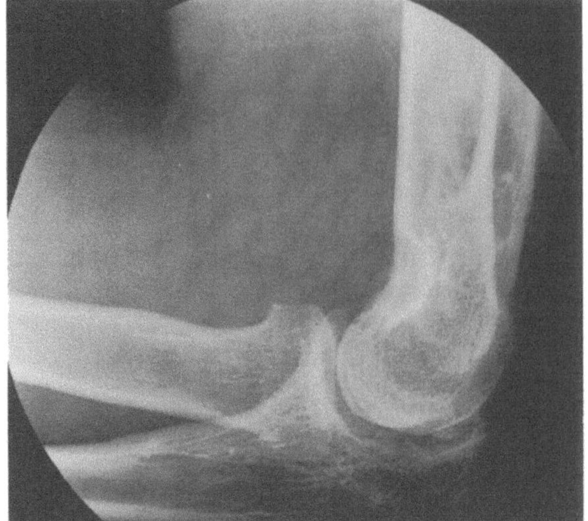

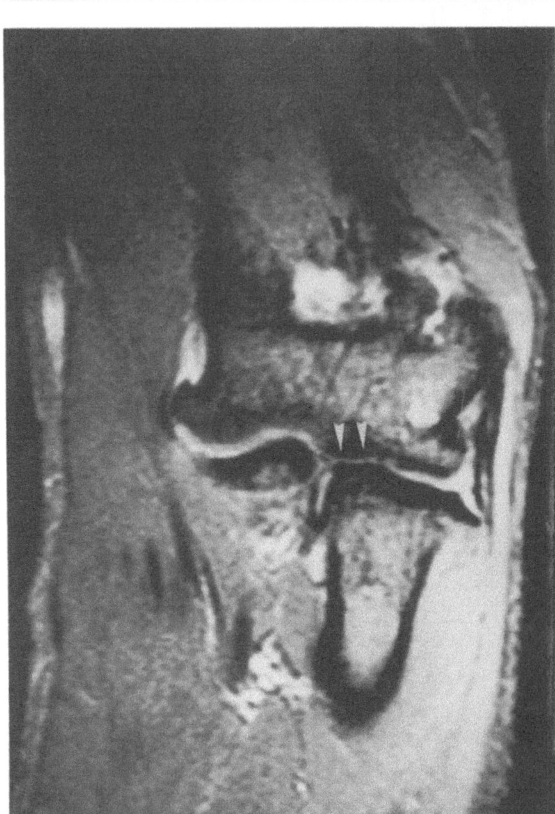

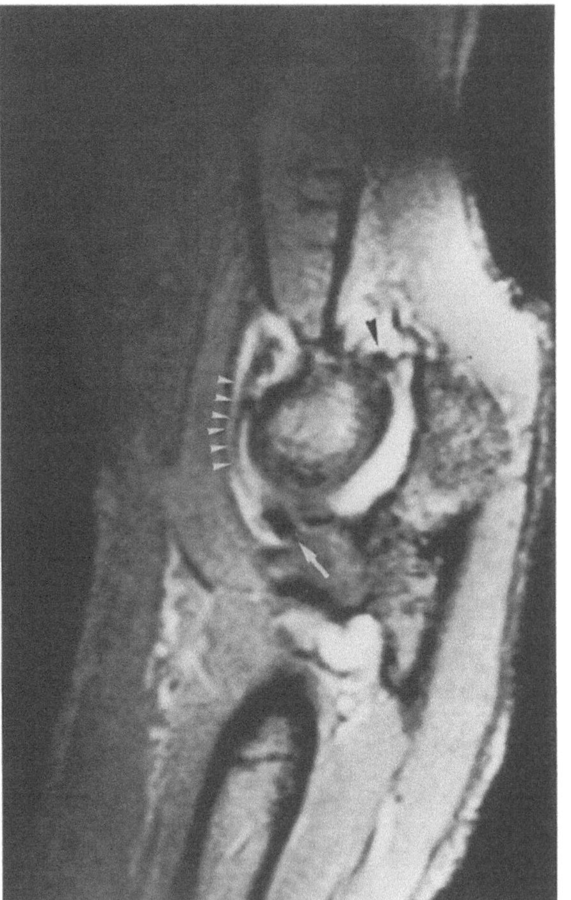

Fig. 11.39a–e. Elbow dislocation after 10 years. Routine X-ray **a** AP and **b** lateral view; ossification in the anterior part of the joint. **c** MRI, coronal plane in T2 with cartilage loss (*white arrowheads*) and osteophytes. **d** Sagittal plane in T2, linear low signal intensity (*white arrowheads*); central (*white arrow*) and posterior (*black arrowhead*) consistent with loose cartilaginous bodies **e** Axial plane in T2, low signal intensity (*black arrow*) of the same origin

Fig. 11.39a–e. *Continued*

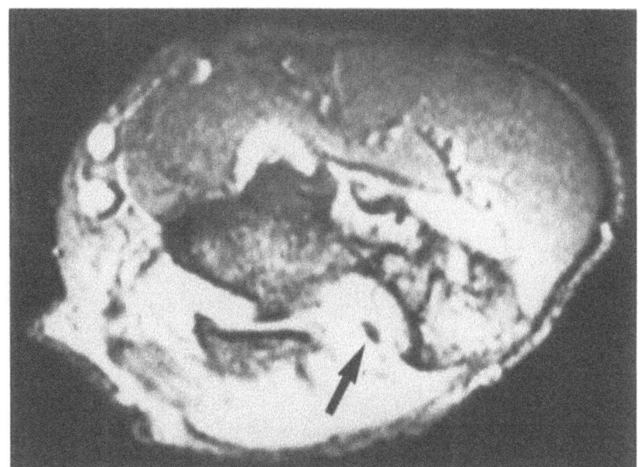

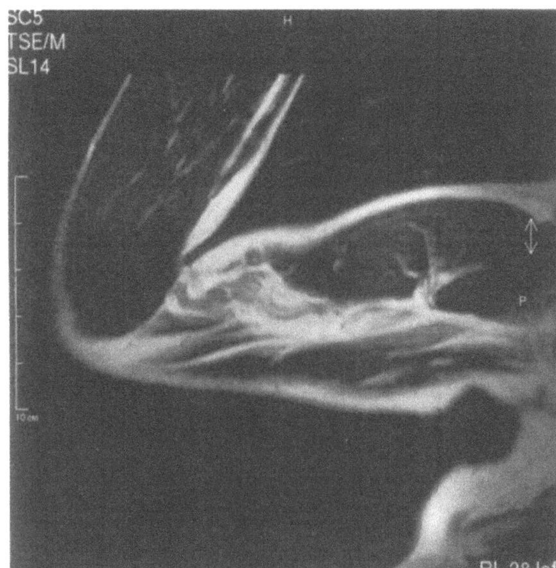

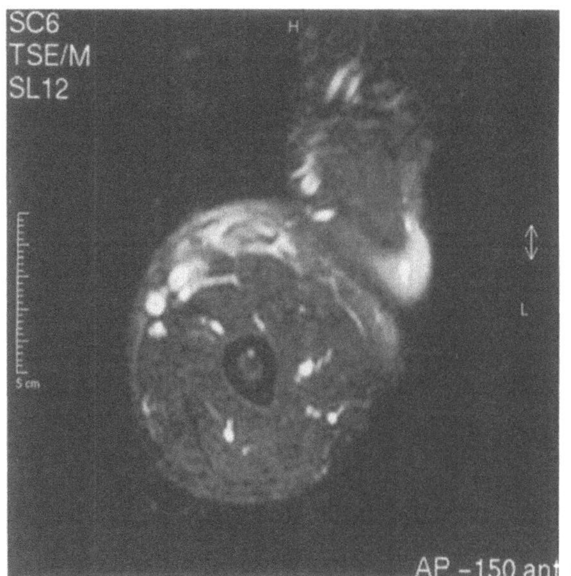

Fig. 11.40a–f. Anterior impingement. Acute tear of the musculo-tendinous junction of the biceps brachialis anterior in **a** T2 sagittal and **b** T2 axial plane. Impingement (*arrowheads*) of the distal biceps brachialis tendon near its insertion with bursitis; **c** axial T1-weighted image and **d** gradient-echo T2-weighted image. **e** Ossification of the brachialis anterior muscle and tendon related to impingement. **f** Classification of radial density around the elbow after injuries

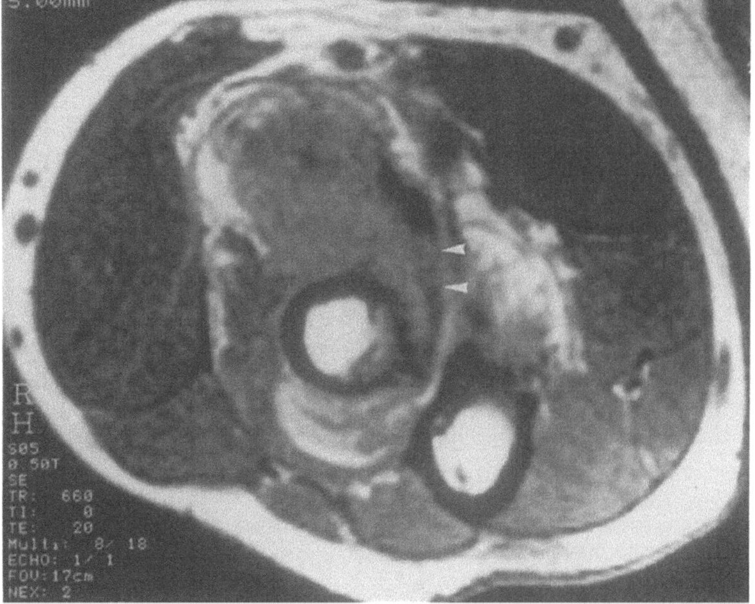

(d, e, f, see next page)

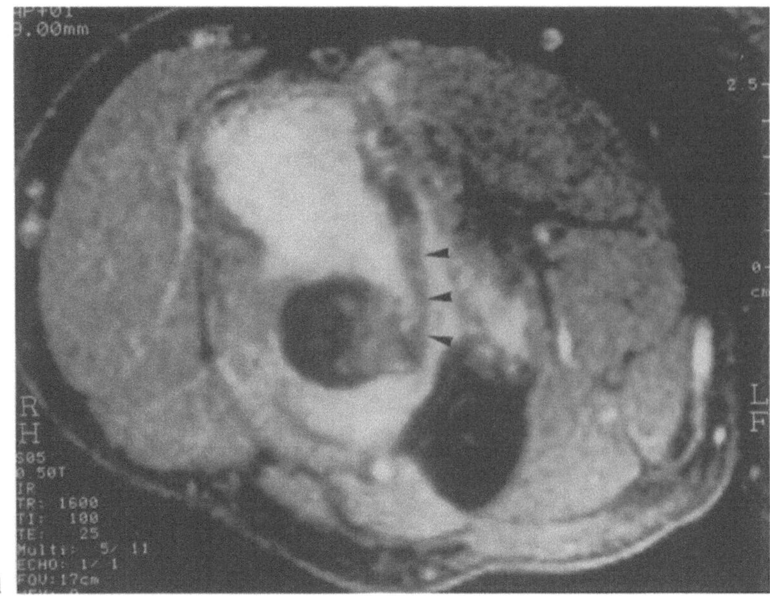

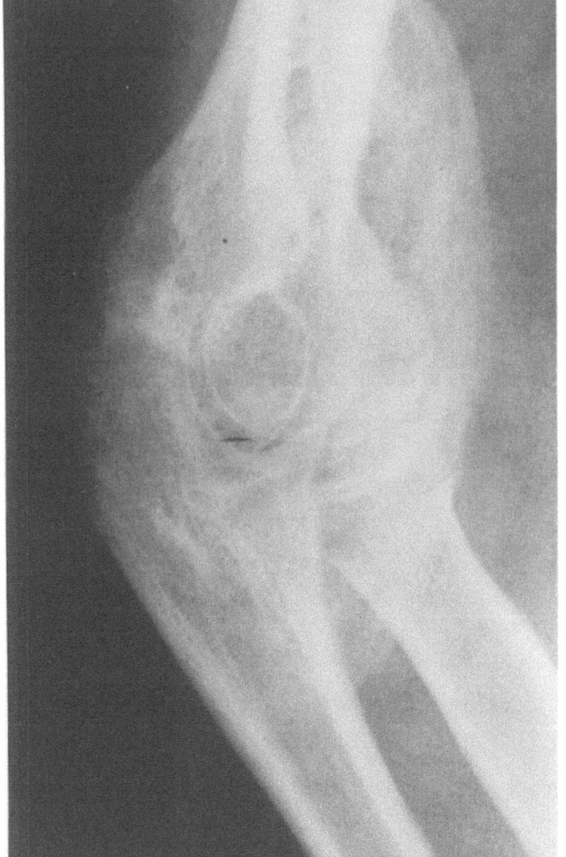

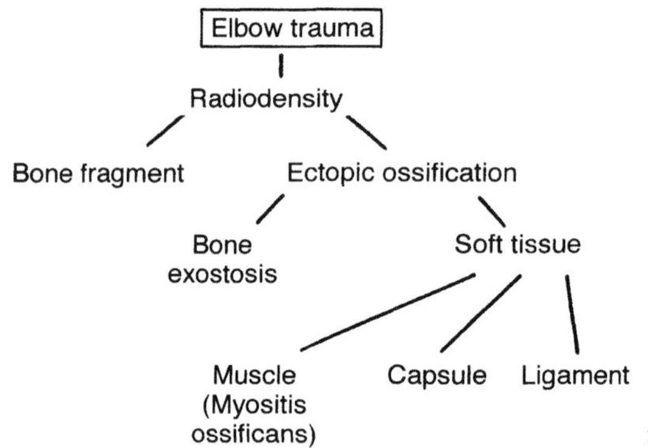

Fig. 11.40a–f. *Continued*

osteophyte formation and/or the presence of an os styloideum, an accessory ossification center that occurs during embryonic development. When this condition is symptomatic, patients present with complaints of pain and limitation of motion of the affected hand. The symptoms of carpal boss may result from an overlying ganglion or bursitis, an extensor tendon slipping over this bony prominence,

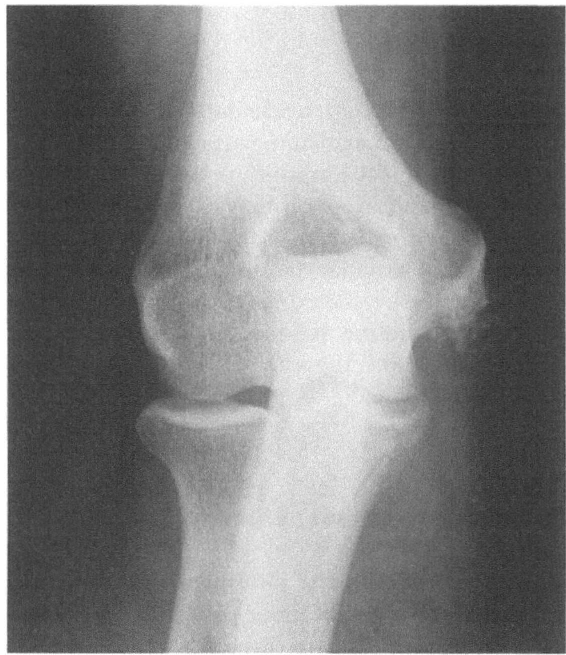

Fig. 11.41. Periosteal avulsion of the medial epicondyle; nerve and tendon impingement

or from osteoarthritic changes at this site. Radiographically, the view that best profiles the separate os styloideum is a lateral view with 30° of supination and ulnar deviation of the wrist. Once a diagnosis has been made, treatment can range from the use of nonsteroidal antiinflammatory medication and limited use of the wrist to surgical excision of the anatomic abnormality (CONWAY 1985).

Subluxation of the extensor carpi ulnaris has been noted in athletes (Figs. 11.43, 11.44). A painful snap over the dorsoulnar aspect of the wrist occurs with pronation and supination. This injury results when the ulnar septum of the sixth dorsal compartment is ruptured, allowing the extensor carpi ulnaris tendon to subluxate during supination and to reduce during pronation.

11.3.5
De Quervain's Disease

De Quervain's disease is a tenosynovitis of the abductor pollicis longus and extensor pollicis brevis at the first dorsal compartment (Fig. 11.44). Sports activities that require repetitive ulnar deviation place an athlete at risk of the syndrome.

De Quervain's tenosynovitis affects the tendons in the radial styloid region. Inflammation is related to overuse due to pinch, grasp, or radial and ulnar deviation of the wrist. The extensor pollicis brevis and abductor pollicis longus are affected in the region of the fibroosseous tunnel. The condition is most common in racquet sports. Patients typically present with pain in the anatomic snuffbox with associated swelling.

11.3.6
Intersection Syndrome

The intersection syndrome (squeaker's wrist; Fig. 11.44) is an overuse syndrome that occurs slightly proximal to De Quervain's syndrome. There is a potential bursa located between the extensor carpi

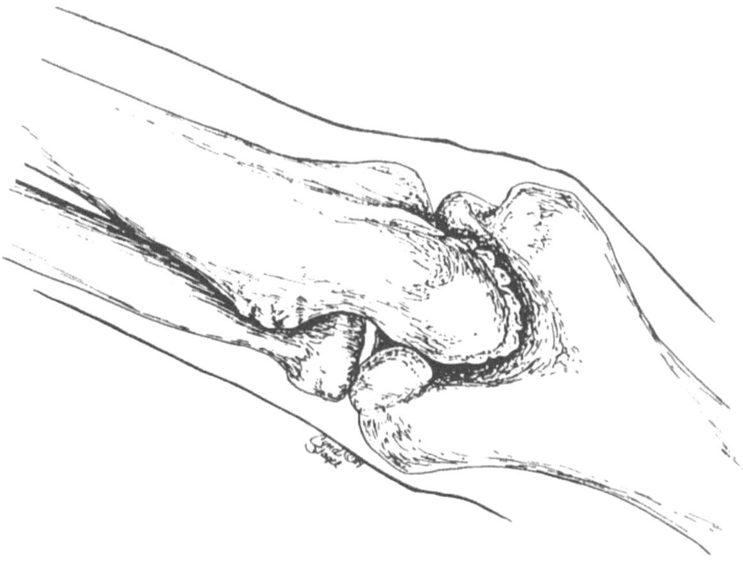

Fig. 11.42. Typical location of posterior and posteromedial osteophytes of the olecranon associated with extension overload

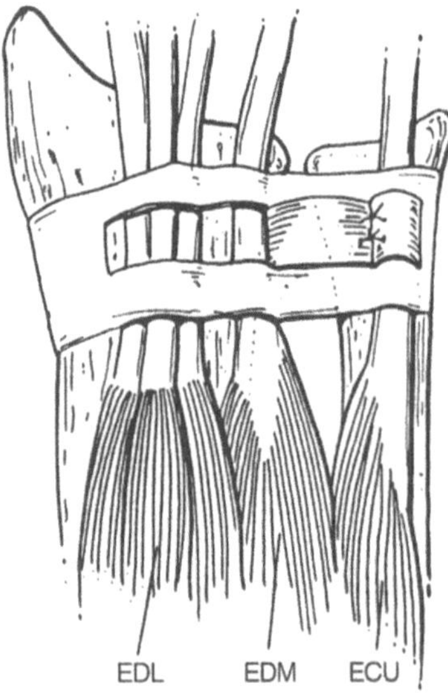

Fig. 11.43. Extensor carpi ulnaris (*ECU*) stabilized with flap of retinaculum. *EDM*, extensor digitorum minimi; *EDC*, extensor digitorum communis

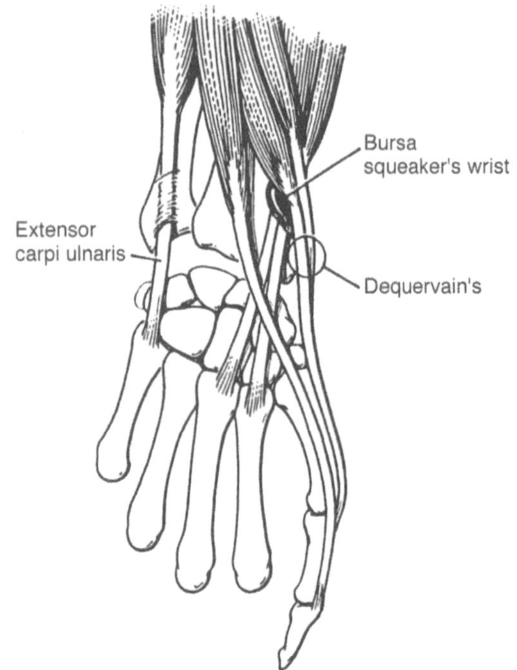

Fig. 11.44. Illustration of sites of De Quervain's tendinitis, squeaker's wrist, and extensor carpi ulnaris tendinitis or subluxation

radialis longus and brevis and the abductor pollicis longus and extensor pollicis brevis. Irritation occurs with repetitive extension and radial deviation and is most frequently noted in rowers, weight lifters, and participants in racquet sports. Patients present with pain, weak grasp, and crepitation.

11.3.7
Imaging Modalities

Routine radiographs provide important information in cases of tendon avulsion, carpal boss, and calcifying tendinosis. Ultrasonography may be useful in identifying tendon pathology, but MRI is more frequently performed in practice. Osseous and soft tissue (neural, vascular, tendon, or ligament) abnormalities can be evaluated. Contrast agent injections are useful to define tendon sheaths for purposes of diagnostic and therapeutic injection, ensuring proper localization.

11.3.8
Ulnolunate Abutment Syndrome

Patients with ulnolunate abutment syndrome most frequently present with ulnar pain that may be confused with pain due to injury to the triangular fibrocartilage complex or some other pathology. Usually, overuse or stress syndrome is responsible for this condition. Radionuclide scans demonstrate focally increased tracer uptake in the ulnar region. Tomography is most useful for demonstrating the characteristic features of positive ulnar variance with sclerosis, erosion, or cystic changes in the ulnar aspect of the proximal lunate. Surgery may be indicated if conservative therapy fails (BERQUIST 1992b).

References

Adams JE (1965) Injury to the throwing arm: a study of traumatic changes in the elbow joints of boy baseball players. Calif Med 102:127–132

Anzel SH, et al. (1989) Disruption of muscles and tendons: analysis of 1014 cases. Surgery 45:406–414

Berquist TH (1992a) Elbow and forearm. In: Kricun ME (ed) Ligament, tendon and osteochondral fractures. (Imaging of sports injuries, vol 10) Aspen, Gaithersburg, p 282

Berquist TH (1992b) Hand and wrist. In: Kricun ME (ed) Ligament, tendon and osteochondral fractures. (Imaging of sports injuries, vol 10) Aspen, Gaithersburg, p 350

Bigliani LU, Morrison DS, April EW (1986) The morphology of the acromion and its relationship to rotator cuff tear. Orthop Trans 10:228

Brodgon MD, Crow NE (1960) Little leaguer's elbow. AJR Am J Roentgenol 83:671–675

Brown C (1983) Compressive, invasive referred pain to the shoulder. Clin Orthop 173:55–62

Burk DL (1989) Rotator cuff tears: prospective comparison of MR imaging with arthrography, sonography and surgery. AJR Am J Roentgenol 153:87–92

Codman EA (1931) Rupture of the supraspinatus tendon. Surg Gynecol Obstet 52:579–586

Conway WF (1985) The carpal boss: an overview of radiographic evaluation. Radiology 156:29–31

Coonrad RW (1986) Tennis elbow. Instr Course Lect 35:94–101

Cotty PH, Fouquet D (1994) Rupture de la coiffe des rotateurs. Valeur diagnostique du cliché standard en abduction contrariée (manoeuvre de Leclercq) dans l'épreuve douloureuse chronique. Rev Imag Med 6:43–47

Crass JR, Craig EV, Fainberg SB (1988) Ultrasonography of rotator cuff tears. A review of 500 diagnostic studies. J Clin Ultrasound 16:313–327

Dreyfus U (1978) Snapping elbow due to dislocation of the medial head of the triceps. J Bone Joint Surg [Br] 60:56–57

Edelson JG (1995) The "hooked" acromion revisited. J Bone Joint Surg [Br] 77:284–287

Erickson SJ, Cox IH, Hyde JS (1991) Effect of tendon orientation on MR imaging signal intensity: a manifestation of the "magic angle" phenomenon. Radiology 181:389

Fourcade D, Railhac JJ (1996) Les clichés dynamiques: mesure du pincement sous acromial. In: Gazielly D (ed) The cuff. Elsevier, Paris, in press

Fowler PJ (1988) Shoulder injuries in the mature athlete. Adv Sports Med Fitness 1:225–238

Garth WP, Allman FL, Armstrong WS (1986) Occult anterior subluxation of the shoulder in non-contact sports. Orthop Trans 10:214

Gerber C (1985) The role of the coracoid process in the chronic impingement syndrome. J Bone Joint Surg [Br] 67:703–708

Gilcrest EL (1925) Rupture of muscles and tendons. JAMA 84:1819–1822

Goupille P, Anger C (1993) Valeur des radiographies standard pour le diagnostic de rupture de la coiffe des rotateurs de l'épaule. Rev Rhum 60:440–444

Green DP, Strickland JW (1994) The hand. In: DeLee JC, Drez D Jr (eds) Orthopaedic sports medicine, vol 1. Saunders, Philadelphia, pp 945–1017

Hawkins RJ, Kunkel SS (1990) Rotator cuff tears. In: Torg JS (ed) Current therapy in sports medicine. Mosby, St Louis

Hawkins RJ, Mohtadi MD (1994) Rotator cuff problems in athletes. In: DeLee JC, Drez D Jr (eds) Orthopaedic sports medicine, vol 1. Saunders, Philadelphia, pp 623–656

Haygood TM, Langlotz CP, Kneeland JB, Iannotti JP, Williams GR, Dalinka MK (1994) Categorization of acromial shape: interobserver variability with MR imaging and conventional radiography. AJR Am J Roentgenol 162:1377–1382

Hill JA (1983) Epidemiologic perspective on shoulder injuries. Clin Sports Med 2:241–245

Jobe FW (1983) Serious rotator cuff injuries. Clin Sports Med 2:407–412

Jobe FW, Bradley JP (1988) Rotator cuff injuries in baseball: prevention and rehabilitation. Sports Med 6:378–387

Leclercq R (1950) Diagnostic de la rupture du sus-épineux. Rev Rhum Mal Osteoartic 10:510–515

Mack LA (1988) Sonographic evaluation of the rotator cuff. Radiol Clin North Am 26:161–177

Meyer AW (1934) Chronic functional lesions of the shoulder. Arch Surg 35:646–674

Middleton WD (1986) Ultrasonographic evaluation of the rotator cuff and biceps tendon. J Bone Joint Surg [Am] 68:440–450

Morrey BF, Regan WD (1994) Tendinopathies about the elbow sports injuries of the upper extremity. In: DeLee JC, Drez D Jr (eds) Orthopaedic sports medicine, vol 1. Saunders, Philadelphia, pp 860–872

Neer CS (1972) Anterior acromioplasty for the chronic impingement syndrome in the shoulder: a preliminary report, vol 2. J Bone Joint Surg [Am] 54:41–50

Nicholas JA, et al. (1977) The importance of a simplified classification of motion in sports in relation to performance. Orthop Clin North Am 8:499–532

Nirschl RP (1985) Muscle and tendon trauma: tennis elbow. In: Morrey BF (ed) The elbow and its disorders. Saunders, Philadelphia, pp 481–496

Nirschl RP (1988) Prevention and treatment of elbow and shoulder injuries in the tennis player. Clin Sports Med 7:289–308

Pappas AM, et al. (1985) Biomechanics of baseball pitching. A preliminary report. Am J Sports Med 13:216–222

Patte D (1990a) Classification of rotator cuff lesions. Clin Orthop 254:81–86

Patte D (1990b) The subcoracoid impingement. Clin Orthop 254:55–59

Resnick D (1995) Rotator cuff tears. In: Resnick D (ed) Diagnosis of bone and joint disorders, 3rd edn. Saunders, Philadelphia, pp 2964–2969

Rigal A (1994) Intérêt de la radiographie de l'épaule de face strict en décubitus dans la rupture de la coiffe des rotateurs. Thesis, University of Toulouse

Welfling J (1965) Le diastasis omo-huméral inférieur provoqué. Rev Rhum 32:588–592

Zlatkin MB, Iannotti JP, Roberts ML (1989) Rotator cuff tears: diagnostic performance of MR imaging. Radiology 172:223–229

12 Impingement Syndrome of the Lower Limb

C. Faletti[1] and N. De Stefano[2]

CONTENTS

12.1
Introduction

The term "impingement" means the presence, in the joint area, of a formation originating from one of the components in that same joint and limiting function by effecting the biomechanics of movement. The impingement syndrome in the shoulder is defined as friction between skeletal components due to articular disequilibrium caused by injury to the tendons and ligaments.

In the lower extremities, this type of syndrome is secondary mainly to synovial hyperplasia which determines interaction in the joint spaces, between the articular surfaces and the synovia. Bone, tendon, and cartilage lesions in the lower extremities are due to overexertion and therefore are considered to be pathologies related to biomechanical overload. This chapter thus excludes degenerative joint diseases with marginal osteophytes, as well as osteochondral lesions due to trauma or overload that cause limited joint function.

12.2
Etiology and Pathogenesis

During sporting activities, on an amateur level and above all on a professional level, workloads are increased without any consideration of articular me-

chanics and the physiological differences among people. This leads to overuse of the various articular structures submitted to biomechanical stress. Such overuse evokes reactions of these structures and especially of the synovia, which provides proper lubrication for articular mechanics.

Many athletes, such as runners, cyclists, aerobics enthusiasts, volleyball players, and basketball players, develop painful disorders of the lower extremities without any acute injury. In a runner, for example, the examiner should ask whether there was an increase in the distance run or a change in the running surface, at what point the pain was felt, and what home remedies were tried before the runner sought advice from a physician. The physical examination should include not only the affected area but also evaluation of the back, pelvis, leg lengths, varus or valgus knee, femoral and tibial torsion, and cavus or flatfoot deformities.

Impingement syndrome may also manifest itself when the recovery phase for a joint injury due to sprain or trauma is too early and full recovery of the articular structure is not permitted. These structures tend to cause chronic phlogistic reactions with a tissue hypertrophy mechanism. The reactions are authentic neoformations which act on articular mechanics by reducing function and are the cause of a painful symptomatology.

A period of rest followed by gradual return to activity is often the best treatment.

12.3
The Hip

The hip joint is used in all types of sports activities, but it is in athletics and in cycling that it undergoes the most use, and overuse injuries are therefore particularly frequent in these sports. The injuries can lead to an impingement, which manifests itself in the form of the so-called *herniation pit.*

A localized hyperplastic reaction of the articular synovial membrane can determine erosion of the

---

[1]C. Faletti, MD, Radiology and MRI Service, Institute of Sports Medicine, Via Filadelfia 88, 10137 Turin, Italy
[2]N. De Stefano, MD, Radiology and MRI Service, Institute of Sports Medicine, Via Filadelfia 88, 10137 Turin, Italy

subchondral bone, which may cause hip pain directly over the anterior surface of the femoral neck and on the greater trochanter area.

Stress pain, functional deficiencies, and the "snapping joint" sensation are the most notable symptoms and are evident particularly frequently in patients with a history of sports activities on a competitive level. Radiologically, a small, well-defined area of osteorarefaction with discontinuity of the cortical profile is observed in a typical location, this being an indication of synovial penetration in a bone site (Fig. 12.1). This radiolucent area may occasionally enlarge, perhaps in relation to changing mechanics such as the pressure and abrasive effect of the overlying hip capsule and anterior muscles. Scintigraphy is usually negative but can sometimes be mildly positive (Fig. 12.2).

The most informative examination, which usually allows a precise diagnosis, is magnetic resonance imaging (MRI). It emphasizes a typical fluid collection pattern appearing as a low signal intensity area in the T1-weighted sequences and a high signal intensity area in the T2-weighted sequences (Fig. 12.3).

Another cause of impingement in the hip joint is "*strategic osteophytosis*", so called because it is located in positions where articular functional overload of acetabular profile has occurred. This is not just a typical osteophyte; here we are dealing with oxycalcific metaplasia of the capsular attachment at the coxofemoral level. The suspected pathology is linked to the functional limitation of limb abduction and flexion.

The X-ray examination in anteroposterior (AP) projection does not emphasize alterations, while the axial projection of the hip can demonstrate this type of osteophyte (Fig. 12.4). Computed tomography (CT) and MRI give two different topographic images of the osteophyte. Above all, they can define the phe-

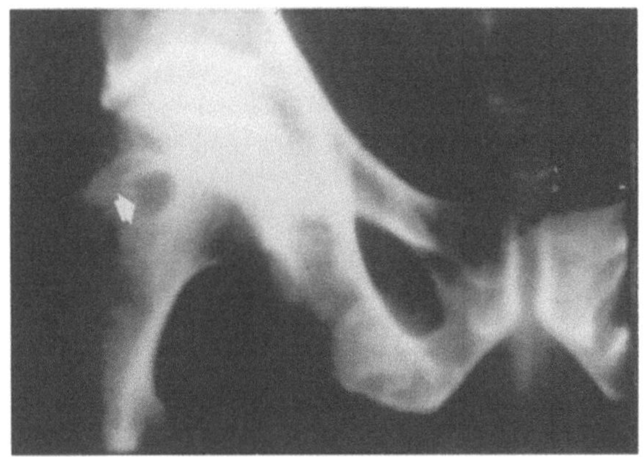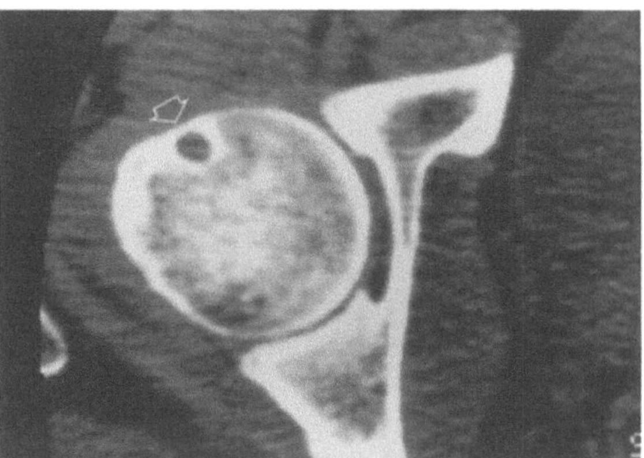

A
B

Fig. 12.1. A AP plain-film projection shows a lytic bone area at the level of the femoral head (*arrow*), well evident also on CT examination (**B**) at the level of capsular insertion (*open arrow*). *AP*, anteroposterior

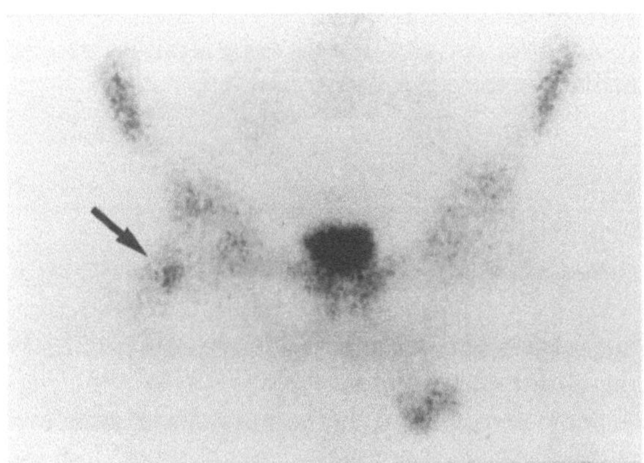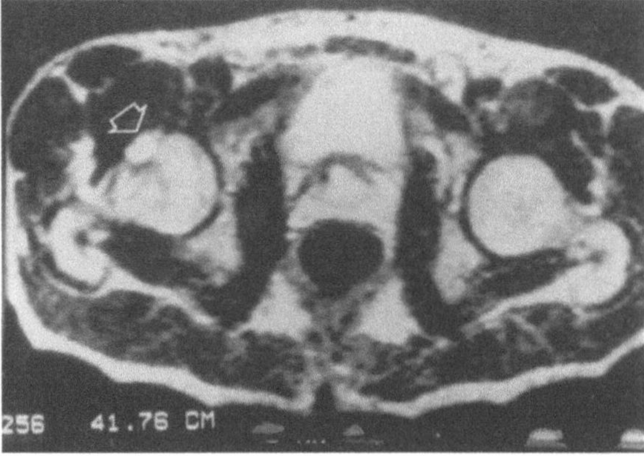

Fig. 12.2. Increased radionuclide uptake in the right hip (*arrow*)

Fig. 12.3. MRI: T2-weighted image in axial plane shows a regular area of high signal intensity at the level of the femoral head as if in presence of fluid collection (*arrow*)

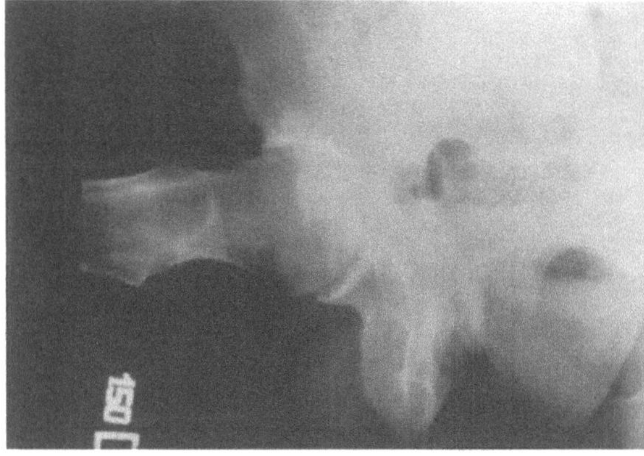

Fig. 12.4. Axial plain-film projection of the hip in which a small anterior osteophytic ridge of the acetabular profile, occurring at the point of capsular insertion, is observed

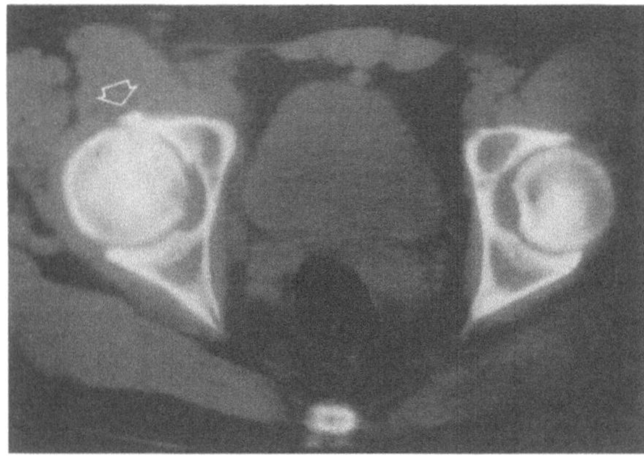

Fig. 12.5. CT evaluation of the same patient as in Fig. 12.4 in which the oxycalcific metaplasia, occurring on the anterior portion of the articular acetabular profile, is confirmed (*arrow*)

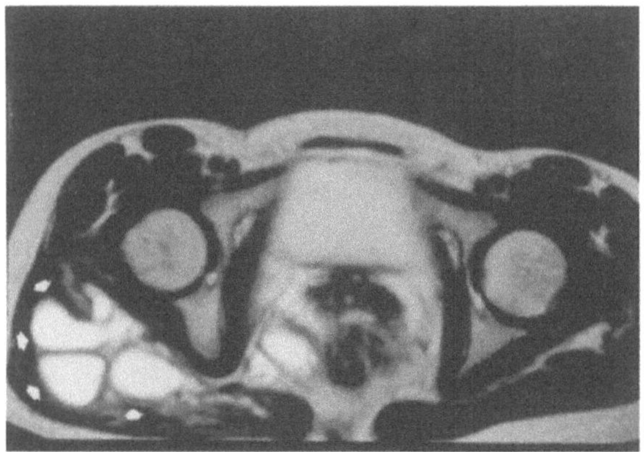

Fig. 12.6. MRI image on axial plane using a T2-weighted sequence. The fluid distension of the iliopectineal bursa, secondary to serous effusion due to phlogistic event of capsular structures, is well evident (*arrows*)

nomenon of impingement linked to articular effusion and synovial hyperplasia exerted in the articular capsule by the osteophyte, which effects flexion and abduction (Fig. 12.5).

In some cases, the situation is complicated by extended inflammation of the ileopsoas serous bursa, which in turn increases the severity of functional limitations. Resolution of the phlogistic process can improve joint function.

Both CT and MRI are able to emphasize bursal distension, defining precisely its boundaries and its relationship to the articular cavity. They are especially useful in monitoring the healing process and rehabilitation (Fig. 12.6).

12.4
The Knee

The knee joint presents a variety of pathologies that can be traced back to the impingement syndrome. These pathologies are especially frequent in sporting activities and are directly linked to movements typically associated with volleyball, basketball, and skiing. These types of syndromes are prevalent in the anterior compartment of the knee involving *Hoffa's adipose body*, the *medial synovial plica*, and the *infra-patellar plica* or supporter ligament of Hoffa's adipose body.

The *thickness of Hoffa's body*, which is secondary to stromal hypertrophy effects an important impingement between patella and femoral trochlea during knee flexion and extension. This may provoke a phlogistic process in the richly vascularized adipose tissue and consequently may lead to symptoms in the central and retropatellar areas. Effusion is unlikely, and if provoked will only be minimal.

Plain radiography, arthrography and ultrasound (US) are not able to recognize these changes. CT shows a thickening of the stromal component in Hoffa's adipose body, yet not in a direct fashion. It is MRI that has allowed the study and codification of this syndrome. In T1-weighted sagittal images, hyperplasia with low signal intensity in the apex of Hoffa's body is observed, indicating phlogistic thickening (acute inflammation; Fig. 12.7). In the T2-weighted sequence, or better still in the "fat suppression" sequences (STIR), this area shows high signal intensity, indicating a phlogistic process in the active phase (Fig. 12.8).

The articular capsule in the knee is subdivided into various chambers. Contact among these chambers is restricted by septa which are covered by the

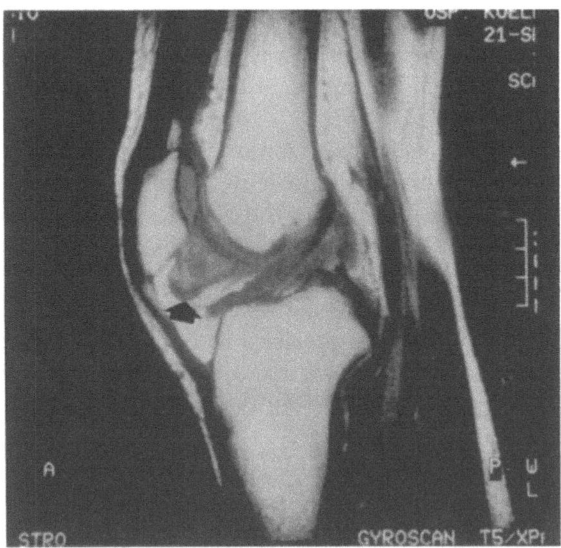

Fig. 12.7. MRI T1-weighted sequence on sagittal plane in which we observe a low signal intensity in the apical portion of Hoffa's body, between the patellar and femoral joint surfaces, corresponding to a hyperplastic process. This indicates the inflammatory reaction of the adipose body due to the friction between the joint surfaces (*arrow*)

synovial membrane. The morphology, the course, and the thickness of these septa may differ physiologically without having any influence on articular mechanics under normal conditions. In situations of particular "overuse," especially in sports such as volleyball, they can undergo hyperplasia and then inflammation. The most common cases involve the medial patellar synovial fold (*medial patellar plica*). Because of its longitudinal course and because it is a particular attachment location, when it undergoes hyperplasia it exerts initial compression and erosion on the anteromedial articular trochlear surface, provoking an authentic case of impingement syndrome.

The symptomatology consists of medial parapatellar pain and a snapping sensation when flexing and extending the knee. This occurs without any significant synovial reaction. Depending on its location, this pathology may be confused with a meniscal syndrome or with medial patellar hyperpressure. Diagnostic imaging seems indispensable in the identification of this type of syndrome. Sometimes, in situations of joint pain in the knee, synovial fold syndrome can represent a "simple" diagnosis. Only in chronic cases is it possible to spot a "sulcus" on the outline of the medial femoral condyle in the axial projection of the patellofemoral joint using standard radiograms. It is easier to spot the medial patellar fold in the same projection while performing arthrography (Fig. 12.9).

The diagnosis of synovial fold hypertrophy is a domain of CT and more recently MRI. On CT, in the various sections, it is characterized by thickening

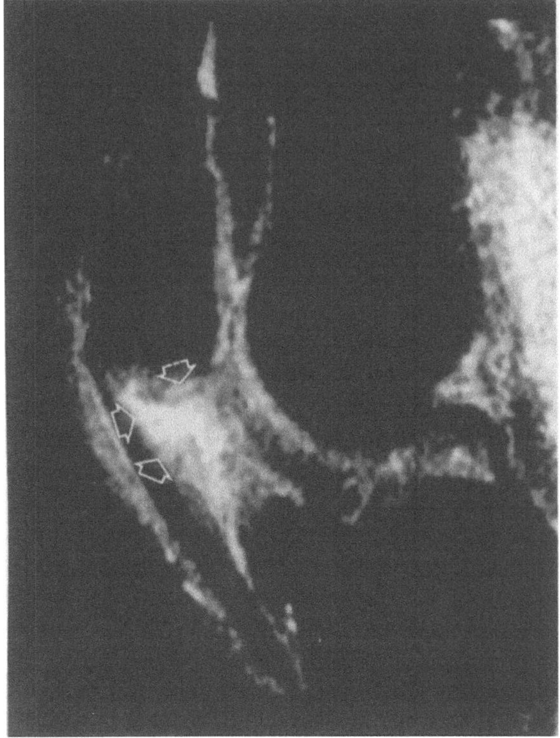

Fig. 12.8. In the same patient as in Fig. 12.7, when using an MRI STIR SE sequence, the area assumes the signal hyperintensity of an inflammatory process (*arrows*)

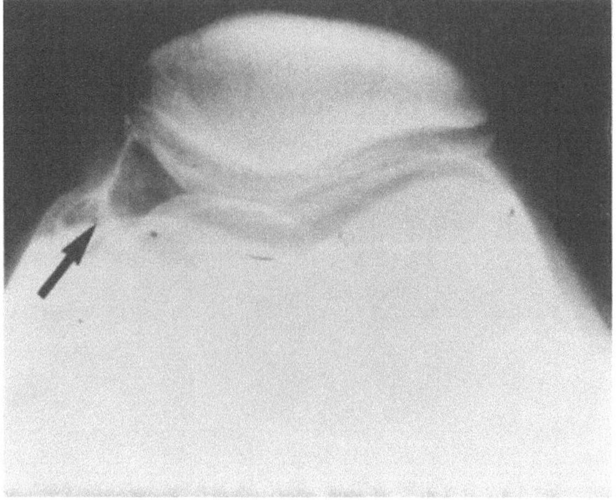

Fig. 12.9. Arthrography of the knee. The axial projection of the patella shows the thickening of the medial parapatellar synovial fold (*arrow*)

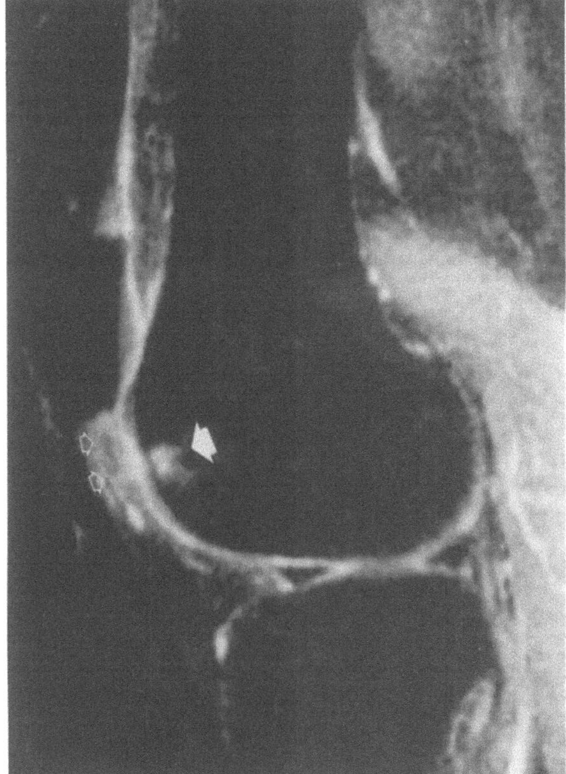

Fig. 12.10. MRI STIR SE sequence on sagittal plane that depicts the presence of a thickened synovial fold (*open arrows*) with a corresponding cartilaginous irregularity. Furthermore, an edemators reaction area at the level of the subchondral bone of the medial femoral condyle is present (*arrow*)

It is difficult to find a clinical regimen for such situations because their occurrence is not isolated to any specific sporting discipline and they come as a clinical surprise during the course of assessment through both diagnostic imaging and arthroscopy.

Only recently, with CT and MRI, have doctors been able to spot such a structure and study its pathology.

In CT this structure presents itself in the various sections as a small area of nodular-like hypodense

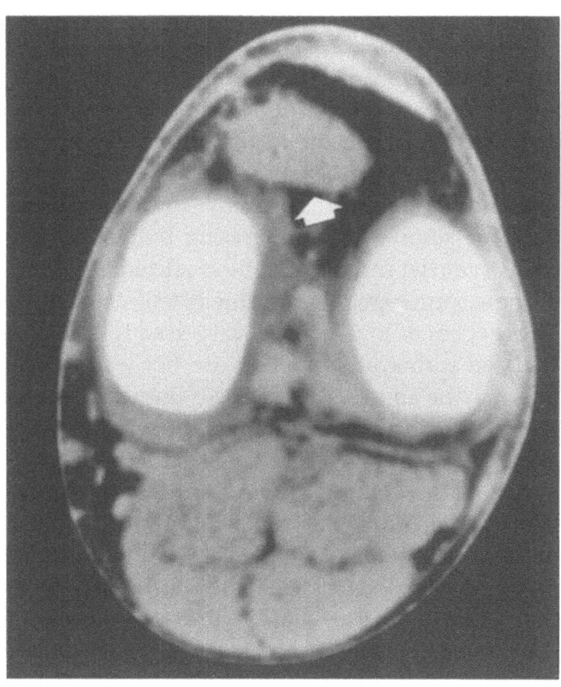

Fig. 12.11. CT section depicting an infrapatellar synovial fold hypertrophy represented by an anterior pseudonodular area with moderately irregular hypodense boundaries (*arrow*)

and hypodensity. During tomodensitometric examination it is shown through both synovial and cartilaginous reactions in which impingement with the femoral trochlea exists. In MRI T1-weighted sequences, the plica appears as distinctly hypointense. In the T2-weighted sequence, it is thickened with a thin peripheral hyperintense halo in the cartilaginous area in addition to morphological irregularity, and it is possible to assess edema in the corresponding subchondral bone during STIR sequences (Fig. 12.10).

Hoffa's adipose body also maintains its position and its functional status thanks to the presence of the *infrapatellar ligament*. This ligament extends from the apex of the adipose body to the femoral intercondylar area where it immediately inserts itself in the front of the anterior cruciate ligament. In some specific situations of functional overload or distortion in which the knee-stabilizing structures are involved, this ligament may become hypertrophic and in turn may provoke impingement syndrome.

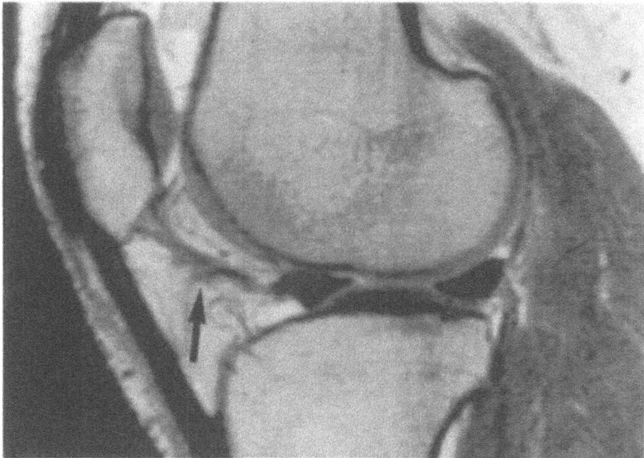

Fig. 12.12. Arthro-MRI (sagittal plane) clearly demonstrates the presence of an anterior central nodular formation extending from Hoffa's adipose body and corresponding to a hypertriphic infrapatellar synovial fold (*arrow*)

accumulation located anteriorly and medially in Hoffa's adipose body (Fig. 12.11). It is MRI that has permitted more accurate study of the ligament. With T1 weighting in the sagittal plane (especially using paramagnetic endoarticular contrast medium), the ligament presents itself as a thin band traveling from the front to the back and from the bottom to the top starting from the apex of Hoffa's body (Fig. 12.12). Whether in T1- or T2-weighted sequences with regular profile, its cuff-shaped thickening is associated with decisive hypointensity. It may also be associated with articular effusion or a reaction having the characteristics of fibrosis of the neurovascular structures contained in Hoffa's body.

In both traumatic and degenerative pathologies, articular effusion is the most common symptom of joint damage. Whether direct or distortive, synovial reaction to trauma is a common occurrence and can often be resolved by eliminating the cause. Sometimes synovial reaction can be localized and become chronic, provoking impingement and causing pain. These types of localizations vary greatly and are associated with symptoms that are not well definable and may be confused with those linked to pathologies of other articular structures, such as the menisci and the cartilage covering the articular joint.

Synovial cysts, though rare, represent a possible cause of functional deficiency and must be detected because the problem can be resolved only by means of surgery. Diagnostic imaging allows detection of the lesion and also enables the morphology and the dimensions to be assessed. CT was the first noninvasive diagnostic method to accomplish this task.

Once considered rare and of uncertain origin, synovial cysts can now be accurately assessed. The anterior area between the articular plane and Hoffa's adipose body represents the most frequent location, although intercondylar location on the central pivot, either between the two cruciate ligaments or between the posterior cruciate ligament and capsule should

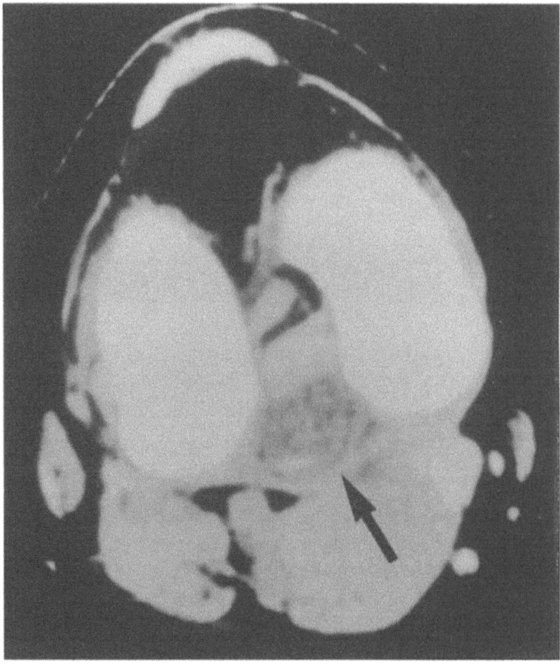

Fig. 12.13. CT examination of the knee depicting a non-homogeneous hypodense nodular area relative to a pseudocystic lesion arising from the synovia between the posterior cruciate ligament and the capsule (*arrow*)

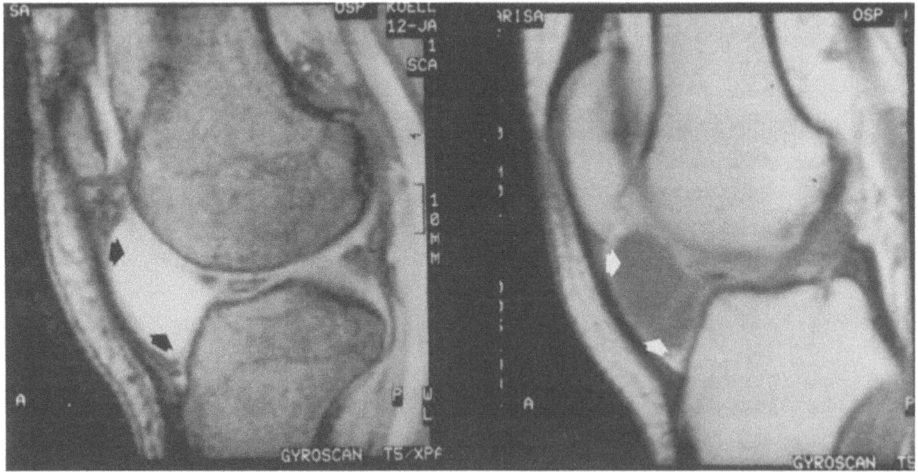

Fig. 12.14. MRI examination of the knee. A cystic lesion in Hoffa's body appears as a hyperintense area on T2-weighted images (*black arrows*) and as a hypointense area on T1-weighted images (*white arrows*)

not be excluded, because the cysts may originate from the synovial membrane covering these structures. In both cases, even if it maintains a certain elasticity, by occupying space the cyst exerts compression on the structures that are related to flexion and extension (Fig. 12.13).

MRI is extremely sensitive when it comes to detecting these formations. Because of the signal characteristics in all the typical sequences for tissues of synovial origin, it allows identification of the formation's origins (Fig. 12.14).

Linked to running, *iliotibial band friction syndrome* involving the lateral and proximal portions of the knee may occur. This ligament represents the last preinsertional segment of the tensor muscle of the fascia lata which extends from the iliac crest to the tibia, where it inserts itself at the level of Gerdy's tubercle (antero-lateral tibial tubercle).

Sporting activities that require repetitive flexion and extension of the knee and put weight on the lateral portion of the joint can create irritation, which may lead to inflammatory reactions. Painful symptomatology is quite common and involves the external part of the joint surface of the knee, which is about 2 cm above the joint space. Based upon the origins of the symptoms and their frequency, a clinical system of classification with four grades, ranging

from pain that arises only after running to pain which makes running impossible, has been proposed.

Through medical examination we are able to easily recognize this syndrome. However, as there is a possibility of confusion with other causes of lateral pain, such as lateral meniscal pathology, femorotibial and femoropatellar pathologies, and that of the popliteal tendon, diagnostic imaging can both rule out the above-mentioned pathologies and detect changes of the iliotibial ligament. During CT examination, the ligament presents itself as a thickened structure surrounded by a halo of hypodensity which is indicative of a phlogistic reaction (Fig. 12.15). With MRI we have been able to detect this type of pathology, unequivocally distinguishing the hypointense fibrosis of the ligament from the inflammatory-type hyperintense halo in axial T2-weighted sequences.

12.5
The Ankle

Bone impingement in the ankle is a pathological entity noted a decade ago, thanks to easy identification by standard radiological examination. In contrast (even though first described in 1942 by Wolin, who called it meniscoid syndrome), the syndrome in which the soft tissues of the joint conflict with each other has only recently been correctly classified, thanks to the advent of arthroscopic techniques. This has been possible through the wide diffusion of participation in sporting activities on both amateur and professional levels, combined with considerable improvement of radiological imaging methods and increased sensitivity in regard to the "smaller" problems in the field of sports traumatology. It is the development and diffusion of surgical techniques such as arthroscopy of the ankle that have allowed physicians to more easily detect and treat this type of pathology.

The root of anterolateral impingement syndrome is usually the occurrence of a distortion due to overuse regarding plantar inversion and flexion as well as of an associated lesion in the tibiofibular and anterior talofibular ligaments. Since these lesions are sectional and incomplete, natural evolution leads to the early disappearance of pain without any residual instability. However, if the reparative process is disturbed by repetitive stress due to premature mobilization, chronic inflammation of the fibrous-scar tissue will occur and will lead to hypertrophy

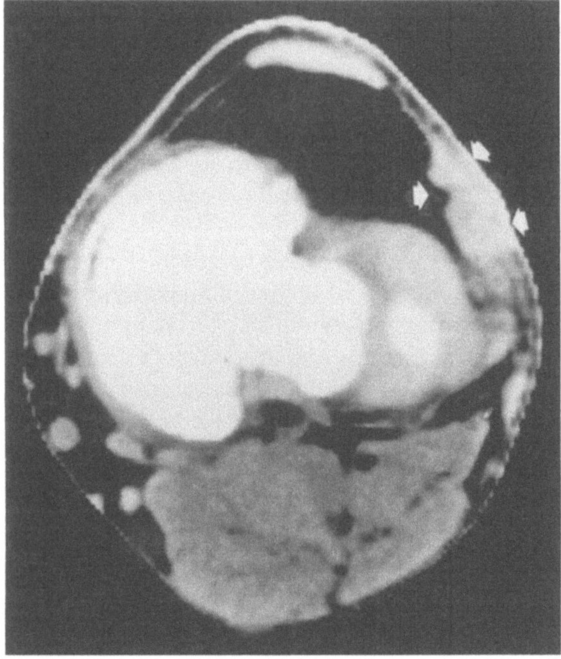

Fig. 12.15. CT examination of the knee depicting a thickened iliotibila ligament with a slight hypodense ring due to an inflammatory reaction (*arrows*)

associated with reactive hyperplastic synovitis. As time passes, these exuberant reparative processes cause the formation of a lamina of scar tissue which tends to insert itself between the outermost portion of the talar dome and the corresponding peroneal articular surface during dorsiflexion of the foot. The impingement that arises is the cause of chronic pain and is sometimes accompanied by a snapping joint sensation.

On arthroscopy the detectable macroscopic aspect is a yellowish-white band of tissue a few millimeters thick with free and irregular margins. This tissue travels towards the talar dome and, when cut, has a slightly denser consistency than synovial membrane.

Sometimes, however, the arthroscope detects the presence of a denser meniscus-like tissue which the histologist sees as cartilaginous shoots that have a more defined fascicular structure and which are probably residues of the injured ligament that originate with the syndrome. Through contrast medium administration, (arthrography and arthro-CT), instrumental diagnostic techniques have been able to detect this entity. Recently, it has been correctly assessed by means of MR.

The possibility of carrying out sequences with high intrinsic contrast (the gradient-echo T2-weighted sequences and the STIR sequences with short interpulse time and selective nulling of the medullary adipocyte component) allows correct identification of hypertrophic synovial tissue by means of thin-layer multiplanar assessment. During these sequences, MRI demonstrates a lamellar synovial coin shape in the classic hypointense anterolateral recess, contrasting with the normal

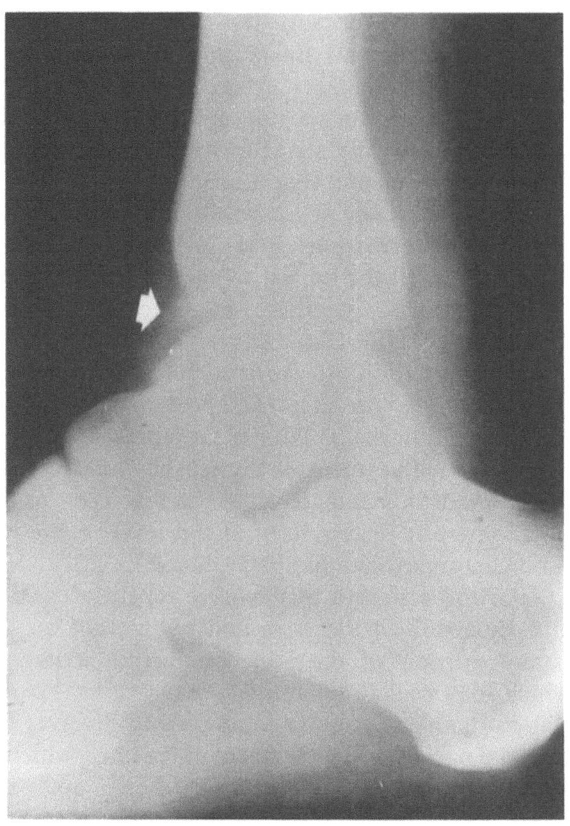

Fig. 12.17. Lateral plain-film projection of the ankle. At the level of capsular insertion on the anterior profile of the tibia, the initial stages of osteophytosis are present (*arrow*)

hyperintensity of the synovial fluid. In addition, such imaging allows for exclusion of the presence of post-traumatic alterations in the osteochondral profile of the tibiotalar and fibulotalar joints (Fig. 12.16).

Arthroscopic excision leads to complete clinical resolution without any evidence of residual instability.

In soccer players, manifestation of exostotic formations on the dorsal region of the foot is common. This may occur at the anterior portion of the tibia the cranial part the talus and the navicular bone. These exostoses are the result of microtraumas due both to contact and to repetitive movements.

The factors responsible for painful syndromes linked to forced dorsal flexion include calcific metaplasia of the anterior capsular profile of the tibia. This is responsible for erosion of the cartilage that covers the talar dome. The consequence is reactive arthrosynovitis followed by painful symptoms.

Clinical diagnosis is facilitated by detection of the osteophytic formation responsible for impingement during the X-ray examination (Fig. 12.17). However, it is MRI that, in addition to detecting osteophytes,

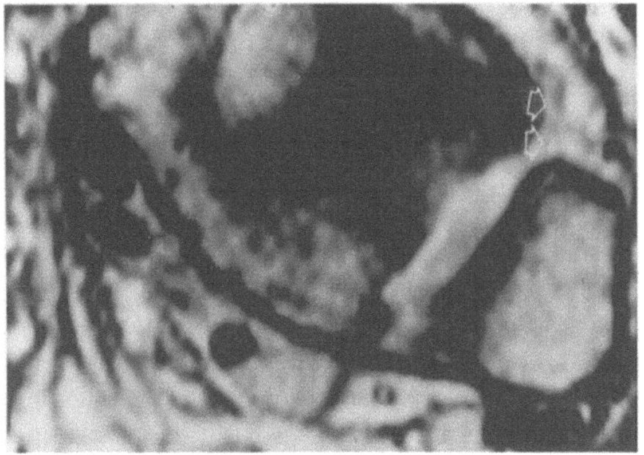

Fig. 12.16. MRI GE T2-weighted image on axial plane of the ankle demonstrates an anterolateral synovial thickening appearing as meniscus-shaped offshoots (*arrows*). *GE*, gradient echo

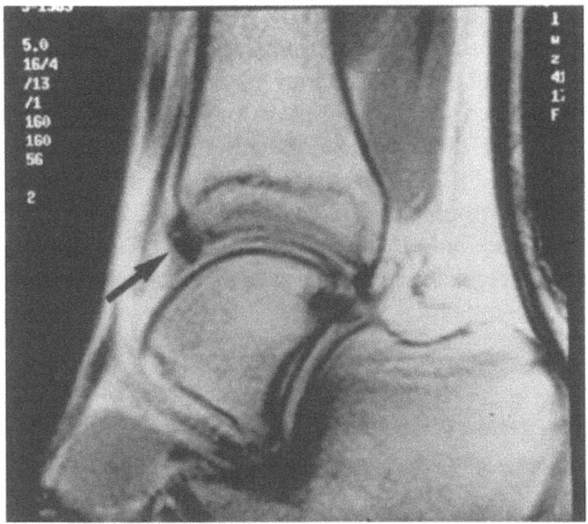

Fig. 12.18. In the same patient as in Fig. 12.17, when using a sagittal T1-weighted sequence, anterior oxycalcific metaplasia in the capsular insertion area with inflammatory capsular distension is observed (*arrow*)

also detects synovial reaction, above all the alterations of the subchondral bone that are the real cause of the pain (Fig. 12.18).

It is also possible to have *posterior impingement* with a pathology similar to that of anterior impingement. In this case, impingement is linked to plantar hyperflexion with contact between the posterior profile of the tibia and the talus. Although also common in soccer and in high jumping, this type of impingement syndrome is known as dancer's heel because of its frequency in dancing.

This syndrome involves the posterior zone consisting of the sulcus of the hallucis longus flexor tendon with its two tubercles, medial and lateral, and the possible presence of an os trigonum. When submitted to overuse, these structures may undergo a phenomenon of hyperplasia with secondary inflammation.

Diagnosis is not always easy, and above all it is difficult to assess the severity of the lesion and the structures involved, even for therapeutic purposes. In the lateral projection, X-ray examination can detect the presence of an os trigonum with an irregular profile and minor geodic reaction (Fig. 12.19). CT and particularly MRI can provide useful information regarding the various components of the ankle.

T2-weighted and fast field echo (FFE) T2-weighted sequences, in both sagittal and axial planes, are able to detect both synovial reactions and the signal alteration of skeletal components and carti-

lage, especially in the posterior portion of the talus (Fig. 12.20).

Physical therapy using specific suitable corrective tools and weight modification has led to favorable results in the treatment of both anterior and posterior impingement syndromes. Only in extreme cases is it necessary to resort to surgical intervention, which is usually arthroscopic.

MRI has proved useful and has found a vast field of applications in the area of sports pathology dealing with *impingement of the sinus tarsi*. This important anatomic area serves a double function with regard to joint mechanics in the ankle. The ligaments

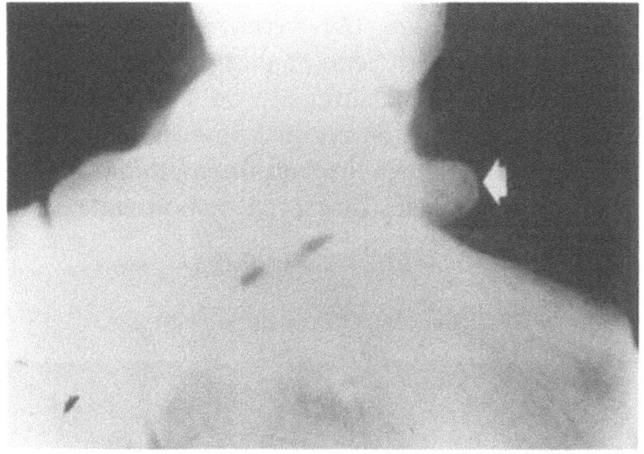

Fig. 12.19. Lateral plain-film projection of the ankle in which the presence of an os trigonum, with irregular borders and an ongoing initial sclerogeodic reaction, is observed (*arrow*)

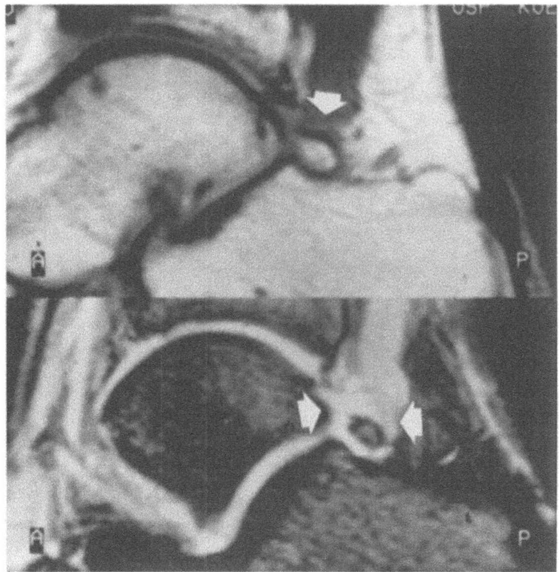

Fig. 12.20. MRI T1- and T2-weighted sequences on sagittal plane in which a synovial reaction involving the joint between the os trigonum and the talus is observed (*arrows*)

and the neurovascular structures contained in the sinus tarsi allow proper stabilization of the subtalar joint, by acting as a pivot, and play an active role in the proprioceptive reflexes of the joint itself.

Occasionally, a small synovial bursa is found in the peripheral part of the sinus, and sometimes a synovial recess, projecting from the posterior subtalar anterior to the sinus tarsi, is also present.

If inflammation or microtrauma due to biomechanical overload occurs, these structures may turn into pseudocystic hyperplasia which will affect the contents of the sinus tarsi. Compression on the ligaments and neurovascular tract causes stimulation of the proprioceptive receptors and therefore impingement of the sinus tarsi.

MRI demonstrates the presence of cystic or lobular formations with regular margins, which appear with medium signal intensity on T1-weighted and hyperintense on T2-weighted images (Fig. 12.21). Differential diagnosis includes hematoma and synovial sarcoma, which, however, demonstrate a more marked bone reaction.

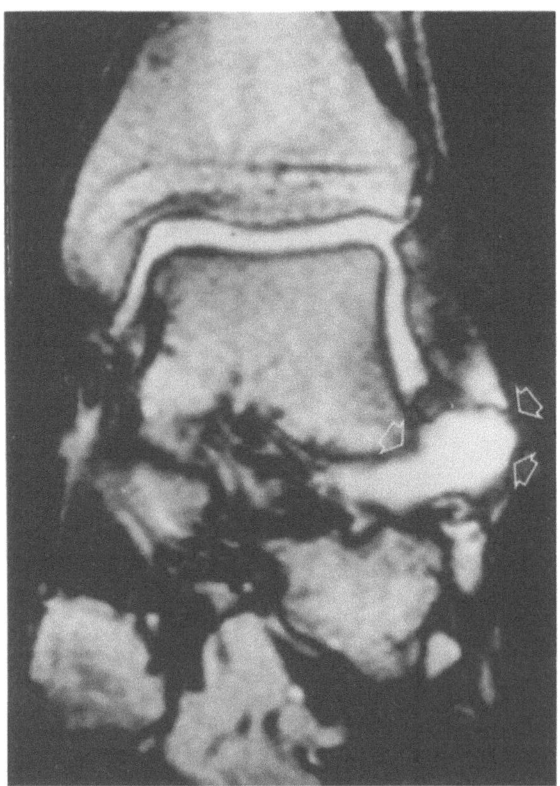

Fig. 12.21. MRI GE T2-weighted image of the ankle in coronal plane. A cystic reaction, due to synovial inflammatory events, appears as a hyperintense area at the level of the sinus tarsi (*arrows*)

Impingement syndrome of the sinus tarsi may also be caused by inflammation of the adipose tissue within the sinus. This may be characteristic of systemic rheumatic diseases or may be a consequence of severe distortion of the mid-foot which causes cellulo-adipositis, increased edema, and consequent compression of the subtalar ligaments.

The advent of "fat suppression" sequences in MRI has increased diagnostic reliability in the assessment of the sinus tarsi.

Suggested Reading

Hip

Crabbe JP, Martel W, Matthews LS (1992) Rapid growth of femoral herniation pit. AJR Am J Roentgenol 159:1038

Dihlmann W (1981) Koxale Computertomographie (KCT). ROFO 135:333

Dihlmann W (1982) CT analysis of the upper end of the femur: the asterisk sign and ischemic bone necrosis of the femoral head. Skeletal Radiol 8:251–258

Nokes SR, Vogler JB, Spritzer CE, et al. (1989) Herniation pits of the femoral neck: appearance at MR imaging. Radiology 172:231

Pitt MJ, Graham AR, Shipman JH, et al. (1982) Herniation pit of the femoral neck. AJR Am J Roentgenol 138:1115

Resnick D, Niwayama G (1988) Diagnosis of bone and joint disorders, 2nd edn. Saunders, Philadelphia

Knee

Burk DL, Dalinka MK, Kanal E, et al. (1988) Meniscal and ganglion cysts of the knee: MR evaluation. AJR Am J Roentgenol 150:331–336

Conway WF, Hayes CW, Loughran T, et al. (1991) Cross-section imaging of the patellofemoral joint and surrounding structures. Radiographics 11:195

Deutsch A, Resnick D, Dalinka M, et al. (1981) Synovial plicae of the knee. Radiology 141:627

Lupi L, Bighi S, Cervi PM, et al. (1990) Arthrography of the plica syndrome and its significance. Eur J Radiol 11:15

Murayama S, Hines MR, Manzo RP, et al. (1991) MR imaging of synovial cysts of the knee. Appl Radiol 3:27

Noble CA (1980) Iliotibial band friction syndrome in runners. Am J Sports Med 8:232

Passariello R, Masciocchi C, Fascetti E, et al. (1992) Computed tomography of the knee trauma. MRI and CT of musculoskeletal system: a text atlas. Williams and Wilkins, Baltimore, pp 395–403

Patel D (1978) Arthroscopy of the plica: synovial folds and their significance. Am J Sports Med 6:217

Stoller DW (1993) MRI in orthopaedics and sports medicine. Lippincott, Philadelphia

Tindel NL, Nisonson B (1992) The plica syndrome. Orthop Clin North Am 23:248–252

Zarins B, Nemeth VA (1985) Acute knee injuries in athletes. Orthop Clin North Am 16:285

Ankle

Beltran J (1990) The ankle and foot. In: Beltran J (ed) MRI msculoskeletal system. Lippincott, Philadelphia, pp 8.2–8.30

Berquist TH (1990) MRI of the musculoskeletal system, Raven, New York

Berquist TH (1992) Imaging of sports injuries. Aspen, Gaithersburg, pp 180–186

Chen Y (1985) Arthroscopy of the ankle joint. In: Watanabe M (ed) Arthroscopy of small joints. Igaku-Shoin, New York

Claustre J, Simon L, Allieu Y, et al. (1979) Le syndrome du tarse: existe-t-il? Rheumatologie 31:19–23

Deutsch AL (1992) Traumatic injury and osteonecrosis: MRI of the foot and ankle. Raven, New York, pp 75–109

Erickson SJ, Cox IH, Hyde JS, et al. (1991) Effect of tendon orientation on MR imaging signal intensity: a manifestation of the "magic angle" phenomenon. Radiology 181:389–392

Erickson SJ, Smith JW, Ruitz ME, et al. (1991) MR imaging of the lateral collateral ligament of the ankle. AJR Am J Roentgenol 156:131

Erickson SJ, Quinn SF, Kneeland JB, et al. (1990) MR imaging of the tarsal tunnel and related spaces: normal and abnormal findings with anatomic correlation. AJR Am J Roentgenol 155:323

Ferkel RD, Karzel RP, Del Pizzo W, et al. (1991) Arthroscopic treatment of anterolateral impingement of the ankle. Am J Sports Med 19:440–446

Golimbu CN (1992) Ankle and foot. In: Firooznia HF, Rafii M, et al. (eds) MRI and CT of the musculoskeletal system. Mosby Year Book, New York, pp 817–873

Guhl JF (1993) Foot and ankle arthroscopy, 2nd edn. Slack, Thorofare, NJ, pp 97–99

Kerr R, Frey C (1991) MR imaging in tarsal tunnel syndrome. J Comput Assist Tomogr 15:280

Kneeland JB, Macrandar S, Middleton WD, et al. (1988) MR imaging of the normal ankle: correlation with anatomic sections. AJR Am J Roentgenol 151:117

Liu SH, Mirzayan R (1993) Posteromedial ankle impingement. Arthroscopy 6:709–711

McCarroll JR, Schrader JW, Shelbourne KD, et al. (1987) Meniscoid lesions of the ankle in soccer players. Am J Sports Med 15:255–257

Meislin RJ, Rose DJ, Parisien JS, et al. (1993) Arthroscopic treatment of synovial impingement of the ankle. Am J Sports Med 21:186–189

Mink JH, Deutsch AL (1989) Occult cartilage and bone injuries of the ankle: detection, classification and assessment with MR imaging. Radiology 170:823–829

Nelson DW, DiPaola J, Colville M, et al. (1990) Osteochondritis dissecans of the talus and knee: prospective comparison of MRI and arthroscopic classification. J Comput Assist Tomogr 14:804

Stoller DW (1993) The ankle and foot. In: Stoller DW (ed) Magnetic resonance imaging in orthopaedics and sports medicine. Lippincott, Philadelphia, pp 373–510

Wechsler R, Schweitzer ME, Deely D, et al. (1993) Comparison of CT and MRI in detection and characterization of tarsal coalition. Radiology 189:135

Wolin I, Glassman F, Sideman S, et al. (1950) Internal derangement of the talofibular component of the ankle. Surg Gynecol Obstet 91:193–200

13 Nervous Diseases (Spinal and Peripheral Nerve Entrapments)

F. Rossi[1] and A. Barile[2]

CONTENTS

[1] F. Rossi, MD, Department of Radiology, Sports Science Institute, Italian Olympic Committee, Via S. Agatone Papa 34, 00165 Rome, Italy
[2] A. Barile, MD, Department of Radiology University of L'Aquila Collemaggio Hospital 67100 L'Aquila, Italy

13.1 Introduction

"Entrapment neuropathies," "canal syndromes," or "tunnel syndromes" are terms used to indicate chronic pathological conditions of a peripheral nerve secondary to compression or combined compression and traction exerted on an osteofibrous unextensible arch, orifice muscular notch, or aponeurotic structure. Though presenting peculiar anatomical and histologically differentiated structures which protect both the nerve and perineural connective tissue, the nerves lying in these narrow passages are vulnerable.

Different reactions are possible as a consequence of a compressive syndrome:

- Fibrosis and secondary adhesions among sheaths, epineurium, and bundles, leading to mechanical irritation
- Neural edema, creating conflict with the canal section leading to mechanical pressure
- Secondary decrease in intraneural circulation, leading to hypoxia, anoxia, and ischemia

The damage suffered by the nerve, depending on the compressive action, the duration, the frequency of repetition, and on the caliber and structure of the nerve, can be due to trauma (blunt, sharp, unique, or multiple), tumors, infection, metabolic and vascular diseases, etc. It may also be iatrogenic (cast). Predisposing factors are bone or muscular abnormalities.

The consequences of nerve compression inducing anatomical damage can be:

- Temporary functional alterations with loss of pulse transmission (neuropraxia)
- Axonal and sheath disruption with preservation of connective sheath (axonotmesis)
- Complete interruption of the nerve (neurotmesis)

Clinically, the damage is represented by hypoesthesia and palsy, as well as by tissue superexcitation which causes pain, paresthesia, and muscular tremor.

Depending on the anatomical site and type (motor, sensory, or mixed) of the affected nerve, there are different clinical findings, which, however, are common to all canal syndromes, such as pain, paresthesia, hypoesthesia, motor deficit, and mixed syndromes.

Diagnosis is predominantly based on clinical examination. Of great help, however, is the comparison with neurophysiological findings [electromyography (EMG) and nerve conduction study (NCS)] and the results of the different diagnostic imaging modalities used.

13.2
Peripheral Nerve Entrapments of the Superior Limb

13.2.1
Thoracic Outlet Compression Syndrome (Neurologic and Vascular)

Upper-extremity dysfunctions may be the result of compression of the brachial plexus or of the subclavian vessels.

"Thoracic outlet" refers to the area of the shoulder and thorax where the brachial plexus, together with the subclavian artery and vein, leaves the chest cavity, passing over the first rib and under the clavicle through the "scalenus triangle" to enter the axillary region.

Several well-outlined entities, according to the causative mechanism, have been defined: cervical rib syndrome, anterior scalenus syndrome, the costoclavicular syndrome, the hyperabduction syndrome (including the pectoralis minor syndrome). Combined syndromes are possible. Symptoms are characterized by upper-limb pain, weakness, fatigability, paresthesia, vascular insufficiencies, and secondary motor dysfunctions. The gravity of the symptoms is associated with the frequency, duration, and degree of the compression.

The syndrome has been described in tennis players, baseball pitchers, water polo players, swimmers, weight lifters, and pole-vaulters. Generally, athletes who sustain traction injuries to the upper limb and chest may exacerbate the symptoms.

Diagnostic examination, as well as screening for physical signs, includes routine chest, cervical spine, and shoulder rays in order to evaluate the presence of cervical ribs, the consequences of clavicular fracture, bridges between first and second ribs, and lesions such as tumors or space-occupying aneurysms

(Fig. 13.1). Arteriography, static or dynamic, and venography document compression, occlusion, or aneurysmal formation. Pulse and blood pressure measurements and Doppler studies aid in diagnosis. EMG and NCS evaluate the neurologic compression and differentiate it from other radiculopathies. Computed tomography (CT) may also be indicated as part of the diagnostic protocol. Magnetic resonance imaging (MRI) is preferred for evaluating any soft tissue injuries or abnormalities that may be present.

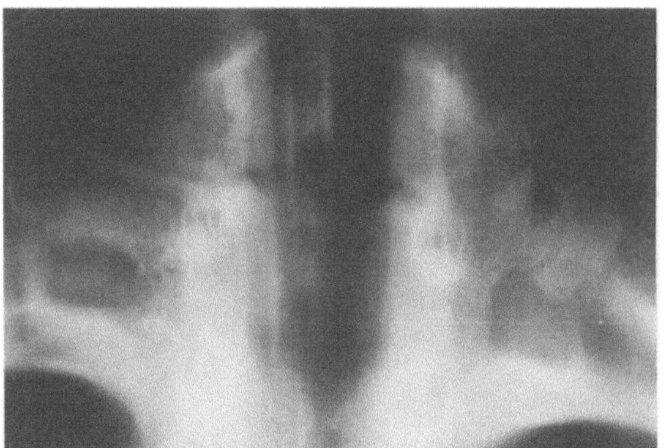

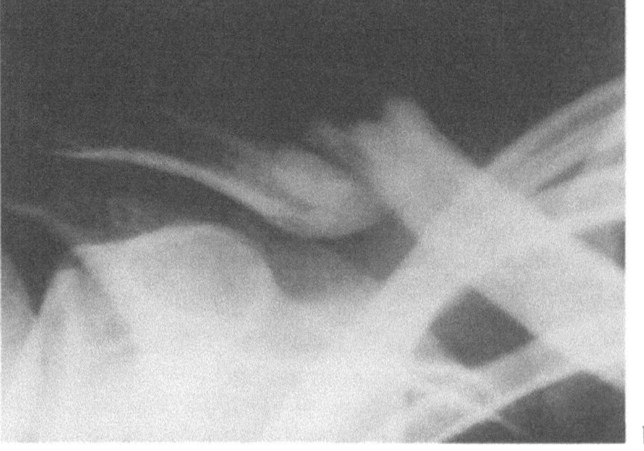

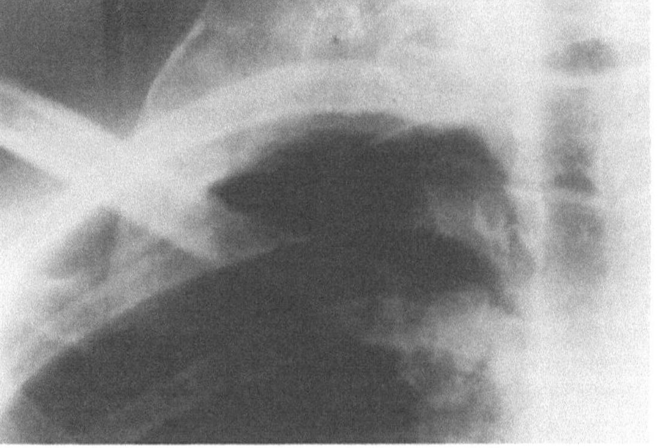

Fig. 13.1. **a** Cervical rib. **b** Clavicular fracture with wide separation of fragments. **c** Bone tumoral mass of the first rib

13.2.2
Suprascapular Nerve Entrapment Syndrome

The nerve originates from either C5 or C6 nerve roots or from the upper trunk of the brachial plexus, courses laterally, superiorly, and posteriorly, and enters the supraspinatus fossa via the suprascapular notch beneath the superior transverse scapular ligament. Here it gives off motor fibers to the supraspinatus muscle and sensory fibers to the acromioclavicular and glenohumeral joints. In the supraspinatus fossa, along the inferior surface of the muscle, the nerve with vessels runs laterally, curves around the base of the spine of the scapula, and enters the infraspinatus fossa through an osteofibrous canal, the spinoglenoid notch, which is often filled by the inferior transverse scapular ligament. After penetrating the infraspinatus fossa, the nerve with its branches arborizes into the muscle belly.

Anatomofunctional studies of the nerve during shoulder movements have led to identification of two critical zones as potential sites of injury: the suprascapular and the spinoglenoid notches. At these sites many different motions of the upper limb can induce compression and traction of the nerve. Cross-body adduction, forward flexion, maximal abduction, and external rotation have been found to place the nerve at greatest risk.

Entrapment at the suprascapular notch (anterior entrapment) will result in palsy of the common trunk of the nerve, explained by atrophy of both the supra- and infraspinatus muscle.

Entrapment at the spinoglenoid notch (posterior entrapment) manifests itself by isolated infraspinatus muscle atrophy, shoulder pain, and loss of strength in abduction and external rotation, resulting from palsy of the terminal branches of the nerve.

The suprascapular nerve entrapment syndrome has been described as a consequence of fracture of the scapula, surgical trauma, bony or soft-tissue pathologies, and mechanical irritation in individuals who work with arms above their head or abduct and rotate them externally. The syndrome has often been associated with sporting activities. Boxers, tennis players, and weight lifters are athletes who frequently suffer from this syndrome.

However, the athletes most frequently affected by posterior entrapment at the spinoglenoid notch are volleyball players. It is estimated that more than 20% of top-level players have a symptomatic isolated paralysis of the infraspinatus muscle of their dominant arm. These findings have been attributed to the re-

peated stress on the nerve during the cocking and follow-through phases of the arm during the serve, especially when performing the "floating service", which is capable of distort the course of the nerve.

Diagnosis is based primarily on the clinical findings, characterized by marked atrophy of the infraspinatus muscle without involvement of the supraspinatus, loss of external rotation strength, and uneven pain localized in the posterior and lateral aspects of the shoulder. EMG and NCS will confirm the diagnosis.

Routine X-ray and CT can provide information concerning scapular fractures (Fig. 13.2) or ossification or abnormality of ligaments and notches. MRI depicts tissue masses such as tumors, ganglion cysts (Fig. 13.3), or muscle traumatic lesions (Fig. 13.4) and dystrophy and conditions of muscular fat degeneration.

13.2.3
Supracondylar Process Syndrome

An atavistic bony spur, the supracondylar process, can arise from the anteromedial surface of the distal humerus shaft. Between the spur and the medial humeral condyle, a fibrous band may be present. In this fibro-osseous canal, the median nerve can be com-

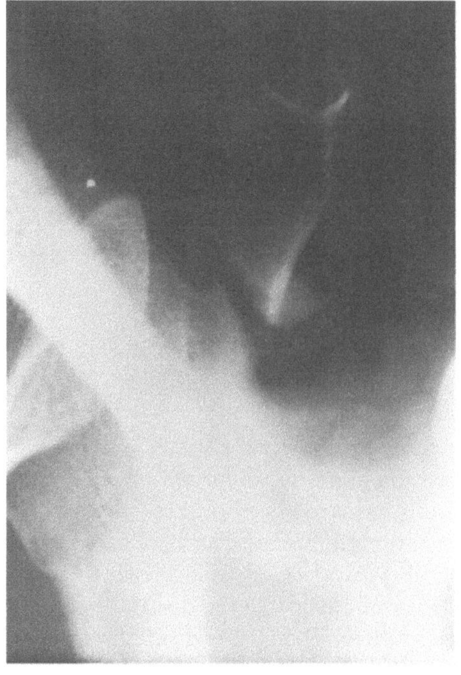

Fig. 13.2. Coracoid process and scapular fracture with separation of fragments

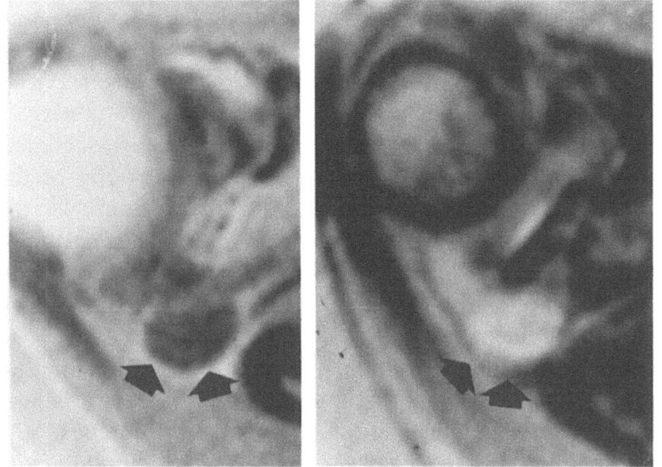

Fig. 13.3a,b. Ganglion cyst (*arrows*) at spino-glenoid notch that causes suprascapular nerve compression, well evident on axial **a** T1-weighted and **b** T_2-weighted images (WI)

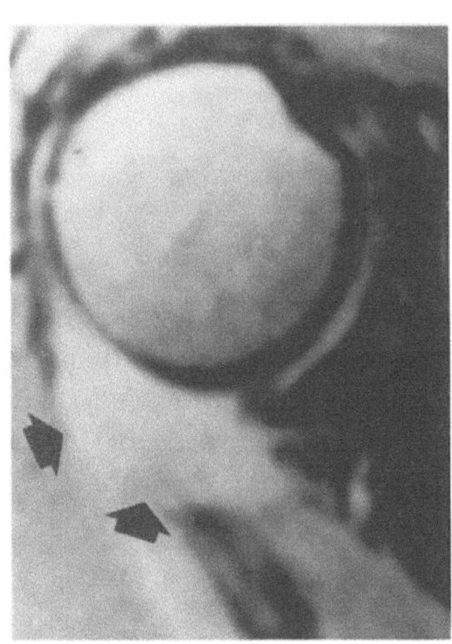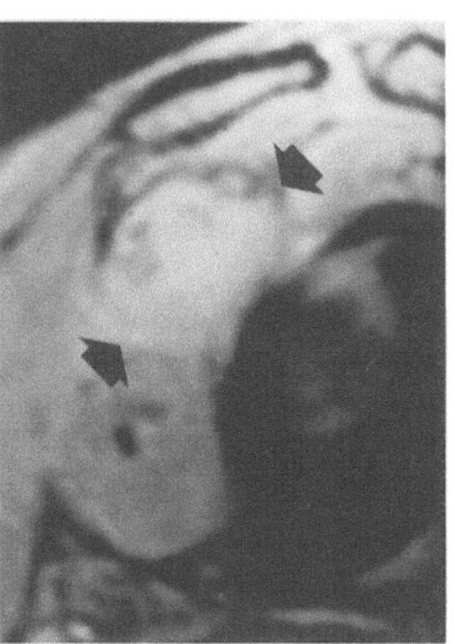

Fig. 13.4a,b. Suprascapular neuropathy provoked by compressive hematoma in isolated lesion of the infraspinatus muscle (*arrows*): axial (**a**) and sagittal (**b**) MRI, T2-WI

pressed, generating symptoms. A fracture of the spur may also be the cause of compression and its symptoms (Fig. 13.5). In slender patients, the spur can be palpated and the percussion produces a Tinel's sign, pain, and paresthesia in the median nerve territory.

13.2.4
Pronator Teres Muscle Syndrome

The median nerve leaves the cubital fossa traversing between the heads of the pronator teres muscle and the tendinous arch of the flexor digitorum superficialis muscles. Sensory and motor symptoms in the whole area of the median nerve result from its compression.

The syndromes has been observed in baseball, weight lifting, gymnastics, rowing, and sports where training programs for development of muscle strength are intense. Usually, there is pain in the

volar forearm pronator surface which worsens during activity involving repeated pronation movements with the elbow in extension.

Paresthesia occurs along the volar and dorsal surfaces of the hand, the palm, and several fingers. Symptoms may be elicited by resistance to forearm pronation and wrist flexion. EMG studies are seldom helpful in this syndrome. MRI may demonstrate a peculiar hypertrophic condition of the pronator teres muscle or possible intrinsic pathology (Fig. 13.6).

13.2.5
Anterior Interosseous Syndrome
(Kiloh-Nevin Syndrome)

The anterior interosseous nerve, the motor branch of the median nerve, can be compressed throughout its course in the forearm. Because of the anatomical

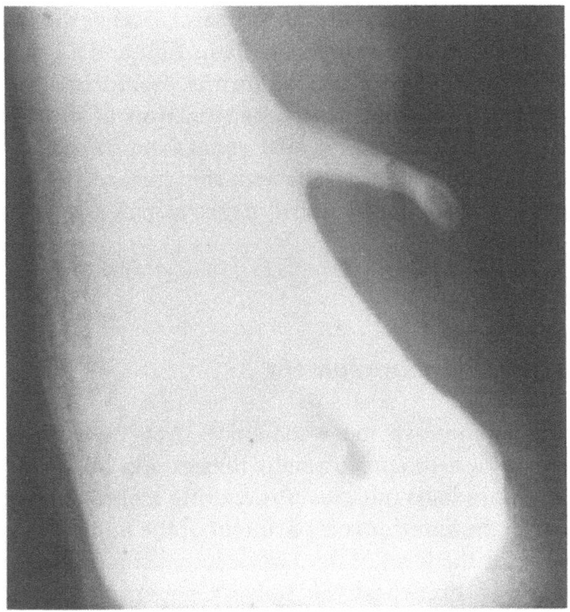

Fig. 13.5. Supracondylar process syndrome. Fracture of a long supracondylar humeral process

The ulnar nerve entrapment syndrome is a neuropathy observed in baseball pitchers, judokas, throwers, gymnasts, and weight lifters, in whom repetitive valgus stress of the elbow plays a key developmental role. Local direct or indirect traumas are often recalled as reasons for repetitive subluxation of the nerve and consequent inflammation and degeneration; osteoarthrosis and chronic lesions of the medial collateral ligament are reported. Hypertrophy of the flexor ulnaris heads inducing a secondary compression of the nerve can also occur in throwers and has been reported in long-distance skiers related to forceful repetitive turns.

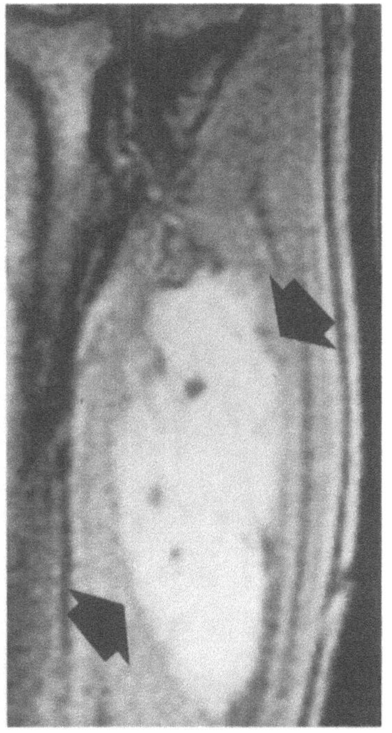
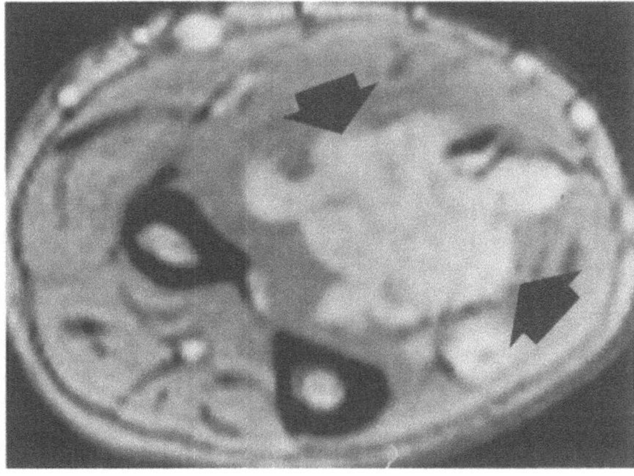

Fig. 13.6a,b. Pronator muscle syndrome due to soft tissue tumor (*arrows*) in a rugby player. Sagittal (a) and axial (b) MRI

relationship to the median nerve, sometimes this syndrome is not differentiated from the pronator teres syndrome. Kiloh-Nevin syndrome, however, is an entirely motor condition without any sensory deficit.

The symptoms involve the flexor pollicis longus, flexor digitorum profundus, and pronator quadratus muscles. The syndrome can be caused by a violent muscle contracture, a forearm fracture, local repetitive microtrauma provoked by excessive exercise, anomalous proximal forearm muscles, enlarged bursae, vasculopathy, etc. Exploration of the anterior interosseous nerve is recommended if spontaneous improvement is not apparent after 2 months.

The clinical findings comprise an inability to pinch thumb and index finger due to impaired flexion of the distal phalanges of the two fingers. Moreover, the subject cannot clench his fist.

13.2.6
Cubital Tunnel Syndrome (Flexor Carpi Ulnaris Muscle Syndrome)

The ulnar nerve leaves the sulcus behind the medial humeral epicondyle and curves between the humeral and ulnar heads of the flexor carpi ulnaris muscle connected by a tendinous arch (arcuate ligament) defining the entrance of the tunnel.

Generally, the subjects complain of pain and paresthesias in the ulnar half of the ring and little fingers. If compression is longstanding, sensory symptoms can occur, including clumsiness and weakness with wasting of muscle of the hand. The elbow flexion test, which consists of elbow hyperflexion for at least 2 min, often reproduces the symptoms.

EMG studies usually confirm and localize the level of ulnar nerve compression. Plain-film and CT studies may indicate signs of former fractures, elbow deformity, osteoarthrosis, calcification of the ligaments, etc. (Fig. 13.7). MRI appears to be the most effective in evaluating the articular surface, the joint space and its content, and neurovascular structure abnormalities.

13.2.7
Radial Nerve Entrapment

The radial nerve above the elbow innervates the triceps, extensor carpi radialis longus and brevis, and brachioradialis muscles. Proceeding from the posterior to the anterior compartment of the humerus, the nerve at the level of the radiocapitellar joint divides into two branches: the sensory superficial branch and the motor posterior interosseous branch.

Traumatic sequelae and osteoarthritic changes can cause symptoms. Strenuous segmentary muscular activities, especially continual elbow extension as in tennis, baseball, rowing, or throwing sports in which rotating movements of the forearm are performed, have been reported in association with entrapment syndromes of the radial nerve.

13.2.7.1
Superficial Branch Syndrome
(Cheiralgia Paresthetica)

Typically, the subject complains of paresthesias without weakness or atrophy secondary to compression in the tunnel region beneath the brachioradialis tendon. Pain – also during the night – burning sensations and other sensory disturbances are referred along the dorsal wrist, thumb and web space. Wearing clothes may be enough to induce paresthesias.

13.2.7.2
Supinator Syndrome (Radial Tunnel
Syndrome; Posterior Interosseous Nerve
Entrapment Syndrome)

The terminal motor branch of the radial nerve, the posterior interosseous branch, may be compressed when it passes under the tendinous arch of the supinator muscle, Frohse's arcade.

Multiple agents, such as trauma, tumors, inflammatory processes, and anatomical conditions, can

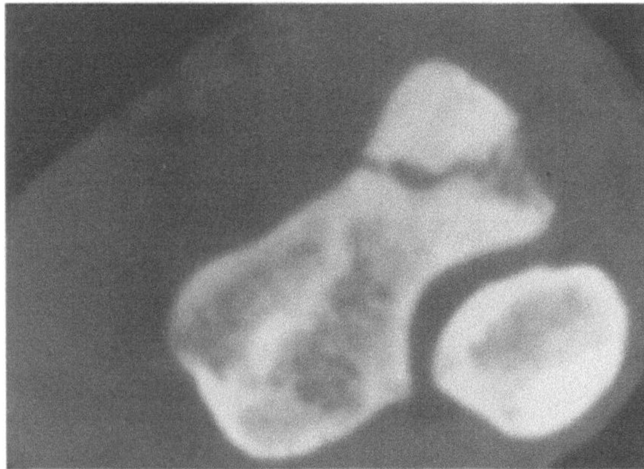

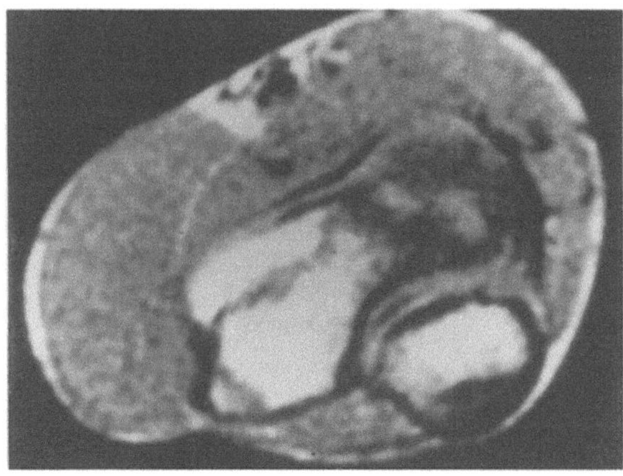

Fig. 13.7. a Degenerative modification of the elbow condyles most evident in the medial compartment. CT (**b**) and MRI (**c**) of epitrochlear fracture in a gymnast with clinical symptoms of cubital tunnel syndrome

compress the radial nerve in the supinator canal. Dynamic compression caused by muscular activity has become one of the most common etiologic factors.

Symptoms are characterized by deep pain in the posterior part of the forearm, followed by fist weakness and local pain on compression to the lateral humeral epicondyle. If the compression lasts longer, the hand takes on the appearance of a hanging hand, typical of radial nerve palsy.

Despite the characteristic clinical findings, the syndrome is often not recognized and diagnosed as radial epicondylitis with which it can manifest together.

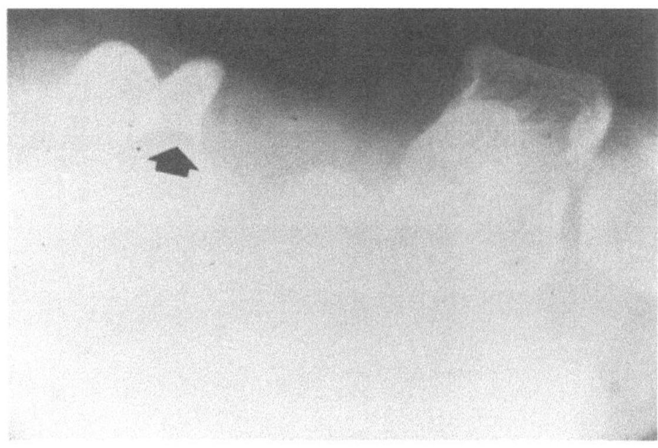

Fig. 13.8. Axial X-ray for the study of the carpal tunnel, where a fracture of the hook of the hamate (*arrow*) can be seen

13.2.8
Median Nerve Compression (Carpal Tunnel Syndrome)

The carpal tunnel syndrome is a chronic entrapment neuropathy reported in cyclists, tennis players, throwers, baseball pitchers, rowers, rock climbers, and rally drivers.

The carpal tunnel is a fibro-osseous canal bordered by the transverse carpal ligament (flexor retinaculum) volarly and the carpal bones dorsally. The transverse carpal ligament attaches to the navicular and trapezium radially and to the pisiform and hamate ulnarly. Nine flexor tendons, including the flexor pollicis longus, digitorum profundus, and digitorum superficialis, all lined by a synovial sheath, traverse the carpal tunnel along with the median nerve.

Prior to entering the tunnel, the nerve gives off sensory branches to the thumb, index finger, middle finger and the radial aspect of the ring finger, and a motor branch to the thenar muscles and to the first and second lumbricals.

Space reduction in the carpal tunnel, usually due to flexor tenosynovitis, can induce compression of the median nerve.

Any sports that involve prolonged wrist extension or repetitive flexion or grasping can provoke mechanical irritation and tenosynovitis of the flexor tendons.

Symptoms include numbness or tingling in the median sensory distribution. Frequently, patients complain of clumsiness and loss of dexterity. Intermittent pain and paresthesias often wake them from sleep.

Physical examination should include sensitivity, motor, and provocative testing. Provocative tests elicite a positive Phalen's sign (pain with maximal flexion of the wrist) and Tinel's sign (pain with percussion over the flexor retinaculum).

EMG can confirm the diagnosis, which must be as promptly as possible to avoid permanent nerve damage. Axial plain-film radiography with the hand in maximal dorsiflexion and the central beam angulated at 30°–40° so that it is directed into the volar surface of the wrist is particularly useful in visualizing bone fractures (Fig. 13.8). CT is helpful and sometimes necessary to obtain or clarify the diagnosis. Ultrasound (US) is very useful in the evaluation of flexor tendon tenosynovitis and allows dynamic evaluation of the carpal structures. MRI gives an optimal representation of the anatomy and its possible variations. It shows objective signs of the median nerve, including swelling as it enters the carpal tunnel, its flattening, the volar bowing of the flexor retinaculum, or the increase of its signal intensity on T2-weighted images. Moreover, nerve compression due to soft tissue pathologies or scar tissue is well defined with MRI (Fig. 13.9).

13.2.9
Ulnar Nerve Compression (Guyon's Canal Syndrome)

Guyon's canal is a triangular space between the pisiform bone and the hook of the hamate, roofed by the palmar fascia and the palmaris brevis muscle. The floor is made up of pisohamate and transverse carpal ligaments. At the canal, the nerve divides into a superficial and deep branch. The former supplies sensation to the ulnar palm and the ulnar skin of the fourth and fifth fingers. The latter innervates the hypothenar muscles, interosseous muscles, third

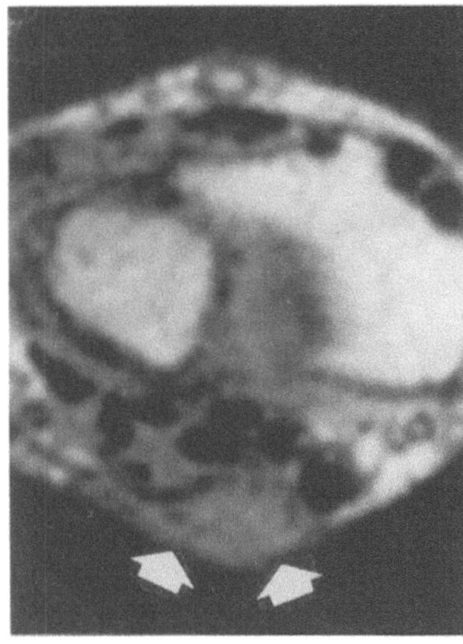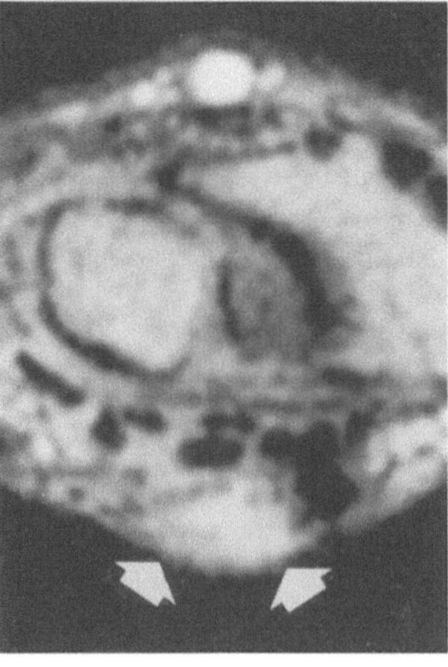

Fig. 13.9a,b. Median nerve compression due to scar tissue (*arrows*) well defined on axial T1-WI (**a**) and T2-WI (**b**)

and fourth lumbricals, and adductor pollicis and flexor pollicis brevis muscles. As a consequence, compression of the superficial branch produces motor and sensory symptoms, while compression of the deep branch causes motor symptoms alone.

The most common form of compression occurs at the terminal branch between the fibrous origin of the abductor and flexor muscles of the fifth finger and the pisohamate ligament against the hook of the hamate (pisohamate hiatus syndrome).

The causes can be intrinsic (ulnar artery aneurysms or thromboangiitis, synovial cysts, lipomas, rheumatoid sclerosis, etc.) or extrinsic (fracture of the hook of the hamate, fracture-luxation of the fifth metacarpal bone, fracture of the pisiform, fibrous sclerosis of the hypothenar perimisium, etc.).

Neuropathy has been reported in persons who use tools that press into the palm of their hands and results in motor weakness and wasting of intrinsic muscles. With a certain frequency, it is found in motorcyclists, bowlers, weight lifters, and long-distance cyclists, who experience constant pressure from handlebars.

The so-called handlebar palsy or cyclist's palsy is characterized by insidious onset of paresthesias in the fifth finger and the ulnar side of the fourth finger. The condition typically develops following heavy training or after a prolonged race. Nerve compression is caused by direct pressure over the hypothenar eminence as the rider supports the weight of the trunk on the handlebars. Hyperextension of the wrist is contributory. The lesion usually affects only the dominant extremity but may be present in both hands. The palsy (electrophysiological testing can help to differentiate it from a proximal ulnar nerve lesion) tends to resolve spontaneously with continuous use of several corrective measures, including well-padded cycling gloves, padded handlebars, correct frame size, correct distance from saddle to stem, and frequent changing of hand position on the handlebars. It the symptoms persist after several weeks in spite of the protective measures suggested, exploration of the nerve should be considered.

EMG is useful in confirming the clinical diagnosis. Plain-film axial views of the carpal tunnel are recommended to evaluate abnormal configurations or fractures. CT is necessary in the diagnosis of the subtle fractures of the hook of the hamate or the pisiform. MRI should prove valuable in carefully selected cases in which compression is caused by tumors, synovial cysts, or ganglia. In these cases, the axial and coronal images on T1- and T2-weighted sequences are well indicated.

13.3
Peripheral Nerve Entrapments of the Inferior Limb

13.3.1
Piriformis Muscle Syndrome

The sciatic nerve can be compressed in the fibro-osseous tunnel present in the proximity of the piriformis muscle.

Many sporting activities may be the cause of this syndrome due to repetitive motion, direct nerve trauma, muscular or bone traumas (Fig. 13.10), or

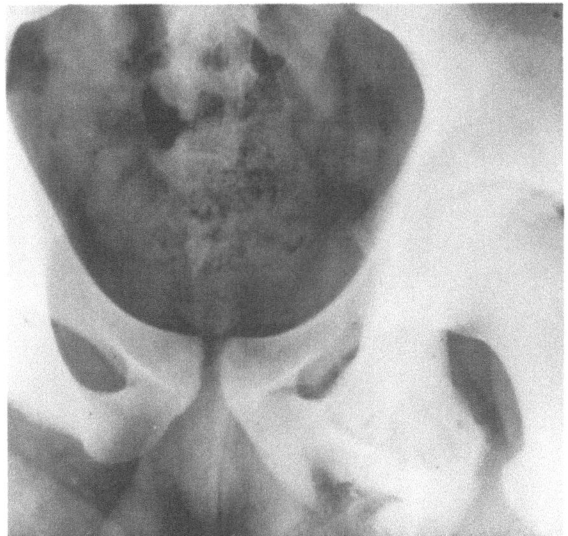

Fig. 13.10. Piriformis muscle syndrome due to ectopic bone overgrowth secondary to ischial apophysiolysis in a young long jumper

muscular hypertrophy. Runners, long jumpers, gymnasts, hurdlers, cyclists, and ballet dancers often complain of pain characteristic of the piriformis syndrome.

The clinical symptoms have many similarities with other pathological conditions such as muscle lesions, acute ischial tuberosity avulsion fracture, or lumbar radiculopathy. A differential diagnosis must be performed with the so-called hamstring syndrome or crossroad ischiatic syndrome in which the compression of the sciatic nerve is determined by the thickened or post-traumatic fibrous flexor tendon of the thigh and clinically characterized by pain and paresthesia along the nerve distribution.

In these cases, MRI is the method of choice in differential diagnosis.

13.3.2
Common Peroneal Nerve Entrapment Syndrome

The peroneal nerve originates from the sciatic nerve at the level of the distal posterior thigh, encircles the head of the fibula, passes below the tendinous origin of the peroneus longus muscle, enters the peroneal tunnel near the fibular neck, and divides into deep and superficial branches.

The common peroneal nerve is entrapped most frequently at the head or neck of the fibula. Knee injuries with associated hematoma, a short leg cast,

acute abduction with peroneal nerve traction, bone fractures, and bone and soft tissue masses may cause the syndrome (Fig. 13.11). Furthermore, nerve pathology such as neurinoma or myxoid intraneural cysts (Fig. 13.12) may have an pathogenetic role. Deep or superficial branches can be of interest for single entrapment syndrome.

Clinically, footdrop with weakness or paralysis of the ankle and foot dorsiflexion are the most common findings. EMG and nerve conduction evaluation may confirm the diagnosis and are useful in differential diagnosis with lumbar radiculopathy or sciatic

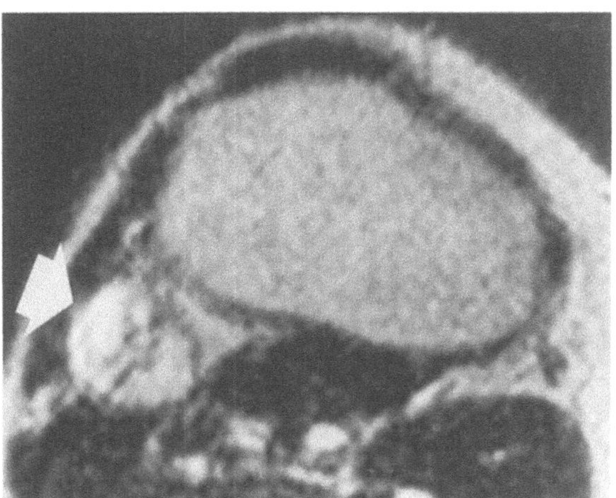

a

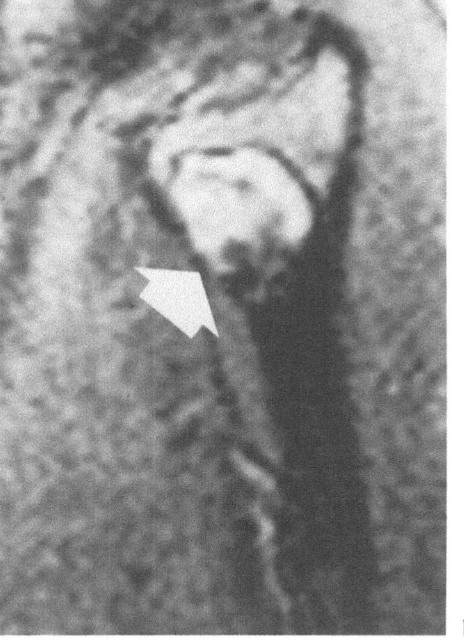

b

Fig. 13.11a,b. Common peroneal nerve entrapment syndrome. MRI axial (**a**) and sagittal (**b**) T2-WI clearly show a chondroma of the head of the fibula (*arrows*) in a symptomatic tennis player

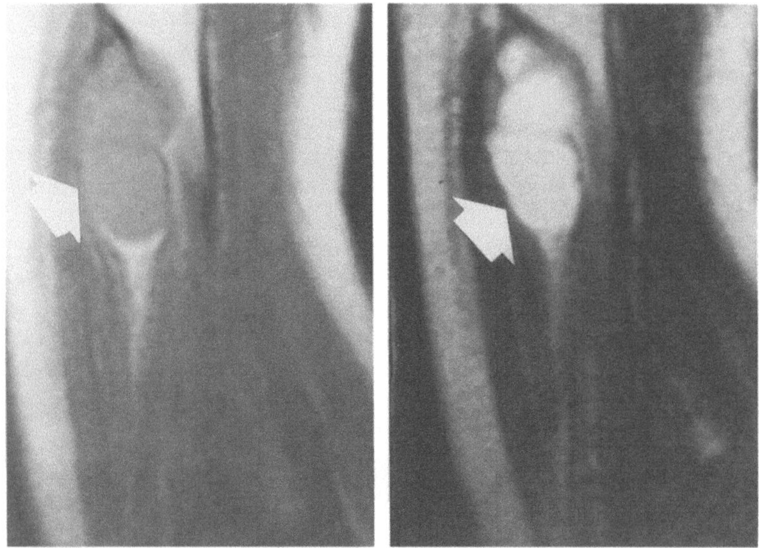

Fig. 13.12a,b. Common peroneal nerve entrapment syndrome due to a myxoid intraneural cyst (*arrows*) well documented by coronal T1-WI (**a**) and T2-WI (**b**)

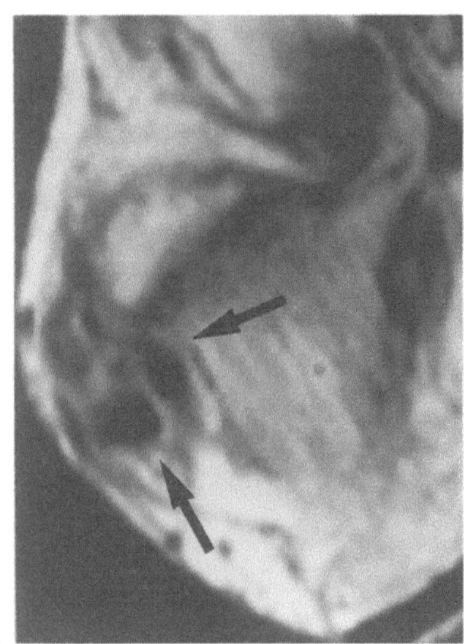
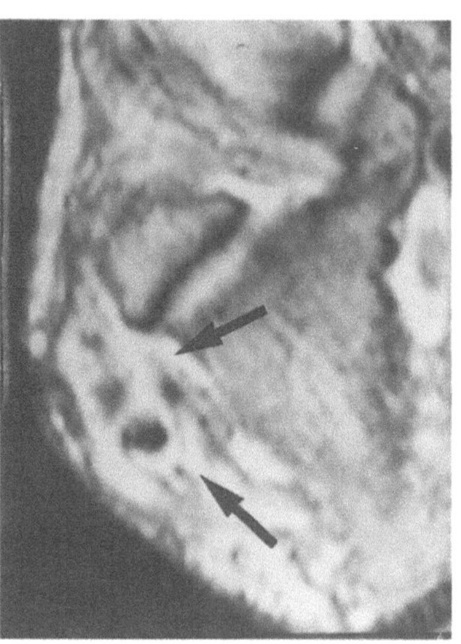

Fig. 13.13a,b. Sural nerve entrapment in a basketball player. MRI axial T1-WI (**a**) and T2-WI (**b**) clearly show the tenosynovitis of the peroneal tendons (*arrows*)

neuropathy. Imaging studies such as US, CT, and MRI can also be useful in demonstrating the lesion that causes the entrapment neuropathy.

13.3.3
Sural Nerve Entrapment Syndrome

The sural nerve is the continuation of the tibial nerve and is formed by the medial sural nerve and the peroneal communicating nerve. It runs along the border of the Achilles tendon next to the short saphenous veins. The nerve provides sensation to the lateral aspect of the ankle and foot.

The sural nerve is generally compressed at the level of the ankle and foot. Several sports injuries may cause sural nerve entrapment. Among these are: peritendinitis of the Achilles tendon, residuals after bone fractures, postsurgical scar tissue, tenosynovitis, ganglia, or tumor-like lesions of the common peroneal tendon sheath, and repetitive ankle sprains that produce fibrosis and nerve reaction.

Clinically, pain and paresthesias along the distribution of the nerve are present. Physical examination and positive Tinel's sign are characteristic. Diagnostic imaging modalities may be useful in detecting the lesion responsible for the clinical symptoms (Fig. 13.13).

13.3.4
Superficial Peroneal Nerve Syndrome (Anterolateral Compartment Syndrome)

The superficial peroneal nerve is the superficial branch of the common peroneal nerve. It penetrates the deep fascia of the leg approximately 10–13 cm above the tip of the lateral malleolus. It presents two terminal branches (the intermediate and the medial dorsal cutaneous) that provide sensations to the dorsolateral aspect of the ankle.

The syndrome, also called "anterolateral compartment syndrome," has been described in ballet dancers due to iterative dorsiflexion of the foot. This syndrome, however, may also occur in athletes with chronic ankle sprains, bone fracture residuals, muscle injuries, or soft tissue masses (Fig. 13.14) that determine a compression of the superficial peroneal nerve or one of its branches.

Clinically, patients report a history of dorsal ankle pain with paresthesia along the distribution of the nerve. Tinel's sign and EMG are useful in diagnosis. Diagnostic imaging modalities can be useful in dem-

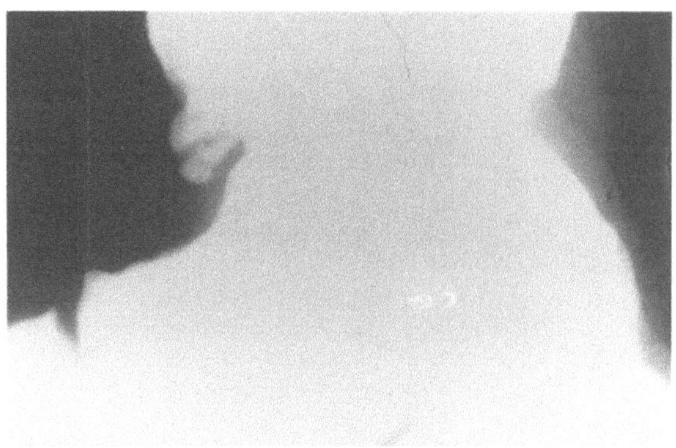

Fig. 13.15. Anterior tarsal tunnel syndrome in a runner due to dorsal osteophytes of the tibiotalar joint

onstrating the causes of this syndrome and making a differential diagnosis with common peroneal nerve entrapment or L5 radiculopathy.

13.3.5
Deep Peroneal Nerve Entrapment (Anterior Tarsal Tunnel Syndrome)

The deep peroneal nerve originates from the common peroneal nerve and, at the level of the inferior portion of the leg, runs between the extensor hallucis longus and the tibialis anterior muscle. At the level of the ankle, the deep peroneal nerve passes underneath the extensor retinaculum, where it generally divides into medial and lateral branches. The entrapment of the deep peroneal nerve at this level is called "anterior tarsal tunnel syndrome."

In athletes, this is the most common site of nerve entrapment and generally occurs in runners, skiers, dancers, and soccer players. Tenosynovitis or tenosynovial ganglia of the extensor hallucis longus tendon or dorsal osteophytes of the tibiotalar joint (Fig. 13.15) can play an important role in determining symptoms. In some cases, the patients report a multiple ankle sprain. The Symptoms are pain in the dorsum of the foot during sports activity and sensory changes that can be revealed in the first web space.

For diagnosis, EMG is useful and reveals an increase in the distal motor latency of the deep peroneal nerve with normal appearance in the proximal portion of the nerve in the ankle. Diagnostic imaging modalities may be very useful in the evaluation of the pathologies that cause this syndrome. Bone fracture residuals and osteophytes are well documented by plain films and CT. In contrast, US and MRI are very useful in evaluating tendons and soft tissue patholo-

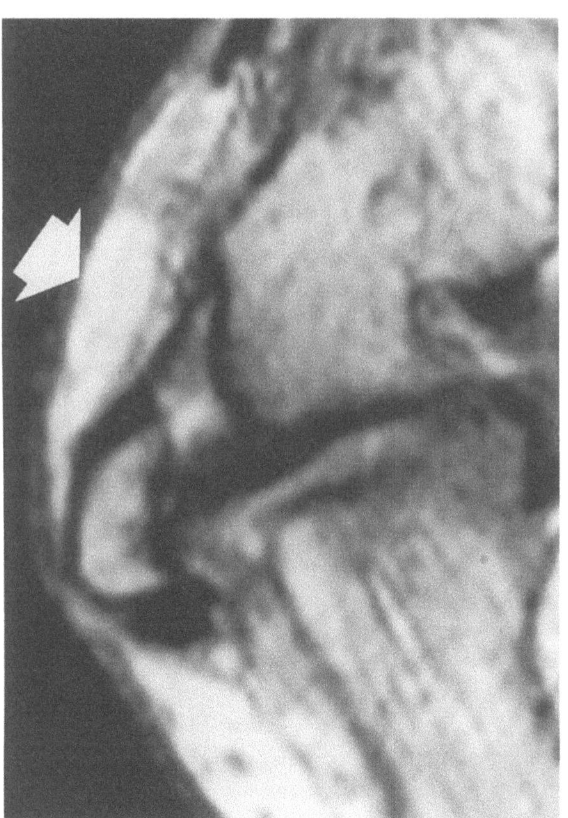

Fig. 13.14. Anterolateral compartment syndrome due to a lipoma (*arrow*), well delineated by axial T1-weighted MRI

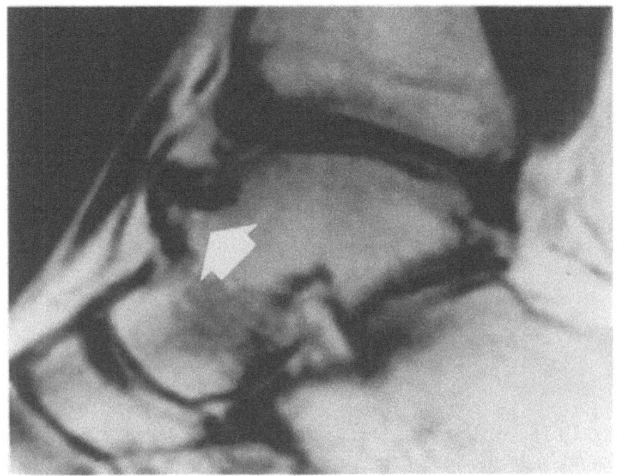

Fig. 13.16. Anterior tarsal tunnel syndrome caused by a pronounced talar nose (*arrow*) in a soccer player, well depicted by sagittal T1-weighted MRI

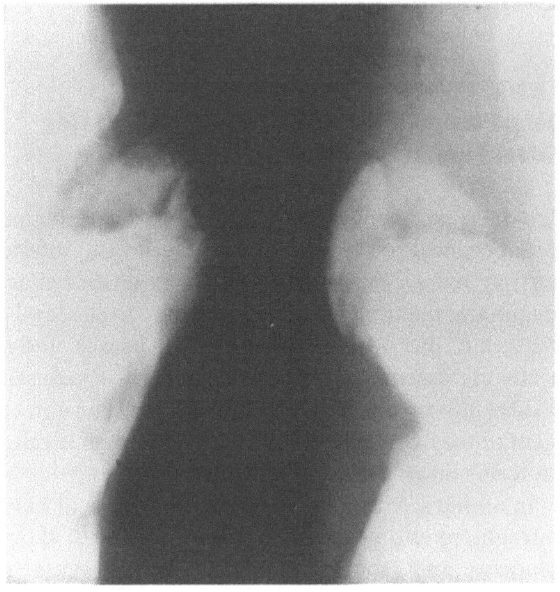

Fig. 13.17. Jogger's foot induced by an osteochondrosis with fracture of the os tibialis externum

gies; MRI also provides information for presurgical planning (Fig. 13.16).

13.3.6
Medial Plantar Nerve Entrapment Syndrome (Jogger's Foot)

The medial plantar nerve is the other terminal branch of the posterior tibial nerve. It courses deep to the abductor hallucis muscle and along the plantar surface of the flexor digitorum longus tendon and

passes through the intersection of the flexor digitorum longus tendon and the flexor hallucis longus tendon, the so-called master knot of Henry. Generally, the nerve entrapment syndrome affects joggers (jogger's foot), and nerve entrapment occurs in the region of the master knot of Henry.

Talar and navicular fractures or abnormalities (Fig. 13.17), heel valgus, sports involving hyperpronation of the foot, or a former ankle injury with chronic hindfoot instability can be considered causative or at least predisposing factors.

13.3.7
First Branch of Lateral Plantar Nerve Entrapment Syndrome

The bifurcation of the posterior tibial nerve generally occurs deep in the flexor retinaculum; the lateral plantar nerve is one of its terminal branches. The first branch of the lateral planter nerve can be compressed between the deep fascia of the abductor hallucis longus and the quadratus plantae muscle. Athletes such as tennis players, runners, and soccer players may be affected by chronic stretching of the nerve.

The most common causes of this syndrome are muscle abnormalities and hypertrophy. Nerve entrapment, however, can frequently occur secondary to plantar fascitis.

Clinically, chronic heel pain exacerbated by running and radiating to the inferomedial aspect of the heel and proximally to the medial ankle region is observed. Heel spurs are sometimes discovered on plain film or CT, but better visualization of the possible causes of this syndrome is provided by MRI (Fig. 13.18).

13.3.8
Tarsal Tunnel Syndrome

Tarsal tunnel syndrome is a compression neuropathy of the posterior tibial nerve or its branches as they pass, along with the flexor tendons and vessels, posterior to the medial malleolus deep to the flexor retinaculum.

The tunnel has an osseous floor (medial malleolus, medial surface of talus, sustentaculum tali and medial wall of calcaneus) and a roof that is formed by the flexor retinaculum. Usually, the tunnel is subdivided by fibrous septa that extend from the undersurface of the retinaculum to the calcaneus.

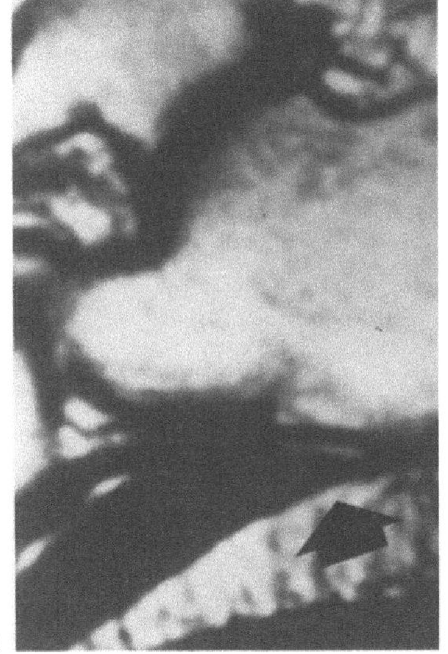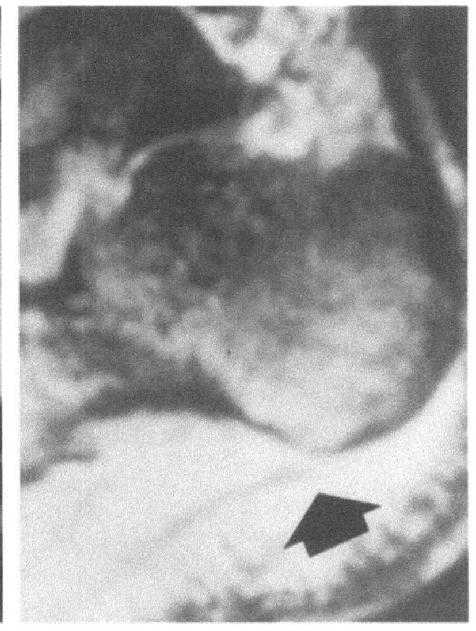

Fig. 13.18a,b. MRI: sagittal T1-WI (a) and T2-WI (b) clearly depict an edema of the plantar aponeurosis (*arrows*) responsible for entrapment syndrome of the first branch of the lateral plantar nerve

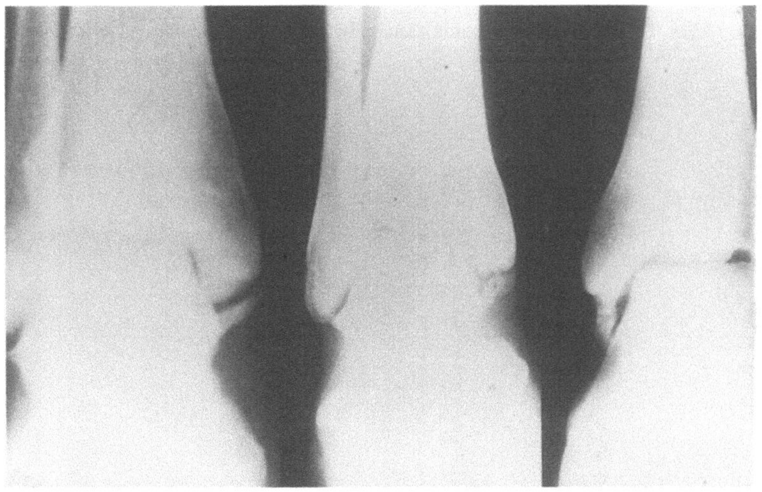

Fig. 13.19. Tarsal tunnel syndrome in athletes caused by post-traumatic exostosis around and deep to the medial malleolus

These separate compartments include, from the anterior to the posterior aspect, the posterior tibial tendon, the flexor digitorum longus tendon, the neurovascular bundle, and the flexor hallucis longus tendon.

The syndrome is idiopathic in 50% of cases; in the remaining cases, a large range of lesions may cause this syndrome, including tumors and tumor-like lesions, fracture deformity, bony exostoses, post-traumatic edema, fibrous scar, ganglion cysts, venous varicosities, tenosynovitis, and accessory muscles.

In athletes, the tarsal tunnel syndrome generally follows an ankle injury and is determined by space-occupying lesions such as tenosynovitis and tenosynovial ganglia of the flexor tendons. It can also be caused by hypertrophied accessory muscles.

The clinical symptoms consist of burning pain and paresthesias in the toes and sole of the foot. These symptoms can also radiate proximally up to the leg. Tinel's sign may be positive. Abnormal condition of the posterior tibial nerve is useful for diagnosis, but normal tibial nerve conduction time does not exclude tarsal tunnel syndrome.

In the study of this syndrome, plain films may be useful in demonstrating osseous bone abnormalities or exostosis (Fig. 13.19). US can well demonstrate tenosynovitis or synovial ganglia of the flexor tendons and venous varicosities. US dynamic studies can be useful for differential diagnosis.

CT (Fig. 13.20) and MRI (Fig. 13.21), however, are the diagnostic techniques that offer the best evaluation of the tarsal tunnel structures. In particular,

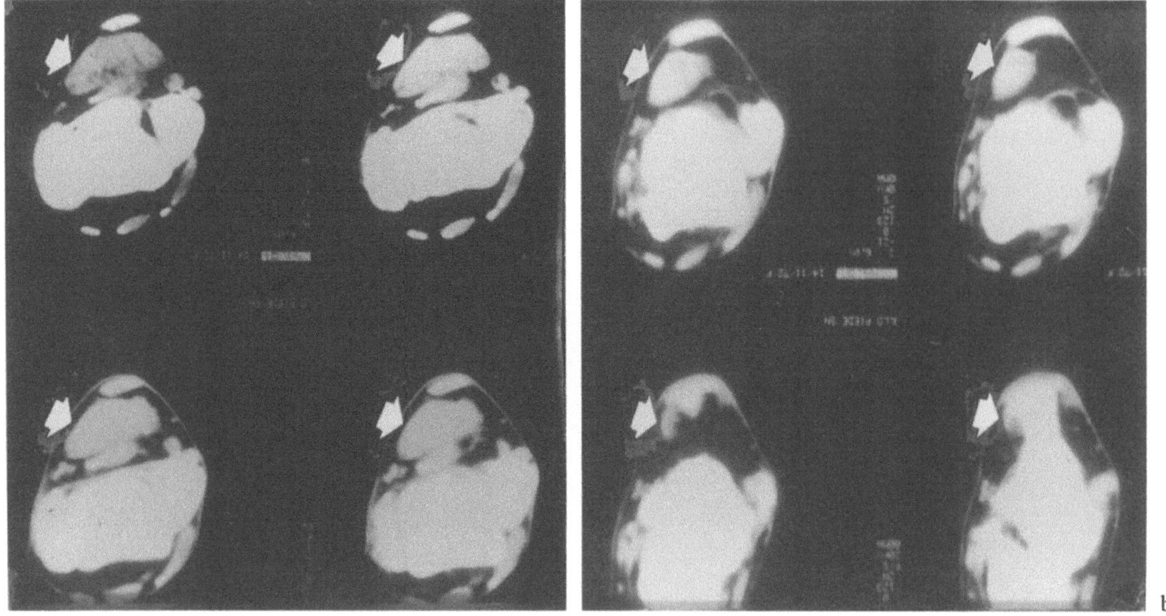

Fig. 13.20. Tarsal tunnel syndrome caused by accessory soleus muscle (*arrows*) well defined with contiguous axial CT scans

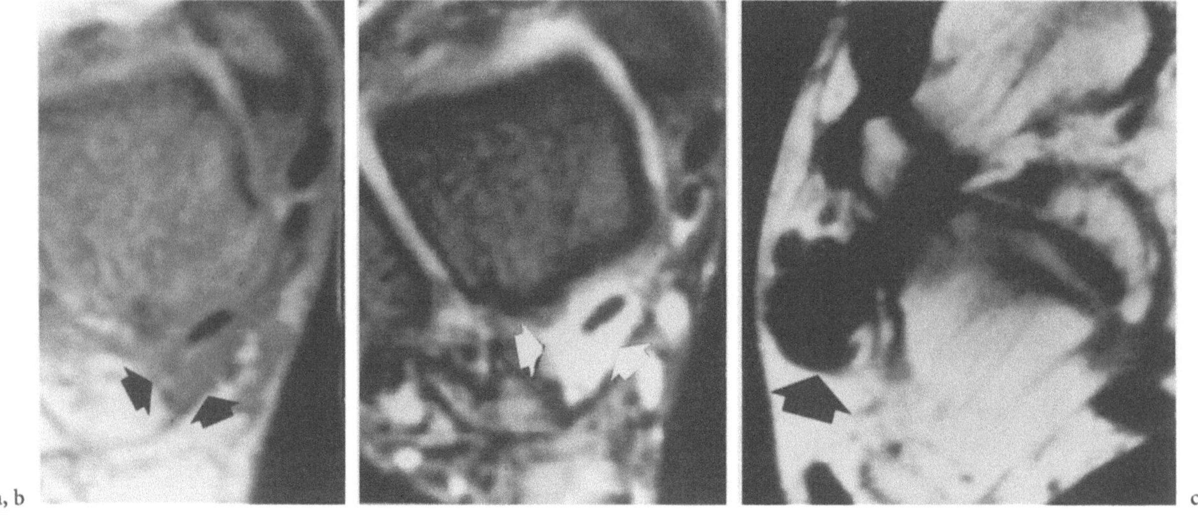

Fig. 13.21a–c. Tarsal tunnel syndrome due to tenosynovitis (*arrows*) of flexor hallucis longus: axial T1-WI (**a**) and T2-WI (**b**). Synovial ganglion cyst of the flexor hallucis longus tendon (**c**, *arrow*)

MRI is useful in localizing a variety of compressive or traction-producing lesions and in determining the lesion extent and its relationship to the posterior tibial nerve and its branches. The information provided by MRI supports surgical planning by indicating the extent of decompression required.

13.3.9
Interdigital Neuropathy (Morton's Neuroma)

The metatarsal tunnel lies between the superficial and deep transverse metatarsal ligaments, which connect the metatarsal heads. The medial and lateral plantar nerves cross the metatarsal tunnel and provide sensation to toes on either side of the web space, producing, with the vessels, the common digital neurovascular bundle. The neuropathy known as "interdigital neuroma," "Morton's neuroma," "Morton's metatarsalgia," "Civinini-Morton disease," or "neuroma plantaris" is a fairly common foot problem in older patients, but it can also present in young subjects, especially if they are engaged actively in long-distance running, basketball, or ballet.

The most accredited mechanism to produce neuromas is compression of the interdigital nerve against the transverse metatarsal ligament by repeated stretching or microtrauma due to continuous dorsiflexion of the toes. The neuroma formed is a non-neoplastic lesion representing perineural fibrosis involving the nerve. The third web space is most commonly involved, followed by the second. Occasionally, two nerves are involved.

Symptoms include forefoot pain brought about by running and sometimes associated with numbness or tingling. The pain is relieved by removing the shoes.

A neuroma can be well identified using ultrasound with a high frequency transducer (7–13 MHz). It appears as a rounded hypoechogenic mass located at the plantar surface of the pathologic web space. With CT, the neuroma appears as a solid lesion with densely fibrous composition. With MRI, the diagnosis of neuroma is well performed in the coronal or axial plane employing a small field of view. The neuroma has low to intermediate signal intensity on T1-weighted images and low signal on T2-weighted images, probably due to its fibrous composition, and medium-high signal intensity on gradient-echo T2-weighted images (Fig. 13.22). The neuroma can be frequently associated with fluid-filled intermetatarsal bursae dorsally situated on the intermetatarsal ligament and prominent at the II-III and III-IV spaces.

13.4
Spinal Nerve Entrapment Diseases

13.4.1
Upper Trunk Brachial Transient Flexopathy (Burner or Stinger Syndrome)

Injuries of cervical nerve roots or to the nerves when they exit the cervical spine foramina can occur during athletic activities. The so-called burner or stinger syndrome or brachial plexus neuropathy due to an upper brachial plexopathy (C5–C6 nerve roots) is reported among rugby players, wrestlers, hockey players, and particularly football players. A blow or jolt to the player's head can cause lateral flexion of the cervical spine with contemporary depression of the shoulder of the opposite side; alternatively, repetitive forced lateral movements (Fig. 13.23) may induce a traction injury to the brachial plexus.

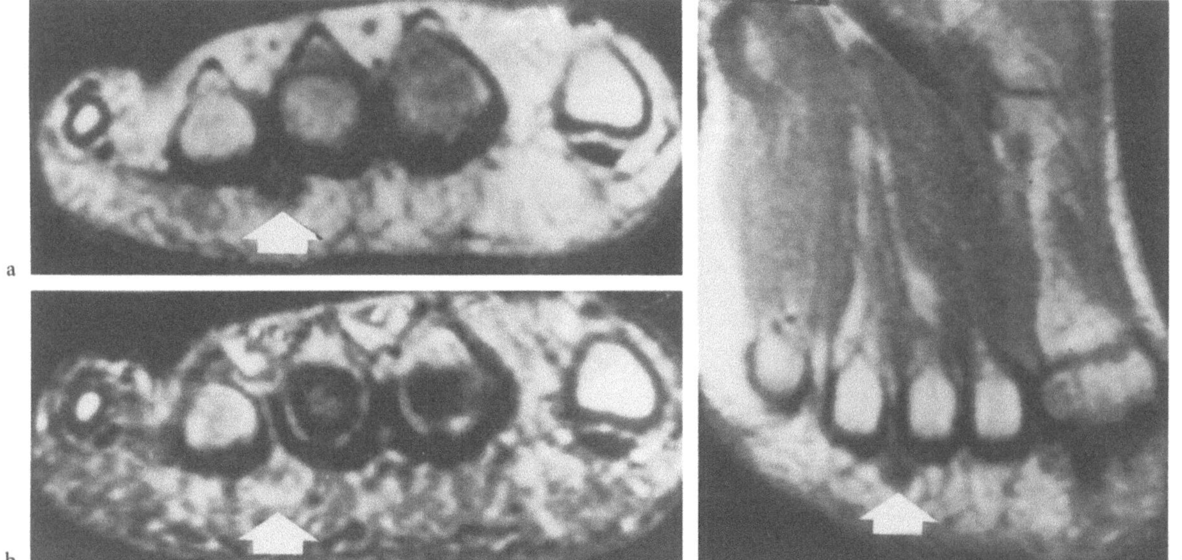

Fig. 13.22a–c. Morton neuroma in a runner. With axial T1-WI (**a**) and gradient-echo T2-WI (**b**) the neuroma (*arrows*) located at the level of the third metatarsal space is well defined. Coronal T1-WI (**c**) confirms the side of the lesion (*arrow*)

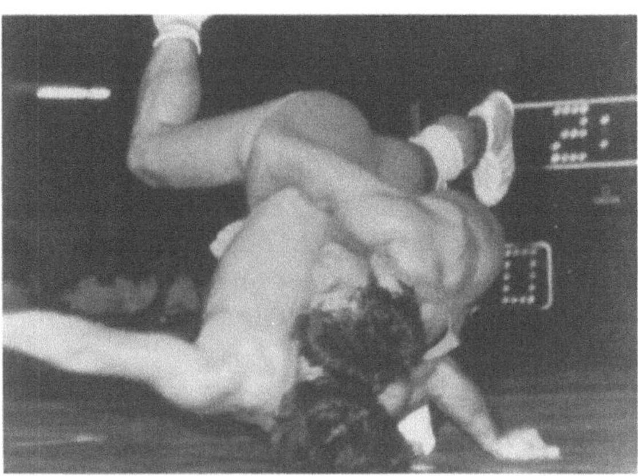

Fig. 13.23. Active cervical traumatic movement during wrestling competition

A sudden and violent blow with lateral flexion of the neck may compress the nerve roots, causing a burning sensation on the side opposite to the blow. Typically, the player experiences a sharp burning pain in the shoulder with paresthesia or dysesthesia radiating into the arm, thumb, and index finger. Associated with this is weakness of shoulder abduction, external rotation, and arm flexion that may be transient, persistent, or late-developing.

EMG, NCS, X-rays, and MRI should be performed as required on a case-by-case basis.

13.4.2
Chronic Thoracic and Lumbar Back Pain

Many athletes of all ages experience chronic thoracic or lumbar pain. Normally, the cause is overuse, in-tervertebral disc disease, or a structural spinal abnormality or deformity. Thoracic and lumbar disc degeneration and herniation are uncommon in athletes. When they are diagnosed, they occur in older athletes at T9/T10, T10/T11, or T11/T12 and at L4/L5 or L5/S1 spaces (Fig. 13.24).

The clinical findings in an athlete with rare thoracic disc degeneration or herniation are variable and normally characterized by pain in the chest wall distributed according to the dermatome pattern of the compressed nerve. Rarely, a thoracic disc may herniate centrally; in such a case there are associated paresthesias and it is possible to observe increased reflexes in the lower limbs or spastic paraparesis.

CT and MRI permit appreciation of degenerative articular signs and provide direct visualization of the thoracic disc, neural elements, and any compressive condition of the spinal cord.

The continuum of degeneration and herniation of lumbar disc that occurs in all people is also evident in athletes. The pain associated with disc degeneration is often located in the paraspinal region and may be excited by activity. The herniated disc compresses and stimulates the nerve roots that leave the spinal canal. The results are pain, numbness, and weakness in the leg corresponding to the area of the compressed nerve. The clinical findings vary with disc degeneration or herniation, and the key in differentiating is a complete and extensive physical examination of the lower limbs.

Anteroposterior and lateral plain films and CT show degeneration signs of the spine, loss of disc height, and pathology of the facet joints (Fig. 13.25). MRI will certainly demonstrate the loss of water con-

a

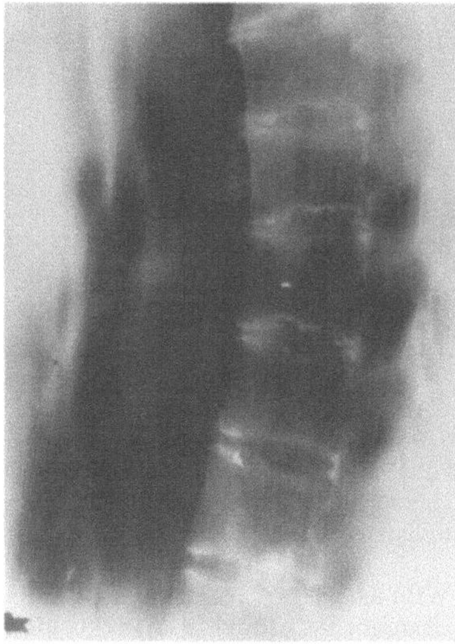

b

Fig. 13.24. Diffuse thoracic spine osteochondrosis in a young athlete with neurological symptoms and kyphotic deformity

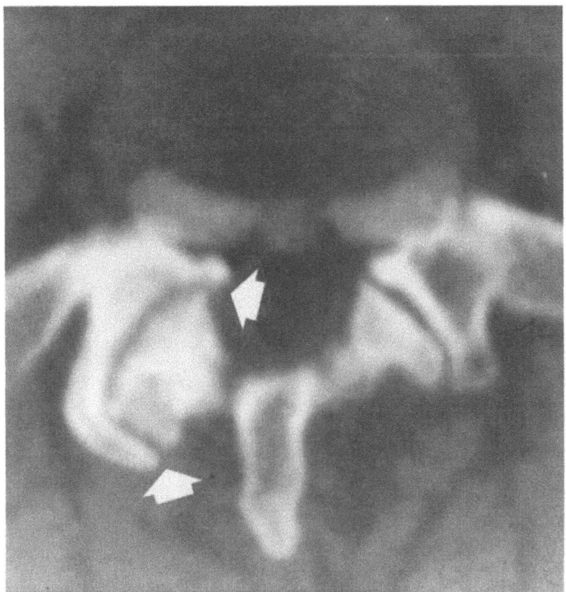

Fig. 13.25. CT scan at the lumbar level. Severe intra-articular arthritis (*arrows*) in an aged rower

tent of the disc. The main diagnostic aids have been myelography, CT, myelo-CT, and MRI. MRI seems to be the most sensitive and specific indicator of lumbar disc problems in athletes (Fig. 13.26).

13.4.3
Lumbar Spondylolysis and Spondylolisthesis

The lumbar radiographic findings of a cleft in the neural arch of a vertebra at the isthmus (spondylolysis) with the consequent ventral gliding of the body over the vertebra beneath (spondylolisthesis) are a not uncommon cause of low back pain in athletes (Fig. 13.27). According to convention, when the term spondylolisthesis is used, it refers to an anterior vertebral gliding in the presence of isthmic lysis.

Several theories have been brought forth to explain the origin of spondylolysis; however, the main etiological and pathogenetical factors advocated in the athletic population are those according to which spondylolysis must be considered as an acquired lesion secondary to a "stress fracture." The mainly provocative mechanisms are repetitive, detrimental movements of flexion and extension of the lumbar spine at isthmic level (Fig. 13.28).

The data from a series of 527 cases of spondylolysis diagnosed in top-level athletes ranging in age from 15 to 27 years affected by low back pain, and submitted to plain-film study offer some interesting considerations:

– The incidence of spondylolysis in athletes (13.54%) is higher than in the normal population (4%–6%).

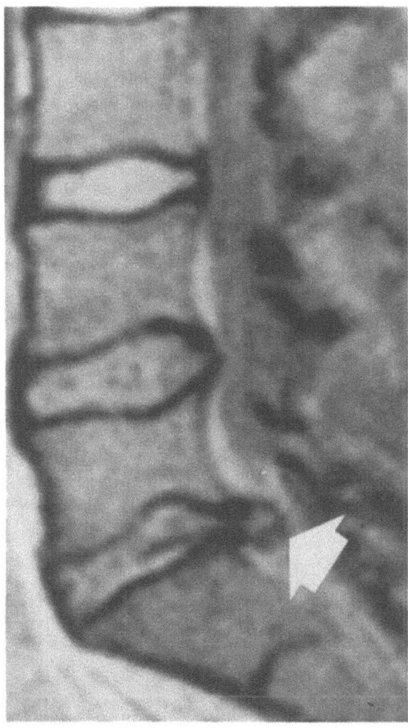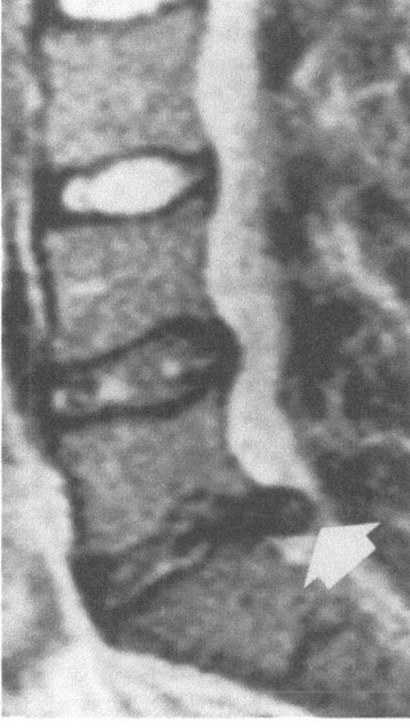

Fig. 13.26a,b. A 16-year-old gymnast with severe herniated L5-S1 disc (*arrows*): MRI evaluation on sagittal T1-WI (**a**) and T2-WI (**b**)

a

b

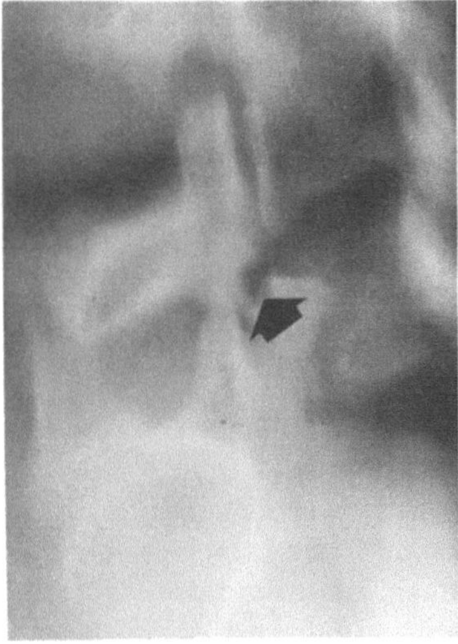 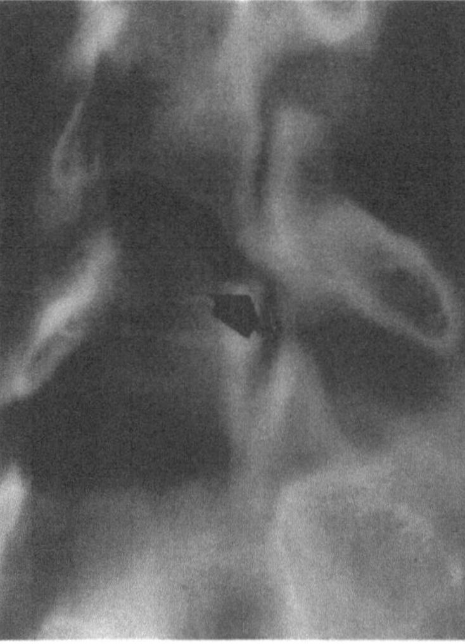

Fig. 13.27. Isthmic spondylolysis of L5 in X-ray oblique projections (*arrows*) in a diver

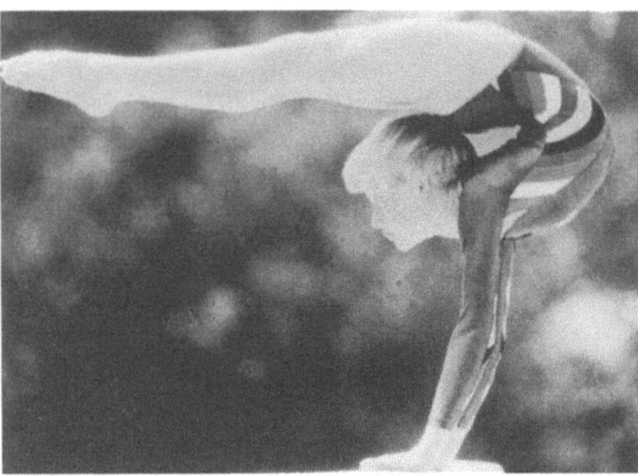

Fig. 13.28. Gymnastic exercise at bar with maximal lumbar hyperflexion: the iterative movement can induce a stress fracture in the ishtmus

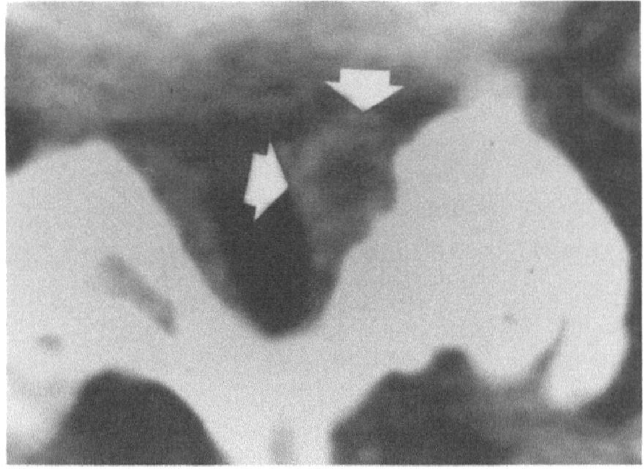

Fig. 13.29. Lumbar intraspinal synovial cyst (*arrows*) of the left facet joint in an old athlete with spondylolisthesis: CT evaluation

- There is considerable variation among the different sporting disciplines with regard to rates of low back pain (41.81% in divers, 28.16% in wrestlers, 22.85% in weight lifters, 16.33% in gymnasts).
- L5 is involved in 435 cases (82.54%).
- In 271 cases (51.50%), low back pain is associated with spondylolisthesis.
- There is a close relationship between the attempt to achieve top-class performances and the onset of lumbar symptoms.
- Analyzing the history and experiences of any athlete, there are multiple episodes of low back discomfort, which, however, are not disabling.
- In each sport practiced, the onset of symptoms in the lumbar area is always referred to and correlated with repetitive, forced, hyperextensive lumbar movements.

Usually asymptomatic and occasionally found on X-ray, spondylolysis is associated with extreme lordosis, contracture of hamstrings, and low back pain. Sometimes, the physical signs indicate disc involvement. This requires treatment if persistent; otherwise, conservative management is appropriate.

Spondylolisthesis is in many cases asymptomatic. When symptoms are present, they depend not on the degree of displacement, but on the degree of instability secondary to disc and ligament degeneration. By the age of 30, stability is usually greater. Whereas low back pain decreases after age 30, facet joint degen-

Fig. 13.30. Grade 2 L5-S1 spondylolisthesis with herniated malacic disc (*arrows*): sagittal T1-WI in a weight lifter

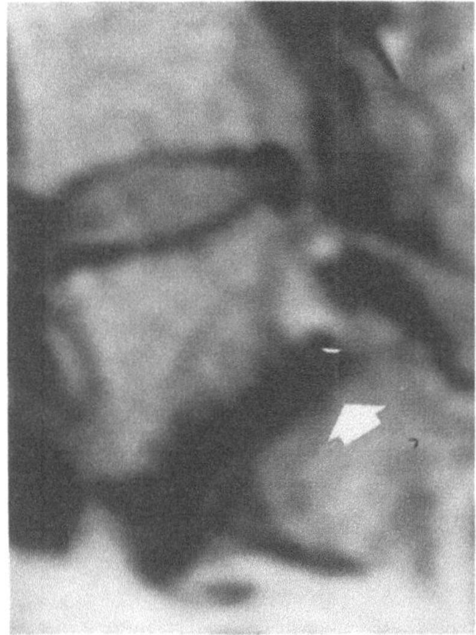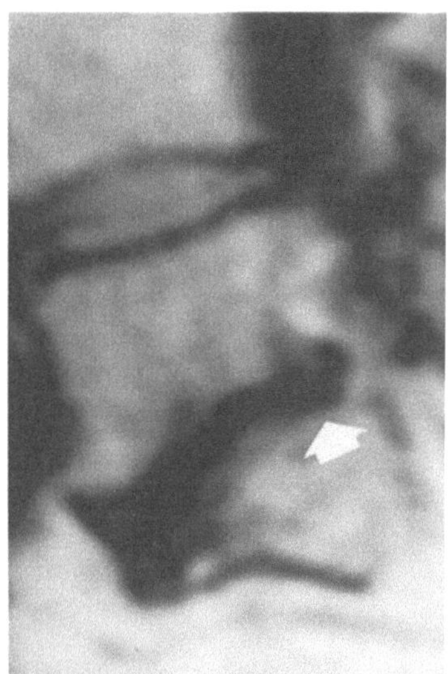

eration increases with age due to the presence of instability. The majority of subjects with elevated displacement (3°–4°, Mayerding measurement) suffer from pressure on the neural elements, provoked by secondary spinal stenosis. A number of long-standing spondylolisthesis complications have been described, including the presence of intraspinal synovial cysts of the facet joint (Fig. 13.29).

While the primary diagnosis of spondylolysis and spondylolisthesis may be obtained by plain-film study in standard and oblique projections (with or without functional rediograms), CT and MRI are very useful, especially in depicting the various complications that may be associated with this condition (Fig. 13.30).

Suggested Reading

Baxter DE (1994) The foot and ankle in sport. Mosby Year Book, St. Louis

Cimino WR (1990) Tarsal tunnel syndrome: a review of the literature. Foot Ankle 11:47–52

Dawson DM, Hallet M, Millender LH (1990) Entrapment neuropathies, 2nd edn. Little Brown, Boston

De Lee CJ, Drez D (1994) Orthopaedic sport medicine. Saunders, Philadelphia

Dussault RG, Lander PH (1990) Imaging of the facet joints. Radiol Clin North Am 28:1033–1053

Erickson SJ, Quinn SF, Kneeland JB, et al. (1990) MRI of the tarsal tunnel and related spaces: normal and abnormal findings with anatomic correlation. AJR Am J Roentgenol 155:323–328

Ferretti A, Cerullo G, Russo G (1987) Suprascapular neuropathy in volleyball players. J Bone Joint Surg [Am] 69:260–263

Fritz RC, Helms CA, Sternbach LS, et al. (1992) Suprascapular nerve entrapment: evaluation with MR imaging. Radiology 182:437–444

Fu HF, Stone DA (1994) Sports injuries. Williams and Wilkins, Baltimore

Griffiths HS (1991) Imaging of the lumbar spine. Aspen, Gaithersburg

Jackson DL, Haglund B (1991) Tarsal tunnel syndrome in athletes. Am J Sports Med 19:61–65

Jobe FW, Nuber G (1986) Throwing injuries of the elbow. Clin Sports Med 5:621–636

Johnson RJ (1993) Low back pain in sports. Phys Sports Med 21:53–59

Karas SE (1990) Thoracic outlet syndrome. Clin Sports Med 9:297

Kerr R, Frey C (1991) MRI in tarsal tunnel syndrome. J Comput Assist Tomogr 15:280–286

Kodros SA, Palumbo RC, Leibman BD, et al. (1994) Neural entrapment in the athlete. Sports Med Arthrosc Rev 2:310–316

Kurosawa H, Nakashita K, Hakashita H, et al. (1995) Pathogenesis and treatment of cubital tunnel syndrome caused by osteoarthrosis of the elbow joint. J Shoulder Elbow Surg 4:30–34

Leach RE, Purnell MB, Saito A (1989) Peroneal nerve entrapment in runners. Am J Sports Med 17:287

Lorei MP, Hershman EB (1993) Peripheral nerve injuries in athletes. Sports Med 16:130–147

Mesgarzadeh M, Schneck CD, Bonakdarpour A (1989) Carpal tunnel: MR imaging. Radiology 171:743–754

Munnings F (1991) Cyclist's palsy. Phys Sports Med 19:113–119

Nicholas AJ, Hershman EB (1990) The upper extremity in sports medicine. Mosby, St. Louis

Pecina MM, Krmpotic-Nemanic J, Markiewitz AD (1991) Tunnel syndromes. CRC Press, Boca Raton

Peri G (1991) The critical zones of entrapment of the nerves of the lower limb. Surg Radiol Anat 13:139–143

Perry J (1983) Anatomy and biomechanics of the shoulder in throwing, swimming, gymnastics and tennis. Clin Sports Med 2:247–270

Puranen J, Orava S (1988) The hamstring syndrome. Am J Sports Med 16:517–521

Rossi F, Dragoni S (1990) Lumbar spondylolysis: occurrence in competitive athletes. J Sports Med Phys Fitness 30:450–455

Schon LC, Baxter DE (1990) Neuropathies of the foot and ankle in athletes. Clin Sports Med 9:489

Stull MA, Moser RP, Kransdorf MJ, et al. (1991) MR appearance of pheripheral sheath tumors. Skeletal Radiol 20:9–14

Sward L (1992) The thoracolumbar spine in joung elite athletes. Sports Med 13:357–364

Wilberger JE, Maroon JC (1990) Cervical spine injuries in athletes. Phys Sports Med 18:57–70

14 Stress Fractures

A. Chevrot[1], J.L. Drape[2], D. Godefroy[3], A.M. Dupont[4], F. Gires[5], N. Chemla[6], E. Pessis[7], L. Sarazin[8], and A. Minoui[9]

CONTENTS

[1] A. Chevrot, MD, Groupe Hospitalier Cochin, Service de Radiologie "B", rue du Fanbourg-Saint Jacques, 75674 Paris Cedex 14, France
[2] J.L. Drape, MD, Groupe Hospitalier Cochin, Service de Radiologie "B", rue du Fanbourg-Saint Jacques, 75674 Paris Cedex 14, France
[3] D. Godefroy, MD, Groupe Hospitalier Cochin, Service de Radiologie "B", rue du Fanbourg-Saint Jacques, 75674 Paris Cedex 14, France
[4] A.M. Dupont, MD, Groupe Hospitalier Cochin, Service de Radiologie "B", rue du Fanbourg-Saint Jacques, 75674 Paris Cedex 14, France
[5] F. Gires, MD, Groupe Hospitalier Cochin, Service de Radiologie "B", rue du Fanbourg-Saint Jacques, 75674 Paris Cedex 14, France
[6] N. Chemla, MD, Groupe Hospitalier Cochin, Service de Radiologie "B", rue du Fanbourg-Saint Jacques, 75674 Paris Cedex 14, France
[7] E. Pessis, MD, Groupe Hospitalier Cochin, Service de Radiologie "B", rue du Fanbourg-Saint Jacques, 75674 Paris Cedex 14, France
[8] L. Sarazin, MD, Groupe Hospitalier Cochin, Service de Radiologie "B", rue du Fanbourg-Saint Jacques, 75674 Paris Cedex 14, France
[9] A. Minoui, MD, Groupe Hospitalier Cochin, Service de Radiologie "B", rue du Fanbourg-Saint Jacques, 75674 Paris Cedex 14, France

14.1 Introduction

Stress fractures (SFs) have become commonplace in the radiologist's practice. Usually SFs are associated with athletic or occupational activity in healthy adolescents and young adults (Keats 1990; Daffneh 1978; Anderson and Greenspan 1996); SFs are also found in elderly patients or in association with other bone pathologies.

The failure of the skeleton to withstand submaximal forces acting over time brings about SFs. Osteoblasts and osteoclasts continuously remodel the bone architecture in a lifelong process, so it can optimally withstand the mechanical environment. Disuse or immobilization cause osteoporosis.

Microdamage related to daily activity is necessary for physiological bone remodelling, stimulating bone reabsorption and formation. SFs develop when bone formation is exceeded by bone resorption.

SFs occur mainly under three conditions:

- Direct repeated impact of the weight of the body (tibial plateau; Fig. 14.1)
- Repeated contraction of antagonist muscles (pubic ramus, ribs, coracoid process; Fig. 14.2)
- Direct and repeated trauma (hamate hook of tennis players or golfers)

Many risk factors have been recognized (Table 14.1). There are two types of SFs: fatigue fractures that occur in normal bone, and insufficiency fractures that occur in abnormal bones, these bones having less elastic resistance and low mineral density. Insufficiency fractures occur with less stress than that causing fractures of normal bone tissue.

Pathological fractures have distinctive features and must be distinguished from SFs. They are induced by a single traumatism and occur on localized destructive bone lesions caused by tumors or infection.

Assessment of SFs is difficult and based on the careful examination of:

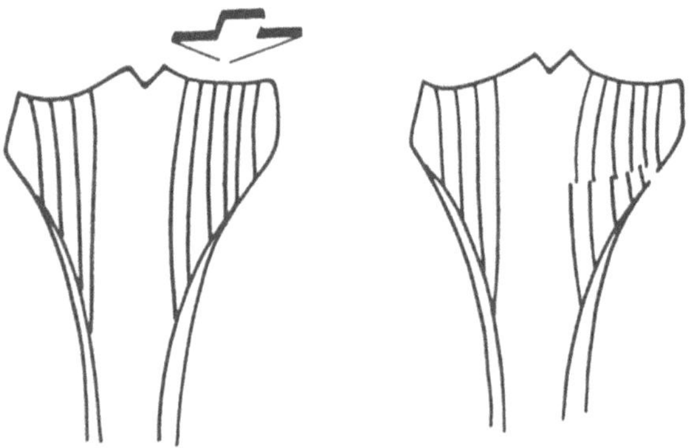

Fig. 14.1. Mechanism 1. Direct action of the weight of the body

Table 1. Risk factors of stress fracture

- Any unusual repetitive activity
- Running
- Wearing of worn-out running shoes
- Leg length discrepancy
- External rotation of the hip
- Caucasian race
- Female sex
- Aging
- Low bone-mineral density
    Age-related osteoprosis
    Corticosteroid treatment
    Low calcium intake
    Fluoride treatment of osteoporosis
    Rheumatoid arthritis
    Paget's disease
    Osteogenesis imperfecta
    Osteopetrosis
    Osteomalacia
    Hyperparathyroidism
    Hyperthyroidism
    Cushing's syndrome
- Altered gait due to tumor, traumatism, surgery, or prosthesis

- Clinical data
- Affected area
- Diagnostic images

14.2
Clinical Data

SFs can be suspected when a patient complains of focal pain that worsens during activity.

Pain most commonly occurs after unusual or prolonged activity and may disappear with rest. However, if activity is continued, pain will increase. Rest relieves pain and allows healing. Most SFs heal very well with the nonsurgical treatment approach (Monteleone 1995).

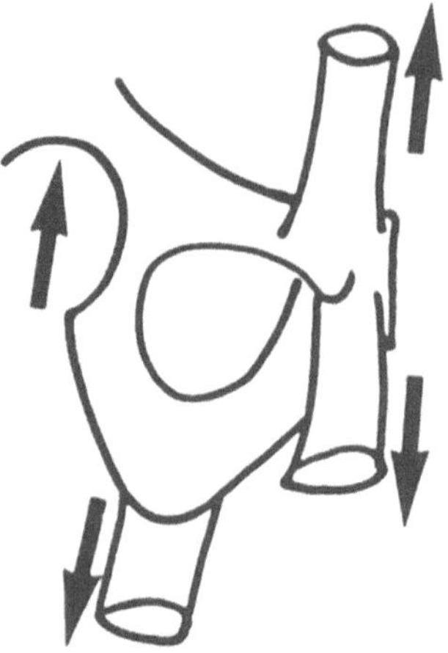

Fig. 14.2. Mechanism 2. Action of antagonist muscles

The physical sign most useful for diagnosis is the point of maximum tenderness, which corresponds well with the site of the fracture. Focal pain must be distinguished from bursitis, tendinitis, and neuromas.

In nonathletic patients, high clinical suspicion is required for the diagnosis of SFs. Often history is vague, and physical features are aspecific. A detailed report should be obtained on any unaccustomed activity engaged in before the onset of acute pain.

14.3
Site of Fracture

Certain activities increase the incidence of SFs. SFs are common injuries in the athletic population. Sports activities and specific points of impact are indicated in Table 14.2.

The most common skeletal areas affected are the metatarsal necks, especially the second, leading to the classical march fracture, often found in military recruits. Other bones regularly affected are the calcaneus and the proximal epiphysis of the tibia, as in long-distance runners and ballet dancers. The pars interarticularis in lumbar vertebrae, which causes spondylolysis and spondylolisthesis, is of concern to athletes. These conditions are occasionally observed as a result of occupational stress or are induced by working on hands and knees (as in carpet layers and miners). Less commonly, SFs occur in the lower ribs and sternum, as a result of chronic coughing, or in golfers; the first rib is involved in patients carrying heavy loads. Bones in the pelvic ring are often involved, especially in aging adults, like the obturator

Table 2. Stress fractures associated with particular activities (from McBryde 1975)

Activity	Site of fracture
Running	Fibula, tibia
Hiking	Metatarsal, pelvis (rare)
Jumping	Pelvis, femur
Tennis	Ulna, metacarpal
Baseball	
Pitching	Humerus, scapula
Batting	Ribs
Catching	Patella, tibia
Javelin throwing	Ulna
Soccer	Tibia
Swimming	Tibia, metatarsals
Skating	Fibula
Curling	Ulna
Aerobics	Fibula, tibia
Ballet dancing	Tibia
Cricket	Humerus
Fencing	Pubis
Handball	Metacarpal

Table 3. Stress fractures in athletes (from Orava et al. 1978)

Bone involved	Total number of cases	Percentage of cases
Metatarsal	88	35.2
Calcaneus	70	28.0
Tibia	60	24.0
Ribs	14	5.6
Femur	8	3.2
Fibula	8	3.2
Spine	1	0.4
Pubic ramus	1	0.4

ring, the neck of the femur, and the sacrum (Table 14.3). Sometimes several sites of different maturation phases are simultaneously seen, which is to be considered as a useful diagnostic factor.

14.4
Medical Imaging Data

14.4.1
Radiography

Depending on the time between symptoms and radiographic examination, radiography often fails to show any abnormality on first examination. Repeat radiography 1 or 2 weeks later may show SFs. In some patients the lag time before the detection of radiographic findings may be as much as several months. Cessation of inciting activity may prevent the development of diagnostic radiographic findings.

Radiographic findings are quite different in cancellous and cortical bone. On cortical bone SF begins with a thin periosteal linear ossification. As the damage increases, a true fracture line may appear. Then, usually after 1 month, a true callus appears on radiography as a hazy zone of increased density across the fracture site (Fig. 14.3). Occasionally, the callus becomes so abundant that it may be confused with an infection or even a bone tumor. In these cases, clinical knowledge and knowledge of the usual SF sites are of great value (Figs. 14.4, 14.5). In long bones, the lesion typically involves the shafts.

On cancellous bones such as the calcaneus, the proximal epiphysis of the tibia, and the neck of the femur, compression fractures generally occur. The fracture line is usually visible as a line of increased density perpendicular to the bone trabeculae (Fig. 14.6).

14.4.2
Computed Tomography

Computed tomography (CT) has only a minor impact on the diagnosis of SFs. There are, however, SFs that are especially difficult to detect with radiography, for instance, longitudinal SFs of the tibia or SFs

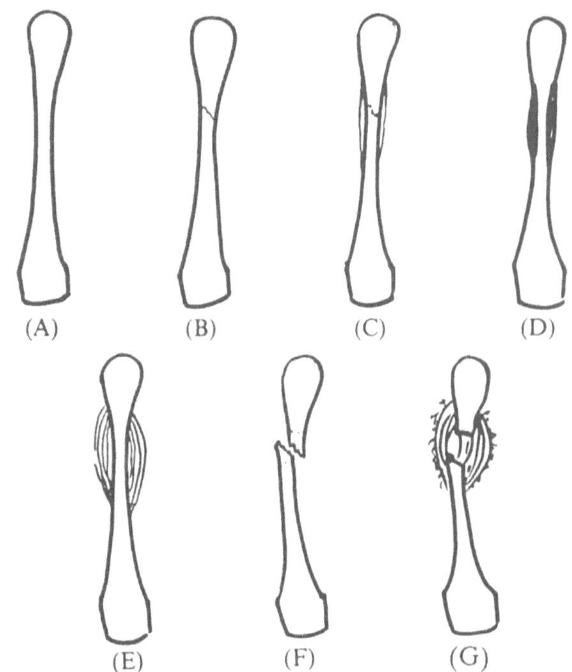

Fig. 14.3A–G. Different patterns of metatarsal stress fractures. **A** Normal, **B** thin radiolucent line, **C** subtle periosteal reaction, **D** small callus, **E** large callus, **F** complete fracture, **G** hypertrophic callus

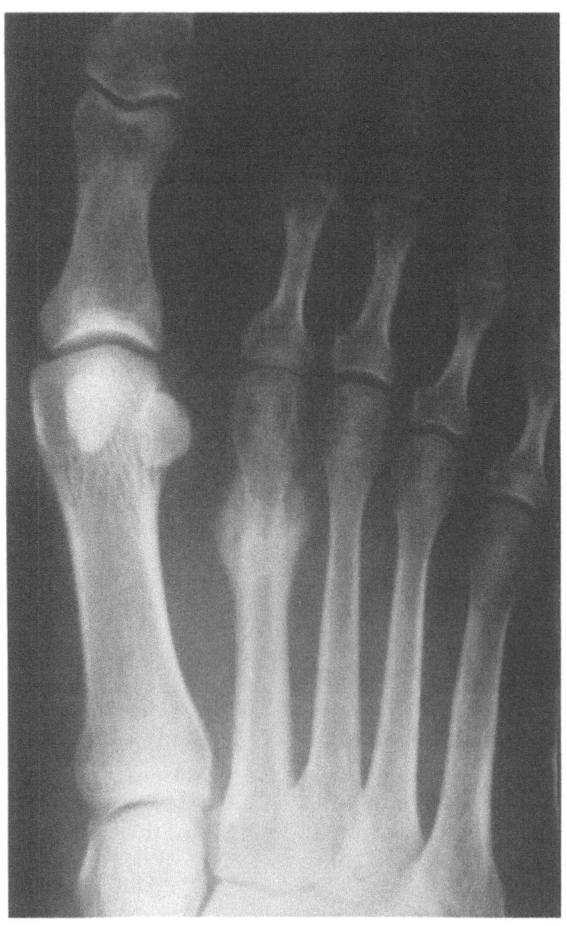

Fig. 14.4. Stress fracture (SF) of the neck of the second metatarsal bone

The scintigraphic evidence of SFs ranges from mild evidence of increased uptake of radiopharmaceutical to well-marginated, very intense areas of uptake. The intensity of the lesion predicts the clinical outcome; higher uptake is correlated

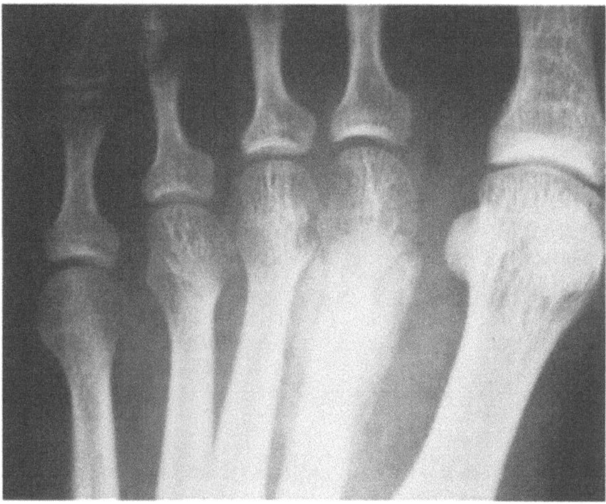

Fig. 14.5. SF of the neck of the second metatarsal bone. Hypertrophic callus

of the tarsal navicular bone. CT is valuable in the diagnosis of these cases.

On CT scanning, difficulties can arise if the slices are not thin enough. It is necessary to use 1 mm slice thickness and good resolution power with a high matrix (512 × 512; Fig. 14.7).

CT is the leading method for distinguishing between tumor masses and SFs with abundant callus.

14.4.3
Radionuclide Bone Scanning

Radionuclide bone scanning is the gold standard for diagnosis of SFs because its sensitivity approaches 100%, although MR imaging and CT may be helpful adjuncts. Scintigraphy is far more sensitive than radiography and also more sensitive than CT. Radionuclide bone scans are positive before typical radiological changes are seen in the days following injury (PATEL et al. 1995).

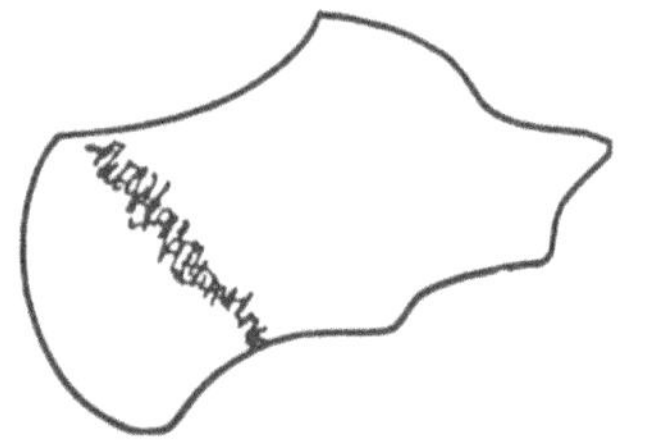

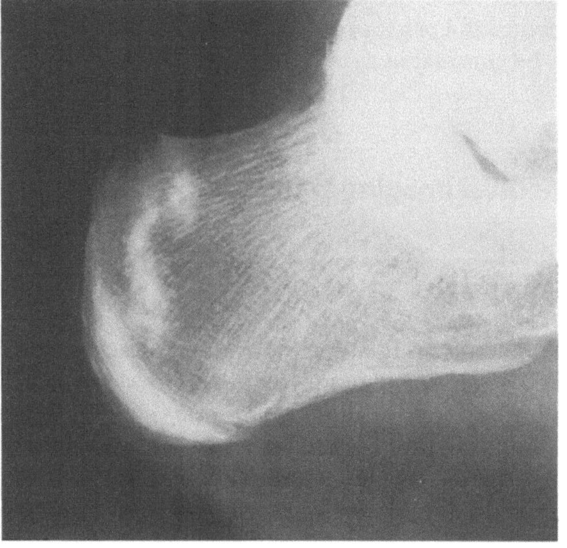

Fig. 14.6. A and B show calcaneus fracture (*dense line*)

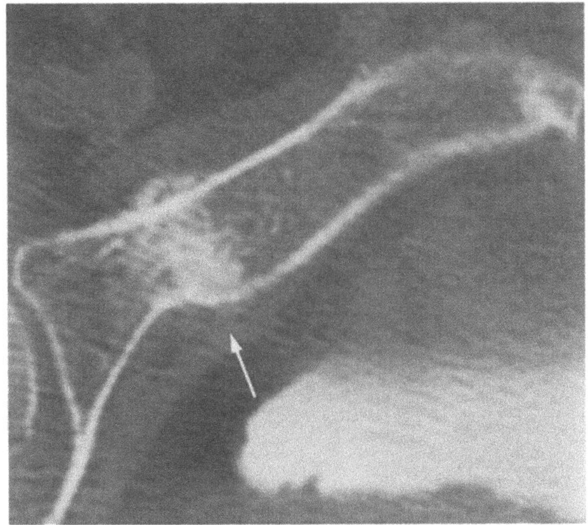

Fig. 14.7. SF of the ischiopubic ramus on CT (*arrow*)

with major bone damage and slower healing (Fig. 14.8).

Radionuclide bone scanning is usually performed on oncological patients while searching for bone metastases; physicians should be aware of the possibility of single or multiple SFs in these patients.

14.4.4
Magnetic Resonance Imaging

Magnetic resonance imaging (MRI) is of growing importance for diagnosing bone pathology. It allows very early diagnosis, with typical findings visible at the same time as on isotopic bone scan. The fracture line is often difficult to identify, but marrow edema or the soft tissue edema surrounding the fractured bone is clearly indicated by signal changes (WAGENITZ et al. 1994):

- On T1-weighted sequences marrow edema and callus appear dark.
- On T2-weighted sequences the same areas become bright (Fig. 14.9).
- If the SF is close to a joint, joint effusion is possible.
- Administration of gadolinium-DPTA contrast medium may allow reliable differentiation of SFs from pathological fractures due to characteristic perifocal contrast enhancement in the T1 sequences. When gadolinium is injected, the dark area in T1-weighted sequences become bright, but the fracture line remains dark. Nevertheless, the MRI appearance is nonspecific because the fracture line is often not identified and because many other diseases can cause marrow edema.

14.5
Differential Diagnosis

Problems are presented by unusual sites of SFs. The main misdiagnoses are:

- Osteoid osteoma
- Chronic sclerosing osteomyelitis

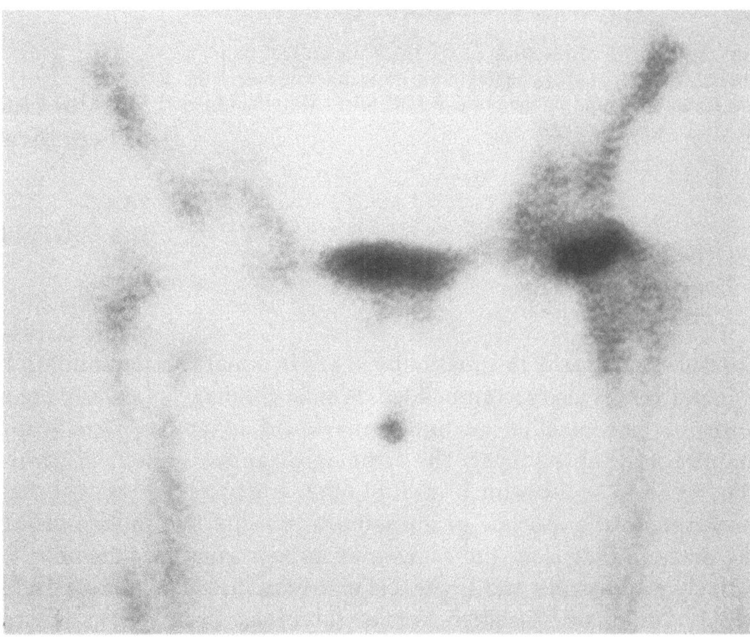

Fig. 14.8. SF of the neck of the left femur. Radionuclide bone scanning. NB: hip prosthesis on right side

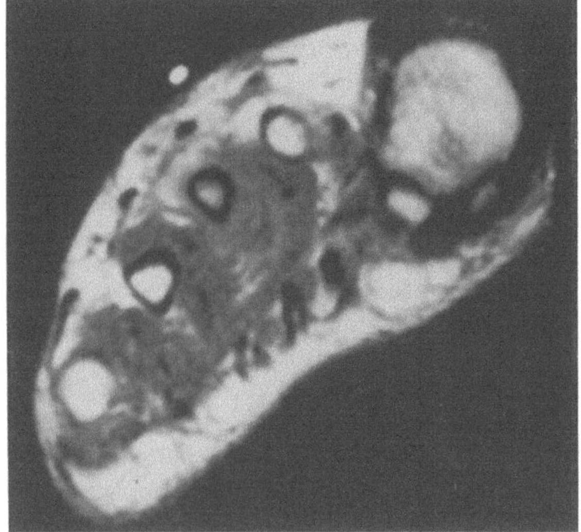

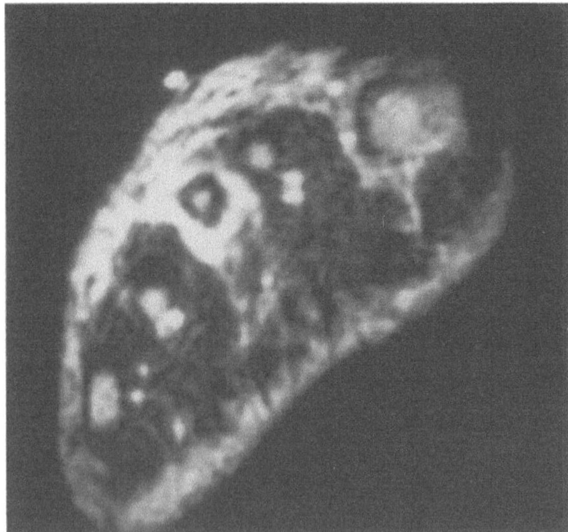

Fig. 14.9A,B. SF of the neck of the third metatarsal bone. A MRI SE T1-weighted low signal in the bone marrow and in the soft tissue surrounding the bone. B MRI SE T2-weighted high signal in the same areas

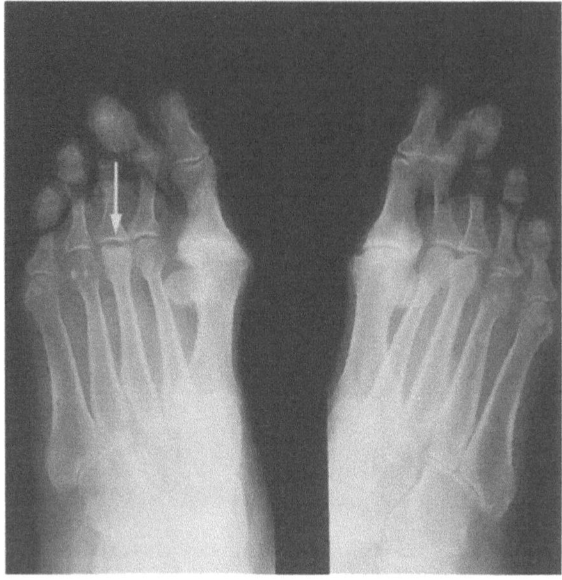

Fig. 14.10. SF of the head of the third metatarsal bone (*arrow*)

- Osteogenic osteosarcoma
- Bone metastasis
- Ewing's tumor

Careful evaluation of the possibility of SFs in nonathletic patients is also recommended. Premature diagnosis of osteomyelitis or tumor may lead to an inappropriate open biopsy. The pathological appearance of an SF is the same as that of other fractures. However, in the absence of immobilization due to the delay in diagnosis, the callus may appear as an actively proliferative and highly cellular bone tissue which could be mistaken for a sarcoma. The presence of mature bony structure, mature cartilage, and endochondral ossification indicates the non-neoplastic nature of the callus. Therefore premature biopsy should be avoided.

The clearest findings are those provided by radiography and clinical observation of the affected area. As in other fractures, the callus displays progressive remodelling and transforms back into mature bone.

14.6
Special Features Related to the Site of Fracture

14.6.1
The Lower Limb

SFs were initially described in military recruits long before X-rays were discovered. March fractures in the military population often involve the foot, particularly the metatarsi and the calcaneus.

Usually the neck of the second or third metatarsal bone is involved (Figs. 14.4, 14.5). Sometimes the SF occurs at the base of the bone, especially of the first or second bone. SFs also frequently occur at the head of the bone (Fig. 14.10).

It is possible to consider "Morton's disease" (Fig. 14.11) as an SF, or at least as a stress remodelling of the second metatarsal, because of the short first metatarsal with hypertrophy of the shaft of the second.

The so-called avascular bone necrosis of the head of the second metatarsal bone is also most likely to be an SF due to the overstress of this bone, which is usually the longest. Furthermore, lesion of the sesamoid bones of the first metatarsophalangeal joint should be considered as an SF.

The calcaneus is the foot bone most frequently affected by SFs. The tarsal navicular has a unique reaction to repeated stress: vertical fracture (Fig. 14.12) or sometimes progressive crush fracture, also called "avascular necrosis" (STEINBRONN et al. 1994). The diagnosis of tarsal navicular SFs is frequently delayed because clinical features are

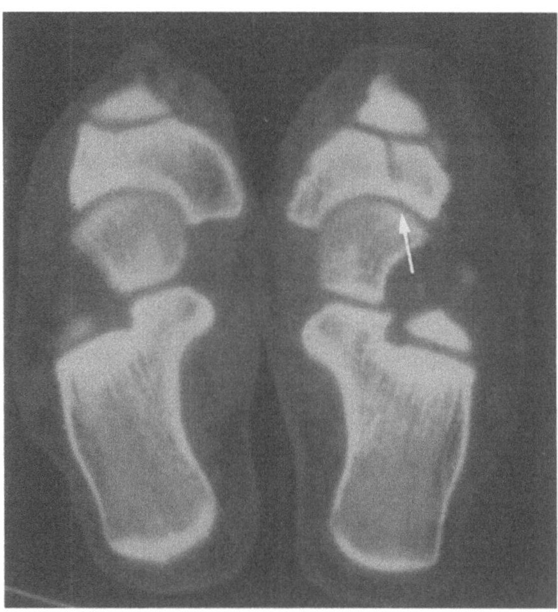

Fig. 14.12. CT scan of tarsal navicular bone SF (*arrow*)

aspecific, and these fractures are usually not evident on plain radiography of the foot.

The initial abnormality due to unaccustomed vigorous activity in athletes and military recruits involves the tibia. SFs involving the tibia arise in the medial proximal plateau, its major weight-bearing portion (Fig. 14.13). Transverse fractures of the tibial shaft are also common (Fig. 14.14). Tibial fractures are equally frequent in elderly patients, in whom fractures are generally associated with abnormality of the same leg. This feature misleads physicians because it provides a ready explanation for the pain.

A special form of SF of the tibia is longitudinal SF. The fracture line is vertical and present on only one side of the tibial shaft; there is also edema in the medullary canal and in the soft tissue surrounding the bone (Figs. 14.15, 14.16). This feature is often mistaken for an infection or a tumor, but the pattern is very characteristic (KEATING et al. 1995; SOUBRIER et al. 1994; MULLIGAN 1995).

SFs sometimes occur on the patella (Fig. 14.17) or tibial tuberosity.

Most insufficiency fractures of the femur are transverse fractures of the femoral neck. Sometimes an SF becomes complete, leading to a true fracture of the neck of the femur. Some authors consider this SF of the neck of the femur as an emergency and perform preventive osteosynthesis of the upper end of the femur.

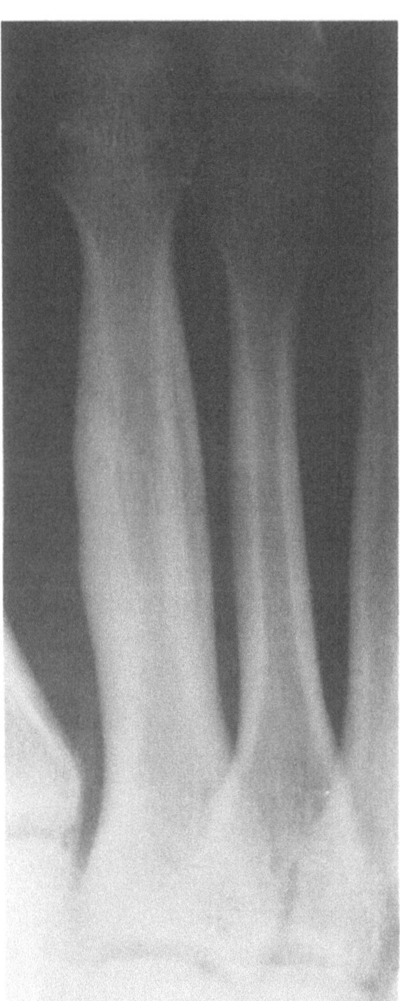

Fig. 14.11. Morton's disease. Hypertrophic reaction of the second metatarsal bone due to overload caused by congenital short first metatarsal bone

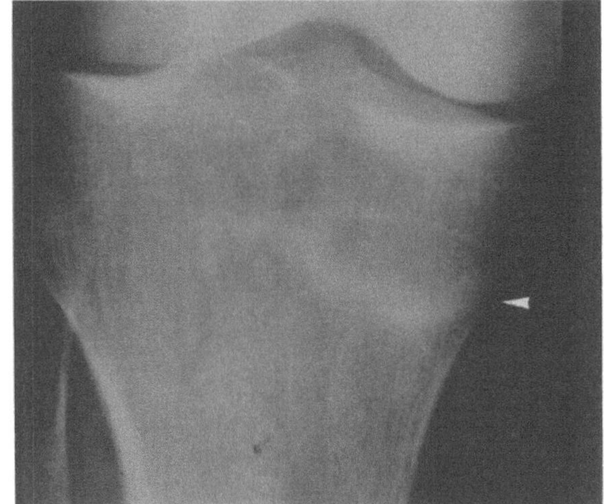

A

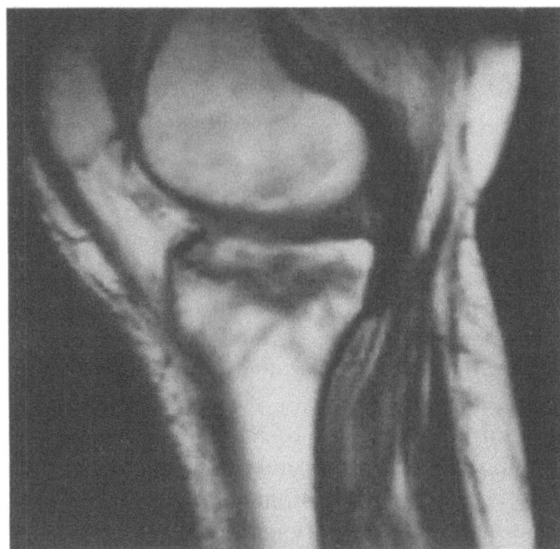

B

Fig. 14.13. SF of the upper tibia. A Radiography (*arrowhead*).
B MRI SE T1-weighted signal

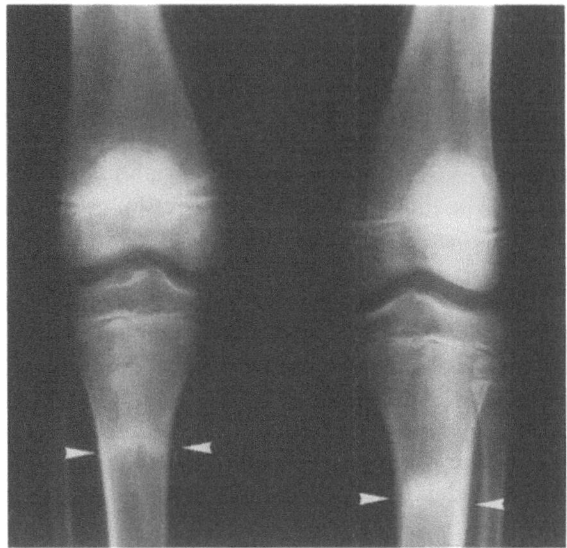

Fig. 14.14. SF of both of the tibias in a young boy (*arrow-heads*)

Longitudinal fractures of the femur are also possible but often escape diagnosis. Hyperactivity on the
bone scan is suggestive of longitudinal fractures but
sometimes so extensive as to be misleading. The callus and, less frequently, the fracture line are sometimes seen on CT sections (SOUBRIER et al. 1995;
SCHUBERT and CARTER 1994).

14.6.2
The Pelvis

SFs of the ischiopubic and iliopubic ramus are not
rare, but sometimes difficult to prove. Vertical SFs of

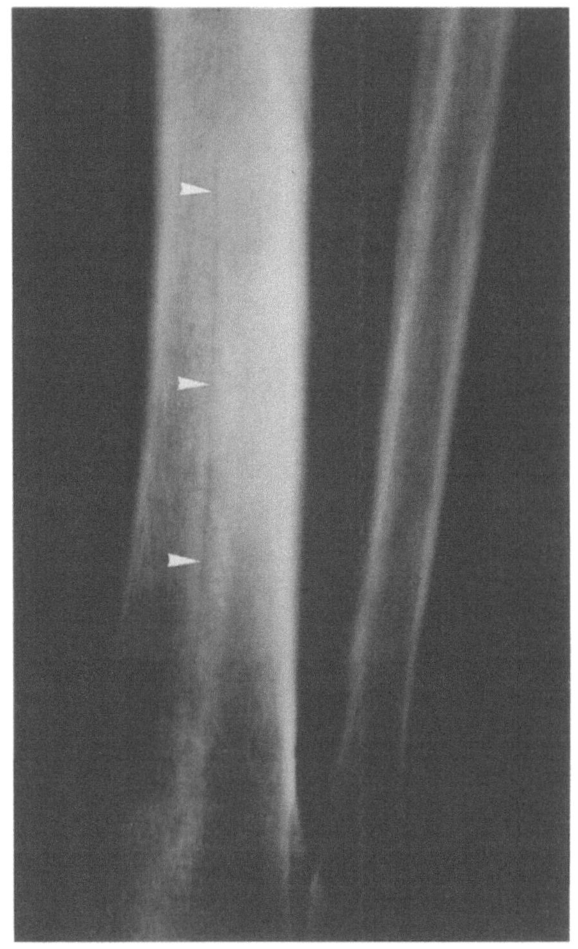

Fig. 14.15. Longitudinal SF of the left tibia in a young boy
(*arrowheads*)

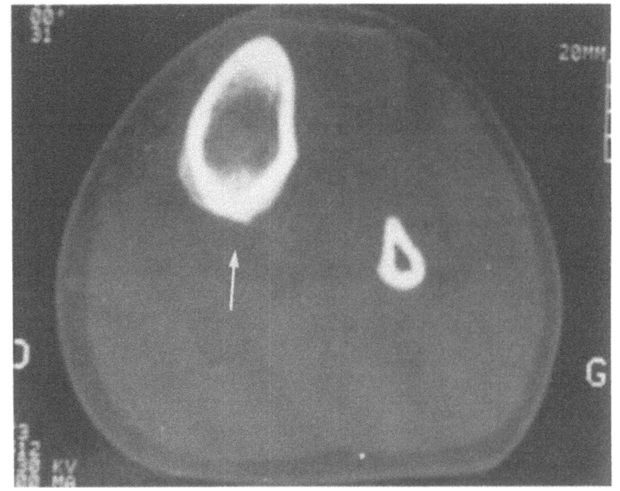

Fig. 14.16A–C. Longitudinal SF of the tibia. **A** CT (*arrow*). **B** MRI SE T1-weighted signal. **C** MRI SE T1-weighted signal after gadolinium injection

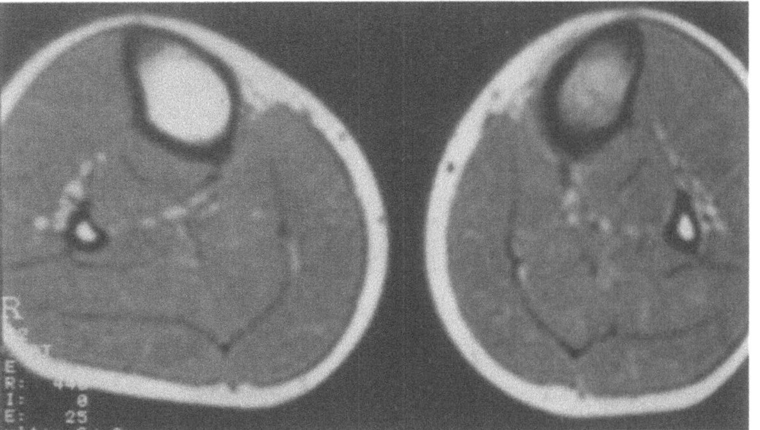

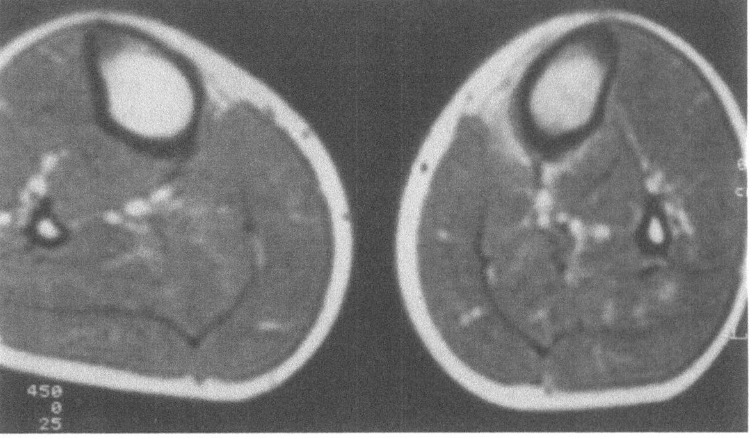

the pubis are often mistaken for an infection (Figs. 14.18, 14.19).

A special type of SF involving the roof of the acetabulum in its upper aspect has been recently described. The fracture line is horizontal, like the fracture line of the tibial plateau.

SFs of the sacrum are frequent and are sometimes mistaken for metastasis or tumor. In fact, they usually have a characteristic pattern:

– Vertical density of the wing of the sacrum on the radiographic front view, uni- or bilateral, is ob-

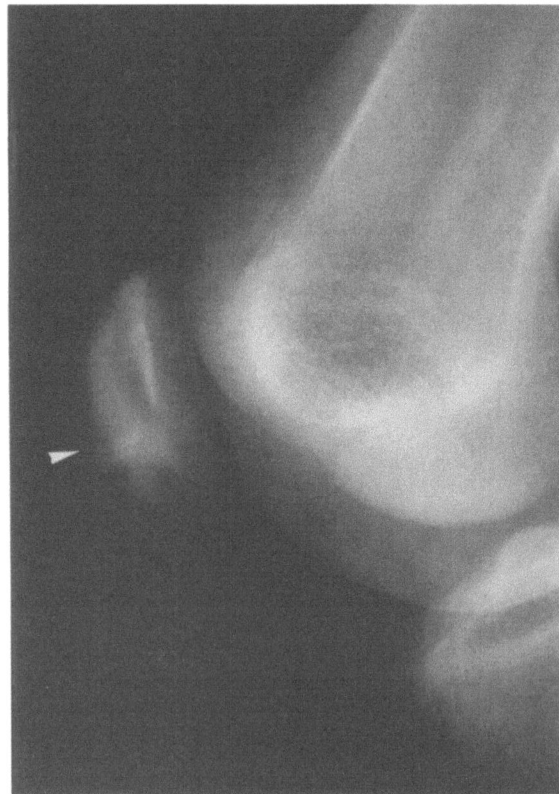

A

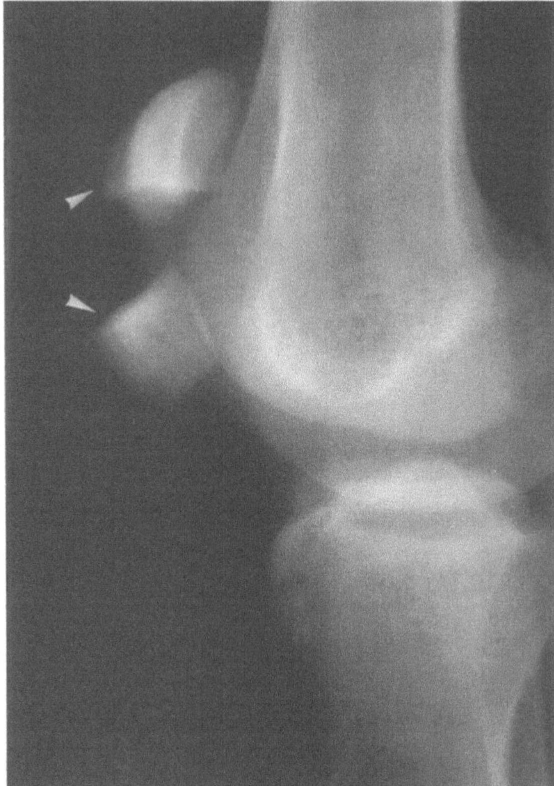

B

Fig. 14.17A,B. SF of the patella, complete fracture with fragment displacement (*arrowhead*)

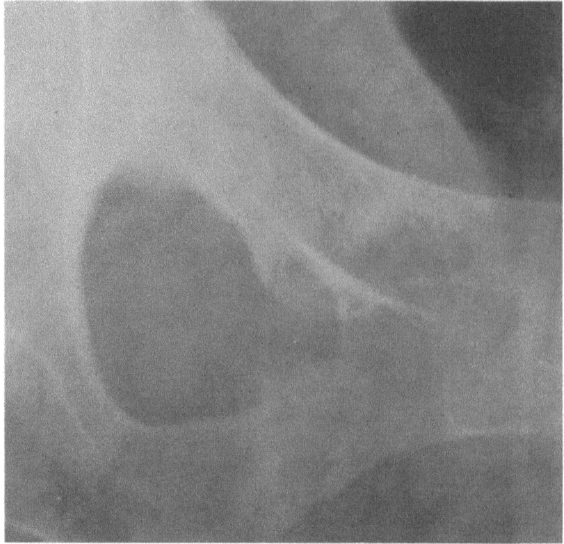

Fig. 14.18. SF of the ischiopubic ramus

served (Fig. 14.20). A horizontal fracture line through the second or the third sacral body may be involved, causing the special scintigraphic pattern.
- The fracture line is easily visible on CT scan (Fig. 14.21).
- H-shaped increased uptake of the isotope is observed on radionuclide bone scanning (Fig. 14.22).

It is possible to differentiate sacral insufficiency fractures from sacral metastases on the basis of their distribution patterns on MRI (NAKAHARA et al. 1995; PEH et al. 1995). Patients with rheumatoid arthritis are subject to insufficiency fractures (Figs. 14.20, 14.21) due to multiple osteoporotic risk factors (WEST et al. 1994).

14.6.3
The Spine

Spondylolysis is considered as an SF due to special stress on the pars intermedia of the L4 or L5 vertebrae (Fig. 14.23).

Crush compression of the body in osteoporotic patients can also be considered as SFs. The problem of distinguishing benign from pathological compression fracture of the vertebral body is common knowledge.

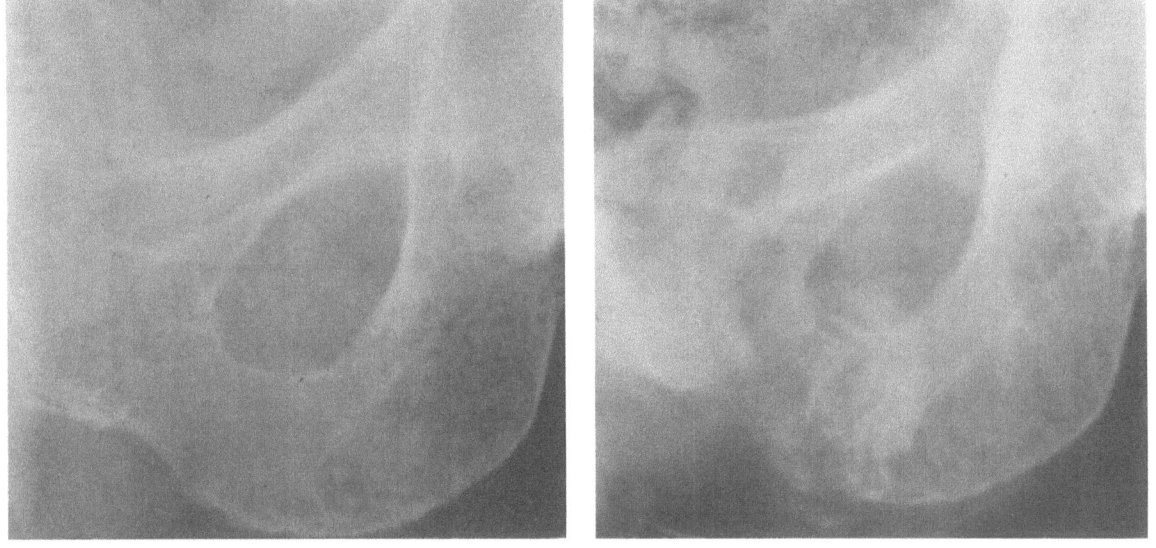

Fig. 14.19A,B. SF of the ischiopubic and iliopubic ramus. **A** Initial radiography. **B** Radiography after 1 month

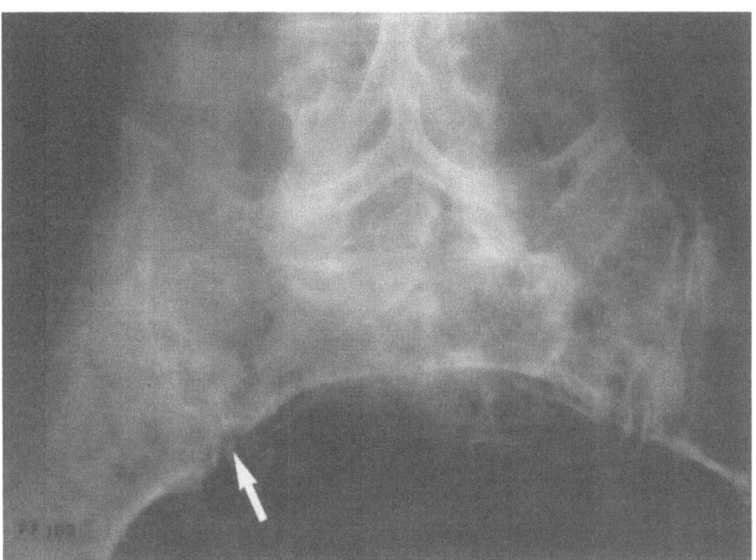

Fig. 14.20. SF of the right wing of the sacrum. Cortex irregularity (*arrow*)

14.6.4
The Head and Trunk

SFs can involve the ribs (READ 1994) or the sternum. The first rib is sometimes of interest and mistakenly diagnosed as "congenital pseudarthrosis" (Fig. 14.24). SFs of the clavicule or the scapula are infrequent. Many sites of SFs are found on the upper limbs (Figs. 14.25, 14.26). The problem of diagnosis is solved if the relationship between the stress and the pain is clear and the setting lesion is easily demonstrated (HORWITZ and DI STEFANO 1995; AHLUWALIA et al. 1994). SFs of the mandibula have been described in patients after prolonged chewing.

14.7
Special Features Related to the Underlying Condition

SFs can arise as a result of postoperative weakness, Paget's disease, or a preexisting local lesion.

Postoperative SFs occur due to loss of balance after certain types of surgery, especially surgery of

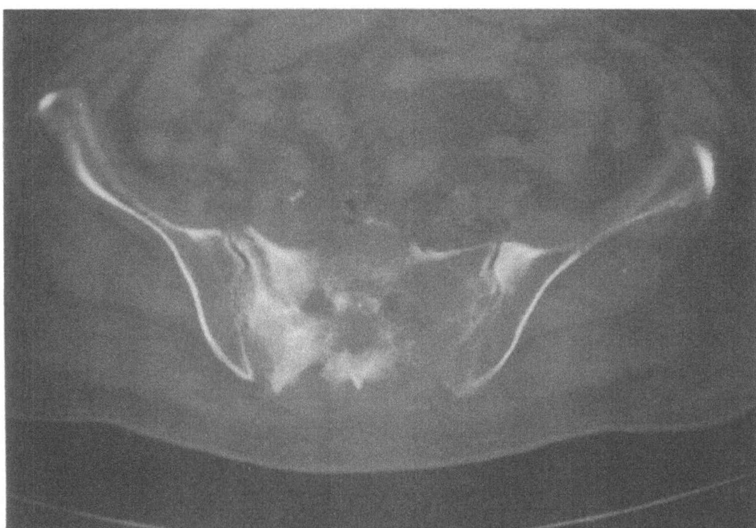

Fig. 14.21. SF of the right wing of the sacrum (same case as Fig. 20). CT densifying reaction and fracture line

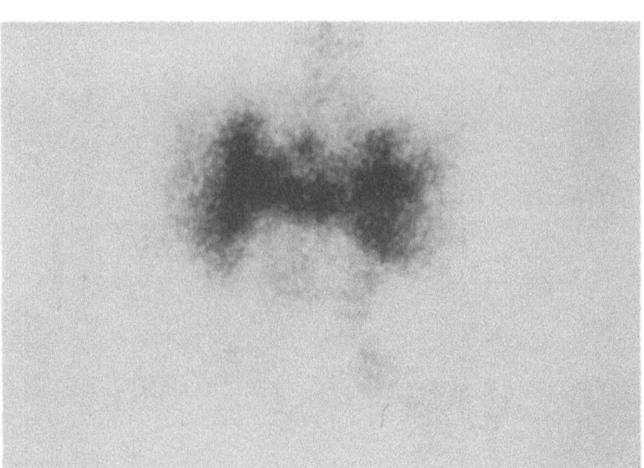

Fig. 14.22. SF of the sacrum. Bone scan, H-shaped abnormal uptake

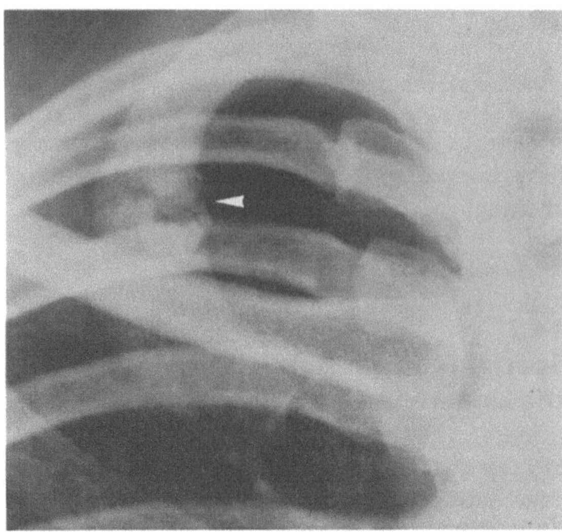

Fig. 14.24. SF of the first rib (*arrowhead*)

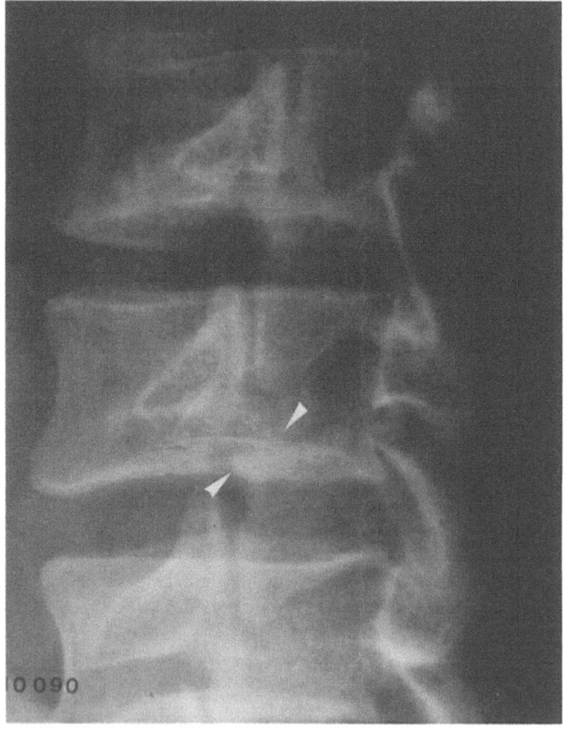

Fig. 14.23. SF of the posterior vertebral arch: spondylolysis (*arrowheads*)

the lower limbs. Postoperative SFs frequently occur on:

- Pubic ramus after total hip replacement (CHEVROT et al. 1986);
- Femoral neck after total knee arthroplasty (PALANCE MARTIN et al. 1994);

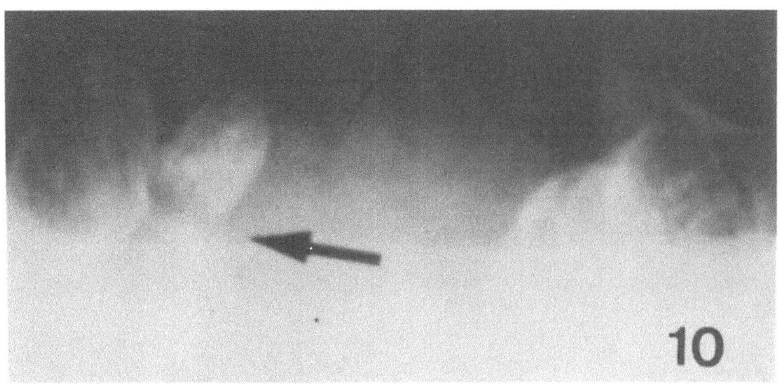

Fig. 14.25. SF of the hook of the hamate (*arrow*). Plain film of the wrist with tunnel view

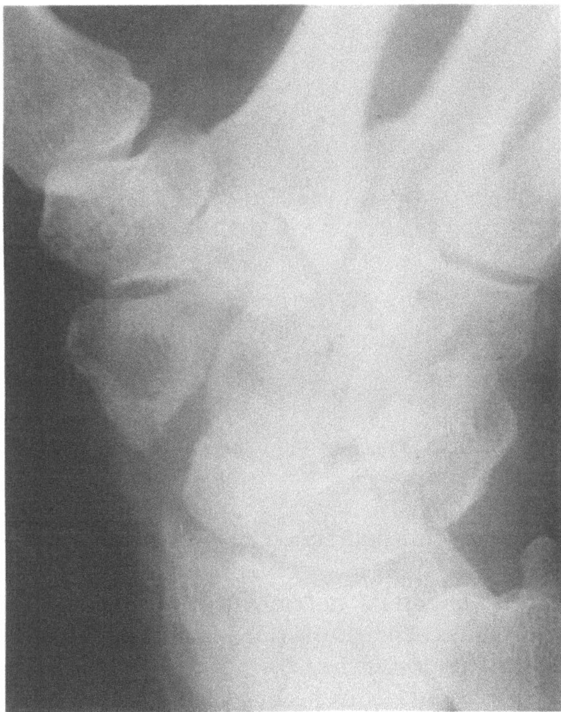

Fig. 14.26. SF of the scaphoid. Oblique view

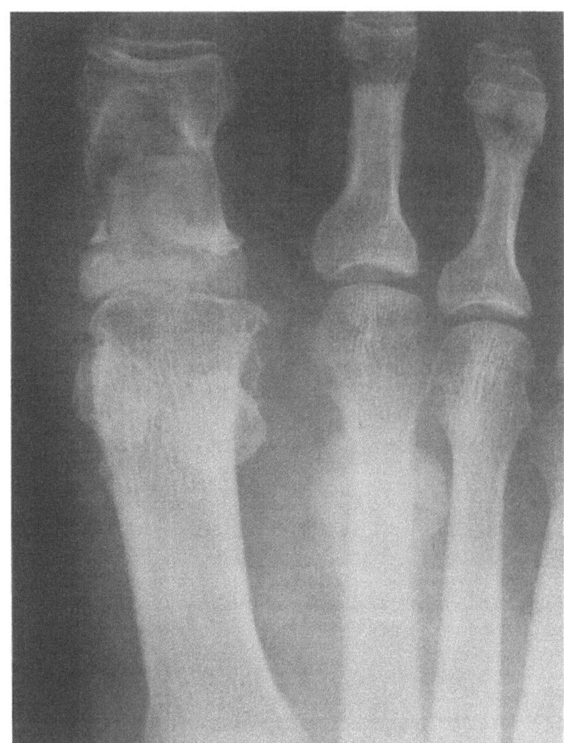

Fig. 14.27. SF of the neck of the second metatarsal bone after surgery on the first ray

– Metatarsal bones after surgery on other foot bones (Fig. 14.27).

Paget's disease can feature SFs in the long bone involved, manifested by radiolucent lines perpendicular to the cortex on the convexity of the shaft (Fig. 14.28).

In Paget's disease it is also possible to observe avulsion fractures without trauma in special areas such as the tibial tuberosity, the iliac spine, the patella, and the calcaneus.

In spite of the definition of SFs as occurring on "normal" bone, similar lesions can be seen on local-ized weakening bone due to a preexisting silent lesion (Fig. 14.29).

14.8
Healing

Most SFs heal very well with nonsurgical treatment, i.e., rest. Depending on the site, healing time is variable, from 4 weeks for a metatarsal bone to 3 months

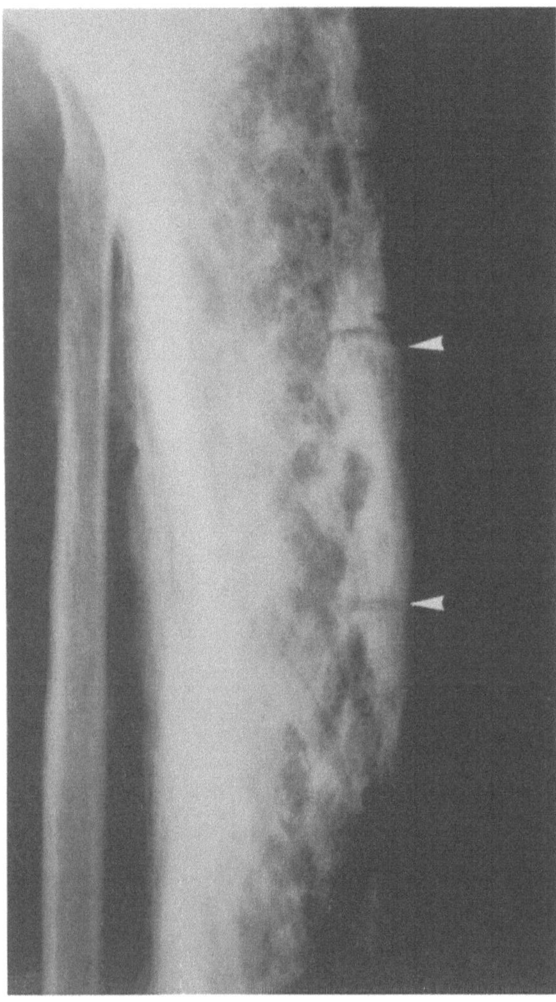

Fig. 14.28. Paget's disease. SF of the tibia on the anterior cortex, Brailsford's line (*arrowheads*)

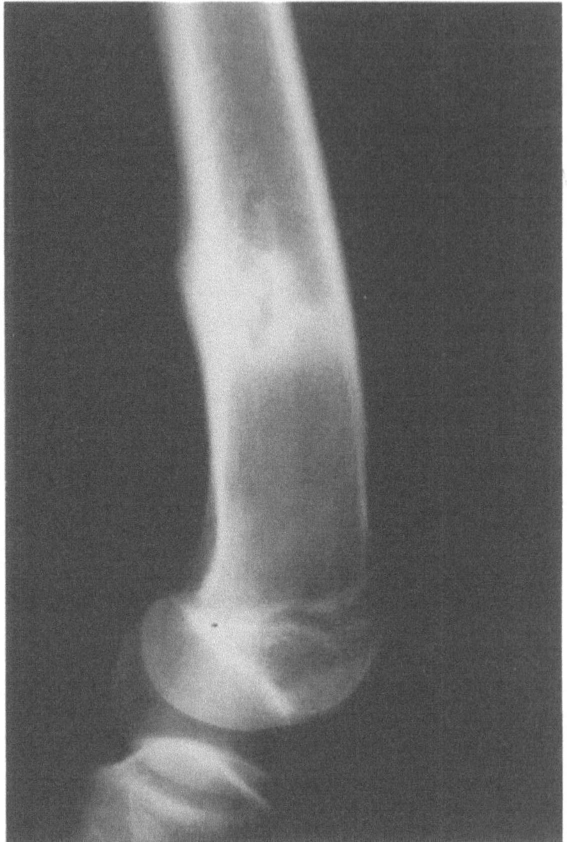

Fig. 14.29. SF of the femur crossing an ossifying fibroma

or more for weight-bearing sites (tibia, femur). Delayed healing is common in the case of stress lesion of the lower limb. Surgery must be reserved for the removal of bone fragments or the treatment of displaced fractures. Sometimes complete fracture occurs following a stress lesion due to the extension of the fracture line. This is particularly severe in lesions of the neck of the femur or the patella, indicating preventive surgery (osteosynthesis). Drilling has been proposed to enhance the formation of bone (ORAVA et al. 1995).

14.9
Conclusion

Diagnosis of SFs is usually simple if the relationship between repeated stress and pain is clear. The special patterns of the findings on medical imaging facilitate diagnosis.

It is important to remember this, because other techniques of diagnosis (for example pathology) are sometimes insufficient.

The spontaneous healing of the lesions and the disappearance of complaints with rest and time are the best proof of SFs. Rest and reassurance are often enough to relieve pain and ensure healing. Thus, such a lesion is a "no touch" condition. Premature biopsy should be avoided.

References

Ahluwalia R, Datz FL, Morton KA, Anderson CM, Whiting JH Jr (1994) Bilateral fatigue fractures of the radial shaft in a gymnast. Clin Nucl Med 19:665–667

Anderson MW, Greenspan A (1996) Stress fractures. Radiology 199:1–12

Chevrot A, Lacombe P, Zenny JC, Auberge T, Vallee C, Gires F, Palardy G (1986) Fracture de fatigue du cadre obturateur après arthroplastie de hanche. Rev Rhum 53:129–132

Daffneh RH (1978) Stress fractures. Current concepts. Skeletal Radiol 2:221–229

Horwitz BR, Di Stefano V (1995) Stress fracture of the humerus in a weight lifter. Orthopedics 18:185–187

Keating JF, Beggs I, Thorpe GW (1995) 3 cases of longitudinal stress fracture of the tibia. Acta Orthop Scand 66:41–42

Keats TE (1990) Radiology of musculoskeletal stress injury. Year Book, Chicago

McBryde AM (1975) Stress fractures in athletes. J Sports Med 3:212

Monteleone GP Jr (1995) Stress fractures in the athlete. Orthop Clin North Am 26:423–432

Mulligan ME (1995) The "gray cortex": an early sign of stress fracture. Skeletal Radiol 24:201–203

Nakahara N, Uetani M, Hayashi K (1995) Magnetic resonance imaging of sacral insufficiency fractures: characteristic features and differentiation from sacral metastasis. Nippon Igaku Hoshasen Gakkai Zasshi 55:281–288

Orava S, Puranem J, Alaketola L (1978) Stress fractures caused by physical exercise. Acta Orthop Scand 49:19

Orava S, Karpakka J, Taimela S, Hulkko A, Permi J, Kujala U (1995) Stress fracture of the medial malleolus. J Bone Joint Surg [Am] 77:362–365

Palance Martin D, Albareda J, Seral F (1994) Subcapital stress fracture of the femoral neck after total knee arthroplasty. Int Orthop 18:308–309

Patel NH, Jacobson AF, Williams J (1995) Scintigraphic detection of sequential symmetrical metatarsal stress fractures. J Am Podiatr Med Assoc 85:162–165

Peh WC, Khong PL, Ho WY, Yeung HW, Luk KD (1995) Sacral insufficiency fractures. Spectrum of radiological features. Clin Imaging 19:92–101

Read MT (1994) Case report – stress fracture of the rib in a golfer. Br J Sports Med 28:206–207

Schubert F, Carter S (1994) Longitudinal stress fracture in the femoral diaphysis. Australas Radiol 38:336–338

Soubrier M, Dubost JJ, Oualid T, Sauvezie B, Ristori JM, Bussiere JL (1994) Fractures de contrainte longitudinales du tibia. A propos de trois observations. Ann Med Intern (Paris) 145(7):474–477

Soubrier M, Dubost JJ, Raml S, Ristori JM, Bussiere JL (1995) Longitudinal insufficiency fractures of the femoral shaft. Rev Rhum Engl Ed 62:48–52

Steinbronn DJ, Bennett GL, Kay DB (1994) The use of magnetic resonance imaging in the diagnosis of stress fractures of the foot and ankle. Foot Ankle Int 15:80–83

Wagenitz A, Hoffmann R, Vogl T, Sudkamp NP (1994) Verbesserte Diagnostik von Stress-Frakturen durch Kontrast-MRT. Sportverletz Sportschaden 8:143–145

West SG, Troutner JL, Baker MR, Place HM (1994) Sacral insufficiency fractures in rheumatoid arthritis. Spine 15;19(18):2117–2121

Subject Index

List of Contributors

ANTONIO BARILE, MD
Department of Radiology
University of L'Aquila
Collemaggio Hospital
67100 L'Aquila
Italy

KLAUS BOHNDORF, MD
Klinik für Diagnostische Radiologie und Neuroradiologie
Zentralklinikum Augsburg
Stenglingstrasse 2
86156 Augsburg
Germany

M. BREITENSEHER, MD
MR and Osteology
Universitätsklinik für Radiodiagnostik AKH
Ludwig-Boltzmann-Institut für radiologische-
physikalische Tumordiagnostik
Währinger Gürtel 18-20
1090 Vienna
Austria

N. CHEMLA, MD
Groupe Hospitalier Cochin
Service de Radiologie "B"
rue du Faubourg-Saint Jacques
75674 Paris Cedex 14
France

ALAIN CHEVROT, MD
Groupe Hospitalier Cochin
Service de Radiologie "B"
rue du Faubourg-Saint Jacques
75674 Paris Cedex 14
France

A. MARK DAVIES, MD
MRI Centre
The Royal Orthopaedic Hospital
Birmingham B31 2 AP
UK

NICOLA DE STEFANO, MD
Radiology and MRI Service
Institute of Sports Medicine
Via Filadelfia 88
10137 Turin
Italy

STEFANO DRAGONI, MD
Istituto di Scienza dello Sport del CONI
Dipartimento di Medicinia dello Sport
Via dei Campi Sportivi 46
00197 Rome
Italy

J.L. DRAPE, MD
Groupe Hospitalier Cochin
Service de Radiologie "B"
rue du Fanbourg-Saint Jacques
75674 Paris Cedex 14
France

A.M. DUPONT, MD
Groupe Hospitalier Cochin
Service de Radiologie "B"
rue du Fanbourg-Saint Jacques
75674 Paris Cedex 14
France

CARLO FABBRICIANI, MD
Department of Orthopaedics
University of Sassari
Via S. Godenzo 175
00189 Rome
Italy

CARLO FALETTI, MD
Radiology and MRI Service
Institute of Sports Medicine
Via Filadelfia 88
10137 Torino
Italy

RUSSEL C. FRITZ, MD
National Orthopedic Imaging Associates
University of California at San Francisco
San Francisco, CA
USA

F. GIRES, MD
Groupe Hospitalier Cochin
Service de Radiologie "B"
rue du Fanbourg-Saint Jacques
75674 Paris Cedex 14
France

D. GODEFROY, MD
Groupe Hospitalier Cochin
Service de Radiologie "B"
rue du Fanbourg-Saint Jacques
75674 Paris Cedex 14
France

ALINA GRECO, MD
Department of Magnetic Resonance Imaging
Princess Grace Hospital
P.O.B. 489
98000 Monte Carlo
Monaco

J. Haller, MD
Roentgeninstitut
Hanusch-Krankenhaus
Heinrich-Collinstrasse 30
Vienna
Austria

Herwig Imhof, MD
MR and Osteology
Universitätsklinik für Radiodiagnostik AKH
Ludwig-Boltzmann-Institut für radiologische-
physikalische Tumordiagnostik
Währinger Gürtel 18-20
1090 Vienna
Austria

F. Kainberger, MD
MR and Osteology
Universitätsklinik für Radiodiagnostik AKH
Ludwig-Boltzmann- Institut für radiologische-
physikalische Tumordiagnostik
Währinger Gürtel 18-20
1090 Vienna
Austria

Luciano Lucania, MD
Department of Orthopaedics
Catholic University
L.go A. Gemelli 8
00168 Rome
Italy

Maria Vittoria Maffey, MD
Department of Radiology
University of L'Aquila
Collemaggio Hospital
67100 L'Aquila
Italy

Carlo Masciocchi, MD
Professor, Department of Radiology
University of L'Aquila
Collemaggio Hospital
67100 L'Aquila
Italy

Marco Mastantuono, MD
Il Cattedra di Radiologia
Università La Sapienza
Policlinico Umberto 1
Viale Regina Elena 324
00161 Rome
Italy

Michael T. McNamara, MD
Chief, Department of Magnetic Resonance Imaging
Princess Grace Hospital
B.O.Box 489
98000 Monte Carlo
Monaco

Giuseppe Milano, MD
Department of Orthopaedics
Catholic University
L.go A. Gemelli 8
00168 Rome
Italy

A. Minoui, MD
Groupe Hospitalier Cochin
Service de Radiologie "B"
rue du Fanbourg-Saint Jacques
75674 Paris Cedex 14
France

Willem R. Obermann, MD
Department of Radiology
Leiden University Hospital
P.O. Box 9600
2300 RC Leiden
The Netherlands

Roberto Passariello, MD
Il Cattedra di Radiologia
Università La Sapienza
Policlinico Umberto 1
Viale Regina Elena 324
00161 Rome
Italy

E. Pessis, MD
Groupe Hospitalier Cochin
Service de Radiologie "B"
rue du Fanbourg-Saint Jacques
75674 Paris Cedex 14
France

Maximilian Reiser, MD
Department of Radiology
Klinikum Großhadern
Ludwig-Maximilians-Universität
Marchioninistrasse 15
81377 München
Germany

Folco Rossi, MD
Department of Radiology Sports Science Institute
Italian Olympic Commitee
Via S. Agatone Papa 34
00165 Rome
Italy

L. Sarazin, MD
Groupe Hospitalier Cochin
Service de Radiologie "B"
rue du Fanbourg-Saint Jacques
75674 Paris Cedex 14
France

Alfredo Schiavone Panni, MD
Department of Orthopaedics
Catholic University
L.go A. Gemelli 8
00168 Rome
Italy

Serge Sintzoff, MD, PhD
Brussels Free University
Department of Radiology and Medical Imaging
Erasmus Hospital
Avenue Prince de Ligne 116
1180 Brussels
Belgium

Marc Steinborn, MD
Department of Radiology
Klinikum Großhadern
Ludwig-Maximilians-Universität
Marchioninistrasse 15
81377 Munich
Germany

Erik R. Tijn A Ton, MD
Department of Radiology
Leiden University Hospital
P.O. Box 9600
2300 RC Leiden
The Netherlands

S. Trattnig
MR and Osteology
Universitätsklinik für Radiodiagnostik AKH
Ludwig-Boltzmann-Institut für radiologische-
physikalische Tumordiagnostik
Währinger Gürtel 18-20
1090 Vienna
Austria

P.N.M. Tyrrell, MD
The Robert Jones & Agnes Hunt Orthopaedic Hospital
Oswestry
Shropshire SY10 7AG
UK

MEDICAL RADIOLOGY
Diagnostic Imaging and Radiation Oncology

Titles in the series already published

DIAGNOSTIC IMAGING

Innovations in Diagnostic Imaging
Edited by J.H. Anderson

Radiology of the Upper Urinary Tract
Edited by E.K. Lang

The Thymus - Diagnostic Imaging, Functions, and Pathologic Anatomy
Edited by E. Walter, E. Willich, and W.R. Webb

Interventional Neuroradiology
Edited by A. Valavanis

Radiology of the Pancreas
Edited by A.L. Baert, co-edited by G. Delorme

Radiology of the Lower Urinary Tract
Edited by E.K. Lang

Magnetic Resonance Angiography
Edited by I.P. Arlart, G.M. Bongartz, and G. Marchal

Contrast-Enhanced MRI of the Breast
S. Heywang-Köbrunner and R. Beck

Spiral CT of the Chest
Edited by M. Rémy-Jardin and J. Rémy

Radiological Diagnosis of Breast Diseases
Edited by M. Friedrich and E.A. Sickles

Radiology of the Trauma
Edited by M. Heller and A. Fink

Biliary Tract Radiology
Edited by P. Rossi

Radiological Imaging of Sports Injuries
Edited by C. Masciocchi

Modern Imaging of the Alimentary Tube
Edited by A. R. Margulis

Diagnosis and Therapy of Spinal Tumors
Edited by P. R. Algra, J. Valk, and J. J. Heimans

Interventional Magnetic Resonance Imaging
Edited by J. F. Debatin and G. Adam

RADIATION ONCOLOGY

Lung Cancer
Edited by C.W. Scarantino

Innovations in Radiation Oncology
Edited by H.R. Withers and L.J. Peters

Radiation Therapy of Head and Neck Cancer
Edited by G.E. Laramore

Gastrointestinal Cancer – Radiation Therapy
Edited by R.R. Dobelbower, Jr.

Radiation Exposure and Occupational Risks
Edited by E. Scherer, C. Streffer, and K.-R. Trott

Radiation Therapy of Benign Diseases - A Clinical Guide
S.E. Order and S.S. Donaldson

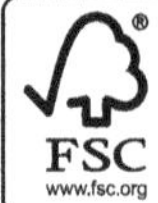

MIX
Papier aus verantwortungsvollen Quellen
Paper from responsible sources
FSC® C105338

If you have any concerns about our products,
you can contact us on
ProductSafety@springernature.com

In case Publisher is established outside the EU,
the EU authorized representative is:
Springer Nature Customer Service Center GmbH
Europaplatz 3, 69115 Heidelberg, Germany

Printed by Libri Plureos GmbH
in Hamburg, Germany